ADVANCES IN

DRUG RESEARCH

VOLUME 13

ADVANCES IN
DRUG RESEARCH

Edited by

BERNARD TESTA

School of Pharmacy, University of Lausanne, Lausanne, Switzerland

VOLUME 13

1984

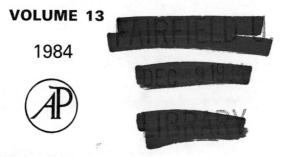

ACADEMIC PRESS

(Harcourt Brace Jovanovich, Publishers)

LONDON   ORLANDO   SAN DIEGO   NEW YORK
TORONTO   MONTREAL   SYDNEY   TOKYO

ACADEMIC PRESS, INC. (LONDON) LTD.
24-28 Oval Road,
London NW1 7DX

United States Edition published by
ACADEMIC PRESS, INC.
Orlando, Florida 32887

LIBRARY OF CONGRESS CATALOG CARD NUMBER: 64-24672

ISBN 0-12-013313-X

PRINTED IN THE UNITED STATES OF AMERICA

84 85 86 87   9 8 7 6 5 4 3 2 1

CONTENTS

Drugs? Drug Research? Advances in Drug Research? Musings of a Medicinal Chemist

BERNARD TESTA

The Binding of Drugs to Blood Plasma Macromolecules: Recent Advances and Therapeutic Significance

JEAN-PAUL TILLEMENT, GEORGES HOUIN, ROLAND ZINI, SAÏK URIEN, EDITH ALBENGRES, JÉRÔME BARRÉ, MICHEL LECOMTE, PHILIPPE D'ATHIS, AND BERNARD SEBILLE

Xenobiotic Metabolism by Brain Monooxygenases and Other Cerebral Enzymes

MARCEL MESNIL, BERNARD TESTA, AND PETER JENNER

Central and Peripheral α-Adrenoceptors. Pharmacological Aspects and Clinical Potential

P. A. VAN ZWIETEN AND P. B. M. W. M. TIMMERMANS

Novel Approaches to the Design of Safer Drugs: Soft Drugs and Site-Specific Chemical Delivery Systems

NICHOLAS BODOR

CONTRIBUTORS

EDITH ALBENGRES, *Département de Pharmacologie, Faculté de Médecine de Paris XII, F-94010 Créteil, France*

JÉRÔME BARRÉ, *Département de Pharmacologie, Faculté de Médecine de Paris XII, F-94010 Créteil, France*

NICHOLAS BODOR, *Department of Medicinal Chemistry, College of Pharmacy, J. Hillis Miller Health Center, University of Florida, Gainesville, Florida 32610, USA*

PHILIPPE D'ATHIS, *Département de Pharmacologie, Faculté de Médecine de Paris XII, F-94010 Créteil, France*

GEORGES HOUIN, *Département de Pharmacologie, Faculté de Médecine de Paris XII, F-94010 Créteil, France*

PETER JENNER, *University Department of Neurology, Institute of Psychiatry and King's College Hospital Medical School, Denmark Hill, London SE5, England*

MICHEL LECOMTE, *Département de Pharmacologie, Faculté de Médecine de Paris XII, F-94010 Créteil, France*

MARCEL MESNIL, *School of Pharmacy, University of Lausanne, CH-1005 Lausanne, Switzerland*

BERNARD SEBILLE, *Département de Pharmacologie, Faculté de Médecine de Paris XII, F-94010 Créteil, France*

BERNARD TESTA, *School of Pharmacy, University of Lausanne, CH-1005 Lausanne, Switzerland*

JEAN-PAUL TILLEMENT, *Département de Pharmacologie, Faculté de Médecine de Paris XII, F-94010 Créteil, France*

P. B. M. W. M. TIMMERMANS, *Department of Pharmacy, Division of Pharmacotherapy, University of Amsterdam, NL-1018 TV Amsterdam, The Netherlands*

SAÏK URIEN, *Département de Pharmacologie, Faculté de Médecine de Paris XII, F-94010 Créteil, France*

P. A. VAN ZWIETEN, *Department of Pharmacy, Division of Pharmacotherapy, University of Amsterdam, NL-1018 TV Amsterdam, The Netherlands*

ROLAND ZINI, *Département de Pharmacologie, Faculté de Médecine de Paris XII, F-94010 Créteil, France*

PREFACE: "SAILING AGAIN"

Advances in Drug Research, under the able captaincy of Drs. N. J. Harper and Alma B. Simmonds, has sailed twelve fruitful voyages, twelve volumes of exploration in the unlimited realm of drug research. Now, after a number of years spent in dry dock, the ship is out at sea again, a fresh captain at the helm.

In recent years, drug research has progressed enormously in several directions. Established therapeutic classes have yielded better analogs, and a number of entirely novel classes of drugs have been discovered. These aspects will of course be given due attention in the series, and specific classes of drugs will be critically reviewed in all future volumes. This is also the case in comparable series, and the point does not need to be emphasized further.

But drug research has also progressed in fields of general significance such as drug metabolism, molecular pharmacology, and drug design. These topics are important, even more in my opinion than specific classes of drugs. Indeed, these general fields are the ones that offer the best promises of understanding how drugs work and of discovering novel and better therapeutic agents. As a result of what may be a personal bias—but it is the captain who sets the course—general topics will be given constant attention in the series. Constant, but not overwhelming: all efforts will be made to offer a good balance between specific and general topics, bearing in mind that this discrimination is not always meaningful. In the first chapter, which is in fact an oversized introduction to the series, some considerations are given on the structure of drug research and on a number of general fields in which impressive advances have been witnessed.

Schematically, and again being aware of the dichotomic trap, drug research has two goals—scientific goals, that is! The first that comes to mind is the discovery of new, more specific, and more active drugs. The second goal, first recognized by clinicians, is to improve the activity of existing drugs by increasing their beneficial actions and by decreasing their unwanted effects. This can be achieved by optimizing the modes and routes of administration, in other words by taking into account the patient's characteristics (age, state of health, etc.), drug interactions, bioavailability, chronopharmacological and pharmacokinetic factors, and many other influences. These two goals are far from being mutually exclusive. Rather, they proceed from approaches that have much in common. To these goals we adjust our compass. But a feedback regulation is needed, which you, the reader, should provide. Comments, suggestions, criticisms, all reactions will be gratefully welcome.

BERNARD TESTA

Drugs? Drug Research?
Advances in Drug Research?
Musings of a Medicinal Chemist

BERNARD TESTA

School of Pharmacy, University of Lausanne, Switzerland

> Knowledge is one. Its division into subjects is a concession to human weakness.
>
> Halford J. Mackinder

What are drugs? How complex and fuzzy a network of theories, concepts, models, findings, assumptions, fictions and errors is hiding behind the simple term "drug research"? Where and how is drug research advancing? Such questions defy complete and explicit answers, but even very fragmentary ones may draw attention to interesting perspectives. In the following pages, a number of rationalizations and of more intuitive views will be offered. Findings and discoveries are not mere data, they also provide the incentive and input for intellectual creations such as recepts, concepts and intuitions.

ADVANCES IN DRUG RESEARCH VOL. 13
0-12-013313-X

These thoughts have inspired the present chapter, which is meant as a general introduction to this and future volumes.

1 Drugs?

Many years ago, workers in drug metabolism realized that they were dealing not only with drugs, but also with many other compounds foreign to the organism. The word "xenobiotics" was thus coined to describe such foreign compounds, i.e. exogenous chemicals of no physiological benefit. A list of xenobiotics is given in Table 1. Drugs make up an important group of xenobiotics, as do other categories in this list. Some cosmetics do find their way into the body, e.g. lipstick constituents.

TABLE 1

Compounds classified as xenobiotics

Drugs
Food constituents devoid of physiological roles
Food additives (preservatives, colouring and flavouring agents, antioxidants, etc.)
Drugs of "pleasure" and of abuse (ethanol, coffee and tobacco constituents, hallucinogens, etc.)
Constituents of cosmetics
Various chemicals (insecticides, herbicides, etc.)
Polluting agents

The difference between xenobiotics and chemicals (of endogenous or exogenous origin) fulfilling a physiological role is far from sharp and well defined (Testa *et al.*, 1981). Thus, where should we categorize the nitrogen gas we inhale? Many examples could be given, but to little avail in the present context. However, to stress the point further, it must be remembered that not all drugs are xenobiotics, no more than all xenobiotics are drugs. This statement is trivial when one considers the therapeutic use of such physiological compounds as vitamins, amino acids, complex lipids, hormones, common salts, and others. From the above, we conclude that it is its use rather than its origin or nature which tells us if a given compound must be considered a drug or not, in close analogy with the well-known fact that the dose makes the poison.

Innumerable drugs exist which are used in a considerable variety of therapeutic indications, not to mention diagnostic and prophylactic agents. In a very schematic manner, these therapeutic indications, and the many pharmacodynamic actions of drugs can be classified into three large therapeutic classes, namely chemotherapeutic agents, neuropharmacological agents, and a less well-defined category of agents acting on regulatory mechanisms (metabolic, hormonal and immunological). Of course all drugs can be considered as metabolic agents in the broadest sense, since in one way or another they interfere with biological processes. This, however, is hardly a classification. On the other hand, too many categories scatter a global view of drug action and therapeutic uses.

Chemotherapeutic agents are meant to inhibit or destroy a parasite while being as harmless as possible for the host—a problem of selectivity. "Parasite" is taken here in the broadest sense, to mean viruses, bacteria, fungi, protozoa, parasitic worms, and also tumour cells. Neuropharmacological agents have various impacts on the central and/or peripheral nervous system, acting directly on receptors or indirectly through neurotransmitters, or by less specific mechanisms as in the case for local or general anaesthetics. The third class includes those drugs acting on various enzyme systems, e.g. several groups of diuretics, or on immunological mechanisms; further, all agents with hormonal or antihormonal activities belong to this class.

Such a general classification cannot be absolute, and overlap exists. For example, there are enzyme inhibitors (metabolic agents) that are chemotherapeutic drugs (e.g. dihydrofolate reductase inhibitors) or neuropharmacological agents (e.g. inhibitors of some amino acid decarboxylases). Overlap between chemotherapeutic and neuropharmacological agents is seen for example with anthelmintic drugs blocking neuromuscular transmission. The above discussion is graphically summarized in Fig. 1.

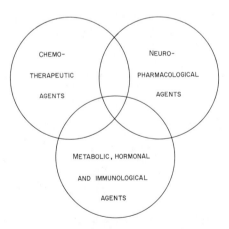

FIG. 1. A broad classification of therapeutic drug classes.

2 Drug research?

Drug research is such a multi-faceted and intricate domain of human activity that any description or discussion of it is bound to remain incomplete. However, a number of salient features exist in the structure of drug research which can usefully be considered.

A scheme summarizing the essence of drug research is presented in Fig. 2; it derives, with a number of additions and modifications, from a simpler scheme published by Kier and Hall (1977). The present section will be devoted to a discussion of various steps in this scheme, each of which corresponds to an important aspect of drug research. The starting point involves examining, in turn, biological and molecular systems. Indeed, essential to drug research is the deepest possible understanding of all relevant properties of drug molecules as well as of the biological systems with which they interact. To "understand" these properties not only means to have unravelled them, but also to be able to determine or measure them, and to express them in a manner suitable for the next steps in drug research.

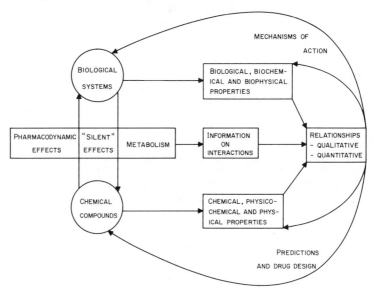

Fig. 2. A schematic view of drug research.

When biological systems and molecular entities interact, it can be in a number of ways: biological effects (pharmacodynamic effects) are elicited by the drug molecules acting on the biological systems, which in turn can handle the former (metabolism) to absorb, distribute, store and excrete them (disposition), as well as to chemically transform them (biotransformation). These two modes of interaction are not independent of each other, but rather are interdependent. Nor are they the only ones which can be characterized: witness "silent" interactions such as non-covalent binding to plasma or tissue proteins. To be useful in terms of drug research, all these types of interactions must be expressed as biological information in the form of qualitative or quantitative data. The discovery of relationships between the latter and some properties of the biological systems and/or the drug molecules is a crucial step in drug research. Indeed, such relationships, often interesting *per se*, are particularly valuable when they deepen our understanding of biological mechanisms and allow improved drugs to be designed.

2.1 BIOLOGICAL SYSTEMS

Biological systems not only interact with drug molecules, but also provide the environment in which these interactions take place. Such a fragmented approach is quite a common one, e.g. in molecular pharmacology, and has often been proven to be of immense value. But taken alone, it provides only a partial understanding of phenomena because any biological system is highly integrated and must also be apprehended holistically. Obviously such topics as biological complexity and levels of organization, biological environment, structure and information, are of capital significance in drug research.

2.1.1 Biological levels of complexity and organization

The targets of drugs, when these are used for therapy and not for research purposes, are always organisms or even populations of organisms (e.g. populations of bacteria in chemotherapy). An organism must be understood as defined by Yates (1982), namely a "complete living system . . . characterized by autonomous morphogenesis, nearly invariant reproduction, and teleonomic behaviour".

In contrast to therapy, drug research deals with biological systems of various levels of complexity, from the simple biological levels of molecules and macromolecules to the higher ones of organisms and populations. The main levels thus encountered are presented in Table 2. Biological complexity, as illustrated in Table 2, is intuitively understandable, but is difficult to explain rationally, as stressed by Yates (1982). Complexity is related to the degree of organization and information content, but also to size, inasmuch as the former depend on the latter. These problems of biological complexity, levels of organization, and biological information are receiving considerable interest (e.g. Cramer, 1979; Pattee, 1979; Ryan, 1980; Arenas *et al.*, 1981; Bolender, 1981; Garfinkel, 1982) and should not fail to interest every worker in drug research. Indeed, it is always recognized in theory, but often forgotten in practice and when assessing results, that in research each biological level of complexity (Table 2) is at best a model of the higher level(s). What is lacking in an isolated system belonging to a given level is the coordination existing in the higher level(s), namely the constraints which regulate the functioning of this system as an integrative part of a larger system.

TABLE 2

Biological levels of complexity encountered in drug research
(expanded from Testa, 1982a)

Entities	Examples
Small molecules	Monosaccharides, amino acids, fatty acids
Medium-sized molecular systems	Oligosaccharides, nucleotides, oligopeptides, lipids
Macromolecules	Polysaccharides, nucleic acids, proteins, enzymes
Supramolecular structures	Multienzymatic systems, membranes, chromosomes, "receptors"
Organelles	Mitochondria, nuclei
Cells	Neurons, hepatocytes, unicellular organisms
Tissues	Epidermis, renal cortex
Organs	Heart, brain
Functional systems	Digestive system
Organisms (pluricellular)	Parasitic worms, human beings
Populations	Intestinal microflora, human populations

Biological models used as tools in drug research take a considerable risk of being irrelevant when non-physiological conditions are applied, or because they bear insufficient relationship to the system on which the model is based. The permanent problem is thus: to what extent are models relevant to the ultimate object of study? There is no doubt that working with membrane preparations containing xenobiotic-metabolizing enzymes or pharmacological receptors has allowed explosive progress in drug metabolism and molecular pharmacology, respectively. But extrapolation to animal or human is far from straightforward as seen in the well-known problem of *in vitro–in vivo* correlations.

In many fields of biological research, the current approach is clearly a reductionistic one, with triumphant successes in great number. In drug research also, the reductionistic approach has been particularly fruitful, as often shown in the following pages. But as stated above, the reduction to models is bound to neglect major aspects of the reality we are investigating. Indeed, biological information is of a completely different nature in the lower (molecular) and in higher levels of organization. This is illustrated by Pattee (1979) in a particularly striking manner:

> ... there is no question that the structure of nucleic acids ... obeys quantum mechanical laws. However, a complete detailed quantum mechanical description of these structures would give no more clue to the meaning of a DNA sequence as biological information than the chemistry of this ink and paper would give a clue to the meaning of these words.

The outcome is obvious; as pointed out by many epistemologists, biology is unique among all sciences in being currently unable to rationally define its object of study—life.

From the above, it should be clear that, while the reductionistic approach to drug research will continue to be followed with success for many years to come, the time now appears ripe for the synthetic, holistic approach to receive more attention. Only by giving comparable importance to these two complementary approaches, like walking on two legs, can drug research expect decisive therapeutic breakthroughs.

2.1.2 Water and hydration; lipophilic environments

A major characteristic of biological systems is the duality or plurality of many of their properties—certainly an important prerequisite of life. Let us consider here the hydrophilic/lipophilic duality of the biological milieu, or better, to avoid the dualistic trap, the plurality or even continuum of properties existing between highly hydrophilic and highly lipophilic ones.

Water is a compound with unique physical properties, particularly in the liquid state relevant to biology (e.g. Symons, 1981; Land and Lüdermann, 1982). But some interactions, particularly with biological constitutents, can modify its properties and behaviour. Conversely, interactions with water can modify some properties of molecules or macromolecules. Witness the fact that a molecule behaves quite differently by a number of criteria depending whether it is studied in isolation (in vacuum) or in solution.

Up to now, much effort has been spent assessing the influence of solvation in general and of hydration in particular on molecular properties. In the field of drug research, this is exemplified by solvent effects on such properties as acidity, basicity, and conformational behaviour (see section 2.2.2.). Much effort has also been devoted to understanding *hydration*, e.g. by defining hydration sites and calculating hydration energies (e.g. Scheraga, 1979; Edmonds, 1980; Mehrotra *et al.*, 1981). Amino acids and small peptides have been favoured objects of investigaton (e.g. Wolfenden *et al.*, 1981). Particularly noteworthy is an extraordinary research paper on the hydration of a dipeptide (Rossky and Karplus, 1979) which reports with exceptional detail the structure of the solute, the structure and dynamics of the solvent, and the influencing factors. Such studies enlarge our understanding of biochemical properties, and as such afford major contributions to drug research. Thus, the thought-provoking book of Lewin (1974) stresses the importance of the displacement of water in the control of biochemical reactions, and this should have implications for the mechanism of action of some drugs. Unfortunately, this aspect of drug research remains essentially unexplored.

Another poorly understood topic concerns the changes in *water properties* caused by the hydration of solutes. A number of solutes have structure-promoting or structure-breaking properties towards liquid water, and this may affect processes occurring in an aqueous environment (Edmonds, 1980; Symons, 1981). Thus, we showed some years ago that, compared with controls, hydrolytic cleavage reactions are notably slowed down in buffered aqueous solutions rendered highly viscous by the addition of small concentrations of a very hydrophilic polymer (Testa and Etter, 1975). The understanding and modelling of the changes in water properties (e.g. Pullman, 1977; Tapia, 1980) have implications for drug research. Long-range ordering of water molecules adjacent to many interfaces, in particular polar macromolecules and various biological membranes, is supported by several lines of experimental evidence (Drost-Hansen, 1971). The role of "bound" water in biology is a challenging object of speculation (Drost-Hansen, 1971; Hazlewood, 1977), and the distinct possibility exists that long-range ordering, by even slightly modifying the thermodynamic properties of water, influences a drug's fate and action—an influence not present in too simple biological models.

The hydrophilic properties of biological aqueous phases are balanced by the *lipophilic properties* of membranes. Constituents such as phospholipids and cholesterol confer their lipid nature on membranes and do not display large variations in their properties. This contrasts with the very broad variations in lipophilicity and other properties existing between various proteins, and between various domains and/or various states of a given protein. The amazing plasticity of proteins in terms of structure and properties is perhaps the best model at the molecular level of the plasticity of organisms. Depending on the proportion of amino acids with polar or non-polar side-chains, a protein will be hydrophilic or lipophilic overall. These properties, however, will not be influenced only by the primary structure, but also by the secondary, tertiary, and quaternary structures, and hence depend on the state of the protein as determined by intrinsic and extrinsic factors. Particularly important is the presence of structural domains in proteins (Wodak and Janin, 1981). Thus, hydrophobic packing will create lipophilic micro-environments in, e.g. an aqueous phase (Ponnuswamy *et al.*, 1980). An illuminating and extensive presentation of the biochemical and biological roles of proteins has been given by Williams (1980).

2.1.3 *Proteins and enzymes*

The numerous functions of proteins such as bio-structural constituents, biochemical effectors (enzymes), and information carriers (hormones), make them privileged partners of drugs in many of the interactions to be considered later (section 2.3). As a consequence, the study of protein structure and function has much relevance to drug research, be it to define binding sites, catalytic sites, or properties of active peptides, among others. These considerations of course do not apply only to simple proteins, but also to complex ones such as glycoproteins, the structures and roles of which have been excellently reviewed (Sharon and Lis, 1981).

Many *structural aspects of proteins* have been extensively investigated, e.g. the conformational aspects of backbone and amino acid side chains, the significance of flexibility, the various types of bends (β-bends, etc.), the stabilization of the three-dimensional structure by H-bonds and other intramolecular interactions, the intermolecular interactions controlling the quaternary structure (e.g. tetrameric proteins), as well as description and representation problems (e.g. Hartley, 1979; Isogai *et al.*, 1980; Milner-White, 1980; Némethy and Scheraga, 1980; Peticolas and Kurtz, 1980; Schwyzer, 1980; Huber and Bennett, 1983). Such studies are important in order to help characterize the chemistry and topography of pharmacological receptors and active sites in enzymes.

The contributions of *enzyme research* to advances in drug research are particularly striking. Indeed, drugs interact with enzymes as substrates (in biotransformation reactions) or as inhibitors (a frequent mechanism of therapeutic action), not to mention inducers, activators, and uncouplers. As regards enzymatic reactions, they are characterized by stereochemical choices (Overton, 1979), electrostatic stabilizations (Warshel, 1981) and thermo-dynamic aspects (Page, 1977; Conrad, 1979; Warshel and Weiss, 1980; Warshel, 1981) which are not apparent in reactions in solution. The reasons for the macromolecular nature of enzymes are thus recognized in the necessity of creating a highly specific stereochemistry and microenvironment at the active site, the necessity of allosteric regulations and particular hydrodynamic properties, and in a number of other demands and justifications. These aspects have been discussed by Luisi (1979) and Williams (1980) and illustrate simpler levels of biological complexity and organization of living matter. From a higher viewpoint, chemical, osmotic and chemiosmotic enzyme catalysis have been formulated by Mitchell (e.g. 1979) in terms of a general ligand conduction principle. This appears as one of the most comprehensive attempts to unravel and model the basic mechanisms of life processes. On a more theoretical plane, we find the conceptualization of cooperative phen-omena and synergistic processes (Haken, 1980), or the theory of hypercycles and hypercyclic regulations (Eigen and Schuster, 1979) with its vertiginous level of abstraction. Someday, it is hoped that fertile minds will take advantage of these or similar approaches in order to formulate new concepts of drug action.

2.2 DRUG MOLECULES

The search for new drugs by synthesis of a random collection and selection of the most active or least toxic compound is an approach which fell into obsolescence long ago. For many decades medicinal chemists have benefited from the powerful paradigm of structure–activity relationships, namely that biological activity varies qualitatively and/or quantitatively as a function of the molecular structure (see section 3.1). The study of molecular structure is thus an important field of medicinal chemistry.

2.2.1 Defining molecular structure

Innumerable scientists speak and write about "chemical structure", but what is understood by this term is anyone's guess and may vary considerably from case to case. More often than not, the term is taken as designating the *geometry of chemical entities*, be it simply the manner in which the constituent atoms are connected (atom connectivity, two-dimensional structure), or their arrangement in space (configuration). At these levels of model construction, molecules are considered as rigid geometrical objects. However, the concept of chemical structure extends far beyond this limited description, since to begin with molecules are more or less flexible. Their three-dimensional geometry will thus vary as a function of time (intramolecular motions, conformation).

The time dependence of molecular geometry is under the influence of *electronic properties*. Such properties are of paramount importance for a more realistic view of chemical structure since it can be stated that the geometric skeleton of a molecule is given flesh and shape in its electronic dimensions. This description, while simplistic, has deep meaning: witness the fact that the morphogenesis and definition of molecular structure and shape is a major problem in quantum mechanics (Wolley, 1978; Bader *et al.*, 1980; Trindle, 1980). In this respect, the theory of quantum topology, which appears as particularly promising, considers molecular structure as the generic property of the distribution of charges in a total system. As a consequence, molecular structure exists in spite of interactions with the environment and not as a result of them (Bader *et al.*, 1980).

Geometric and electronic properties are mutually interdependent. For example, and this is common knowledge for all chemists, the conformational behaviour of a flexible compound is controlled by its electronic properties, and these in turn show some variations as a function of dihedral angle value(s). But geometric and electronic properties also influence, and are influenced by, *interactions with the environment* (e.g. with the solvent). A number of molecular properties which are experimentally accessible result from interactions with the environment or are at least markedly influenced by them, e.g. solvation, partitioning, ionization, complex formation, reactivity. For these reasons, the concept of chemical structure must be extended to include interactions with the environment. Table 3 summarizes the above discussion and may help broaden the intuitive grasp of the concept of molecular structure. This is also presented visually in Fig. 3, where each circle (i.e. each conceptual level or sub-level) is contained in the larger circles (i.e. the higher levels or sub-levels).

TABLE 3

The description of chemical structure (Testa, 1982a)

Conceptual level	Properties considered	Examples of representation
Geometric	2-Dimensional structure (atom connectivity)	Simple diagrams
	3-Dimensional structure (configuration, "steric" properties)	Perspective diagrams, molecular models
+Electronic	Spatio-temporal structure (flexibility, prototropic equilibria, conformation)	Conformational energy diagrams, computer display
	Electronic properties (electron distribution, ionization, polarizability)	Molecular orbitals, electrostatic potential maps
+Interactions with the environment	Solvation, hydration, partitioning, inter-molecular interactions	Computer display

As stated above, the concept of molecular structure must be extended to include interactions with the environment. This is particularly true as far as structure–activity relationships are concerned. Biological activities result from interactions with a biological environment (see section 2.3), whereas a number of structural properties are related to interactions with environments which must thus be restricted to non-biological ones, i.e. none of the systems listed in Table 2. This apparently sharp discrimination (biological versus non-biological) is again an example of a dualistic trap. Consider indeed such simple biological levels as lipids or polysaccharides. Interactions with them will be classified as a biological activity or a structural property (e.g. partition

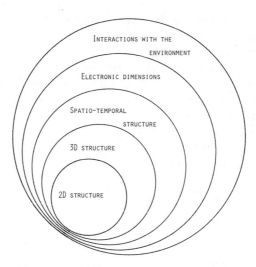

FIG. 3. The concept of molecular structure.

coefficients in water/lipid or in aqueous polymeric biphasic systems) depending on the nature and goals of the study, on the worker himself/herself, and on the door-plate of the laboratory. This discussion simply tends to show that in the expression "structure–activity relationships", the dash navigates on a continuum of possibilities. But no wonder: a molecule tends to interact with any chemical entity it approaches without having first to decide whether the latter is of a biological nature or not; matter is one, and the two chemical partners will interact according to their generic properties and not according to labels attached to them. Yet saying that biological activities are but an additional class of structural properties would be stretching common sense well beyond breaking point.

2.2.2 Stereochemistry and topography of drug molecules

The concept of pharmacodynamic receptors has a corollary, that of pharmacophores. The latter is defined as the three-dimensional distribution of electron density which will fit, and bind with, a given receptor site. This distribution is chemically determined by pharmacophoric groupings arranged in a more or less precise three-dimensional pattern which is itself dependent upon the stereochemistry of the molecule.

At this point, and in view of the overwhelming significance of stereochemical factors in drug action, let us briefly examine the problem of *stereoisomer classification* (Testa, 1979, 1982a). According to the symmetry criterion, stereoisomers can be either enantiomers or diastereoisomers, these two categories being mutually exclusive. There is little controversy in the literature about this rigid discrimination. In contrast, the concepts of configuration and conformation are difficult to apply according to a rigorously defined criterion. The simplest approach is to apply the energy criterion independently of the isomerization process involved. Thus, in qualitative terms, a "high"-energy barrier separates configurational isomers, while a "low"-energy barrier separates conformational isomers (conformers). This classification of stereoisomers lacks a well-defined borderline, and in the continuum of barrier energy values intermediate cases exist which are difficult to label. The boundary between configuration and conformation should be viewed as a broad energy range encompassing the value of 20 kcal mol^{-1} which is the limit of fair stability under ambient conditions. Medicinal chemists ill-at-ease with "fuzzy sets" (Zadeh, 1965) will be reassured by the fact that very few if any stereoisomeric drugs undergo "medium"-energy isomerization. But some future drug molecules may come as surprises.

As a general rule, *enantiomers*—or, to use an empirical and now rather obsolete term, optical isomers—display quantitative differences in their biological activities. This fact has been common knowledge for many years, but it was to the merit of Cushny (1926) to realize that it is caused by one enantiomer fitting the receptor binding site better than the other does. This preferential fit is schematized in a number of publications (e.g. Albert, 1973) by the classical three-point attachment: if three out of four ligands of an asymmetric carbon atom bind to complementary sites of the receptor, only one of the two enantiomers can present to the receptor the three ligands properly positioned. Such a model has been quite useful in allowing preliminary insight into the topography of some receptors.

In many cases, the differences in affinity and in activity between enantiomers is not as large as implied by the above model. In a limited collection of drugs, Pfeiffer (1956) found that enantiomeric potency ratio increases with the potency. This observation has been confirmed by additional examples and rationalized by Lehmann (e.g. 1982, and ref. therein), who concluded that "when a critical chiral centre is involved, in general the stereoselectivity displayed by a biomacromolecule increases with the affinity it has for the more tightly bound isomer". This modern formulation of Pfeiffer's rule is important for two reasons:

1. It allows for stereoselectivity outside the pharmacodynamic phase, and indeed it has found applications in drug metabolism.
2. The development of *in vitro* receptor binding assays allows the rapid screening of large series of enantiomeric pairs; exceptions to the rule may indicate a non-critical role for the chiral centre, or other effects of interest in drug design.

Note that the above discussion mentions only one element of chirality, namely chiral centres. To the best of my knowledge, no drug exists the dissymmetry of which is due to other elements of chirality (chiral axis or a chiral plane), although some axially chiral alkaloid derivatives have been described (Lyle, 1976). Perhaps some imaginative drug designer will one day fill this gap, an invitation for medicinal chemists to brush up less common aspects of stereoisomerism.

As opposed to configurational factors, the influence of conformational factors in drug activity is a more recent object of study, but one which has proven to be of even greater potential. The concept of conformation itself is relatively recent, since it germinated in the 1940s and 1950s owing to the creative contributions of Hassel (1943) and Barton (1950). *Conformational analysis* was soon to become one of the major tools in the search for pharmacophores, for the obvious reason that a compound will display only in a limited conformational range the pharmacophore permitting a given activity.

The search for relationships between configuration and biological activity is a relatively straightforward task; once enantiomers or diastereoisomers have been isolated, their absolute configuration can be established unambiguously and their activity determined. The story is a more complex and difficult one in the case of conformational isomers, and this is what renders this entire topic so fascinating. Theoretical conformational studies face the danger of being mere exercises in numerology if the method of calculation is too crude or unadapted, and/or if solvent effects are neglected when in fact they play an overwhelming role. Illuminating reviews on molecular orbital methods and their application to conformational analysis have been published by Pople (1976), Veillard (1976), and Richards (1977), among others.

The explicit consideration of solvent effects in molecular orbital calculations in general, and in conformational analysis in particular, has been a major challenge for a number of years (e.g. Pullman, 1974; Beveridge *et al.*, 1981; Weinstein and Green, 1981). The amazing progress now being seen in computer hardware and software should largely remove present restrictions on:

1. application of *ab initio* methods to large molecular systems;
2. geometry optimization;
3. number of degrees of conformational freedom;
4. assessment of solvent influences.

Perhaps the not too distant future will permit the calculation of conformational behaviour with highly reliable and realistic results. At present, theoretical results, while indispensable, are nevertheless suspect until they have been confirmed or "calibrated" with results from experimental investigations, in particular spectroscopic studies. The latter have their own limitations in that only some portions of a conformational energy surface or hypersurface can be determined, for example preferred conformations (global and local minima) and transition barriers. As a consequence of these and other limitations, only by taking into account both theoretical and experimental results can the conformational behaviour of a drug be reasonably well understood.

Applications of conformational analysis to drug molecules are innumerable, see for example two extensive reviews (Christoffersen, 1976; Andrews and Lloyd, 1982) and a nice mini-review (Tollenaere, 1981). But in medicinal chemistry conformational analysis cannot be a goal *per se*, only a step leading to the assessment of structure–activity relationships and to the definition of pharmacophores. The problem of finding the active conformation (e.g. van de Waterbeemd and Testa, 1983a) and defining the geometric pharmacophore is an easy one in special cases, but it may be as difficult as finding a needle in a haystack. Indeed, low-energy conformers may be the ones recognized by the receptor, but this is far from being a rule without exception. Defining the active conformation is not a trivial job, but a highly challenging one permitting a number of approaches (Humblet and Marshall, 1980). Activities and conformational behaviour can be compared for large series of compounds. The intuition, insight, imagination and abstraction power of the medicinal chemist shall never be obsolete (for an impressive example, see Portoghese, 1978), but the computer comes as an invaluable tool in allowing storage and retrieval of enormous amounts of data (Wilson and Huffman, 1980), and application of artificial intelligence to pharmacophoric pattern searching (e.g. Cohen, 1979; Gund, 1979; Marshall *et al.*, 1979; Esaki, 1982).

2.2.3 Electrostatic molecular potentials and computer graphics

As outlined earlier, geometric and electronic properties are intertwined, particularly when conformation is considered. But conformational equilibria are not the only processes intimately connected with electronic properties. Indeed, prototropic equilibria (Ganellin, 1977), ionization, solvation, and other intermolecular interactions, can play a role which may or may not be taken into account when electronic features of drug molecules are investigated by theoretical means.

How a drug approaches, "docks", fits to, and reacts with, a receptor site is influenced significantly by its electronic properties; hence the constant interest they are receiving. Some can be measured experimentally (e.g. ionization and dipole moments), while others can be approximated by theoretical means.

Charge distribution within a molecule creates an *electrostatic potential* around that molecule, and this is what a receptor or binding site first perceives.

The calculation of electrostatic molecular potentials appears as a highly interesting and promising step towards a fuller and more realistic description of molecular structures. It is also an invaluable tool in predicting and understanding intermolecular interactions (Peinel et al., 1980). A number of studies have appeared in the literature, in far smaller number, however, than theoretical conformational investigations. This situation may be due, in some places, to an incomplete appreciation of the merits of the method, and/or to some difficulties in interpreting the results. Furthermore, a major difficulty exists in that the degree of confidence to be placed in results is heavily dependent upon the level of sophistication of the quantum mechanical method used, even more so than in the case of conformational analysis. It is indeed the experience of several research groups including our own that electrostatic molecular potentials not obtained by ab initio methods must in general be regarded as suspect. For an example of interesting applications to biomedical molecules, see Kaufman et al. (1981).

Perhaps the greatest problem in practical terms is how to represent electrostatic potentials. When a complex three-dimensional surface is represented in two dimensions, an important loss of information cannot be avoided, be it in perspective drawings or in the representation of successive parallel slices cut through the body defined by that surface. Computer graphics has come as a timely rescuer to liberate electrostatic potential investigations from these limitations.

Several research groups have in recent years developed methodologies to display, view under any angle, superimpose, etc., molecular representations using graphical and screen terminals. When molecules are to be viewed as three-dimensional objects, their surface can be calculated from van der Waals radii (van der Waals surface) (e.g. Cohen, 1971). But it was immediately realized that electrostatic potential surfaces afford a more realistic representation of molecules, and we are currently witnessing an explosive development of computer graphics based on combinations of conformation and electrostatic potential calculations. Much information can be found in a remarkable review by Humblet and Marshall (1981). As an example of the methodology, the reader will find intense pleasure in studying the exceptional paper by Dean and Wakelin (1979) on the docking manoeuvre of ethidium on a DNA fragment. Marvellous colour pictures can be found in, e.g. papers by Langridge and collaborators (Langridge et al., 1981; Weiner et al., 1982).

But the application of computer graphics to drug design is certainly not meant primarily as a source of aesthetic pleasure. If it were, pharmaceutical companies and universities would not be spending millions of dollars in its implementation and development. Computer graphics bears immense hopes for drug research, and is now regarded as the most promising among the rational tools available to the drug designer. Whether the fruits will be up to the hopes, and how long this fascination will last, is anyone's guess. One of the greatest merits of computer graphics, at least in my opinion, is that it provides a much more flexible and dynamic interface between human and computer intelligence than does the QSAR methodology (see sections 3.1 and 3.2).

2.2.4 The parametrization of molecular properties

Linear free-energy relationships (see section 3.1) have led to general models which relate in a quantitative manner biological activities and molecular structures. The first problem one encounters when using this methodology is the description of molecular structures in a suitable language consisting of descriptors (parameters) which quantify properties of entire molecules or parts thereof.

Molecular descriptors can be determined experimentally (e.g. partition coefficient) or by theoretical means (e.g. energy of frontier molecular orbitals), or they can be calculated by adding up group, fragment, or substituent descriptors. The latter procedure raises the problem of energy additivity and of the equivalence of a given group attached to different molecular environments (Fadhil and Godfrey, 1982; Murdoch and Magnoli, 1982). This problem is of central importance in the parametrization of chemical properties, since it should be clear that a molecule cannot be reduced to fragments without loss of information. Assessing and expressing intramolecular interactions must thus be viewed as a second and "constructionistic" step which is aimed at correcting as much as possible the shortcomings of the first, "reductionistic" step. Some attempts already exist (in the form of lipophilic correction terms—see later), but one wonders about the number of published correlations which are of marginal or poor meaning because local descriptors were used irrespective of different intramolecular interactions.

The number of books, chapters and review articles dealing with molecular descriptors is considerable (e.g. Hansch and Leo, 1971; Purcell *et al.*, 1973; Grieco *et al.*, 1979; Osman *et al.*, 1979). In efforts to unravel pharmacophores and to adequately describe those geometric factors which influence activity, many *steric descriptors* have been proposed and used. Cartesian coordinates may be of interest in simple cases (e.g. Testa and Purcell, 1978), but sophisticated treatments exist such as molecular shape analysis (Hopfinger, 1981) or size parameters generated by the Sterimol program (Verloop *et al.*, 1976). An elaborate distance geometry analysis appears highly promising in rationalizing binding data (Crippen, 1979, 1982), and drug designers at large certainly look forward to the publication of future developments and applications.

Recent acquisitions in this active field have been the object of an interesting mini-review by Gund (1982).

Let us also briefly bring to the reader's attention the concepts of general topology and graph theory as used to encode molecular structures (Merrifield and Simmons, 1980). Their application to drug research mainly takes the form of molecular connectivity indices, a field pioneered in particular by Kier (Kier, 1980; Kier and Hall, 1976, 1981). These indices, a number of which can be calculated for each molecular structure, encode such properties as connectivity, placement and type of substituents, and electronegativities. This variety of structural information has proved of value in obtaining many significant correlations, but physicochemical interpretation may be difficult. This promising field will certainly witness interesting developments.

A much studied class of parameters are the ones describing lipophilicity/ hydrophilicity properties, e.g. partition coefficients and hydrophobic constants. This is not fortuitous, for two reasons. First, *lipophilic parameters* are the ones which up to now have yielded the largest number of successful correlations with biological activities, the reason being that distribution processes always, and binding processes very often, involve interactions with lipophilic biological environments. Second, lipophilic properties (as revealed in Fig. 3) result from the contributions, to unassessed degrees, of all other molecular properties, be they geometric or electronic. Lipophilic descriptors thus contain a wealth of structural information, and here lies a problem, as discussed later.

Partition coefficients (Leo *et al.*, 1971) are experimental measures of lipophilicity, as obtained by a variety of techniques (shake-flask method, titration in binary systems, HPLC, etc.) in a variety of solvent systems. In the last two decades values for well over 10 000 compounds have been determined, and large collections of data are available (Hansch and Leo, 1979). Partition coefficients are mostly determined in the *n*-octanol/water system for reasons extensively discussed by Hansch (Leo *et al.*, 1971; Smith *et al.*, 1975).

One fascinating aspect of the partition coefficient, which may lead to significant developments, is its relation to the kinetics of the partitioning process (e.g. van de Waterbeemd *et al.*, 1981). Another field where much remains to be done and unravelled is the thermodynamic study of partitioning (e.g. Dearden and Bresnen, 1982), from which breakthroughs can be expected in our understanding of the fundamental aspects of the phenomenon.

The most fruitful current approach to partition coefficients is their approximate additive–constitutive character, which has led to the development of several substituent or fragmental constant systems (Leo *et al.*, 1971; Rekker, 1977; Hansch and Leo, 1979; Rekker and de Kort, 1979). The hydrophobic substituent constant π conceived and developed by Hansch (e.g. Hansch *et al.*,

1963) is, in my mind, now superseded by *hydrophobic fragmental systems* (Rekker, 1977; Rekker and de Kort, 1979; Hansch and Leo, 1979). These systems are more accurate than substituent constants in calculating the partition coefficient of entire molecules, thus providing the drug designer with a helpful tool to predict lipophilicity of potential drugs before synthesis.

Both the hydrophobic fragmental system of Rekker and that of Hansch and Leo use correction terms in order to take intramolecular interactions into account. The inherent weakness of these approaches lies in these correction terms which in both cases are oversimplified, incomplete, and at times disturbingly arbitrary, as critically reviewed by us (Mayer *et al.*, 1982). More efficient hydrophobic systems should be based on a better understanding of intramolecular interactions and how such interactions affect solvation and hydration. We have recently suggested that a hydration factor could be the common denominator of the correction terms in Rekker's and Leo's systems, and could be used to express a number of perturbative influences (van de Waterbeemd and Testa, 1983b).

This search for improved correction terms cannot be separated from investigations to unravel the molecular properties which are expressed in lipophilicity/hydrophilicity (see above). There have been proposals (e.g. Testa and Seiler, 1981) that the partition coefficient is composed of a purely lipophilic steric term, and a lipophobic (polar) contribution. The most sophisticated treatment currently available is that of Cramer (1980a), who from principal factor analysis concluded that the main contributors to partition coefficient—as well, for that matter, to other properties—are bulk and cohesiveness terms.

Partition coefficient data are accumulating at an accelerating rate. Medicinal chemistry would be a poor science indeed if to this plain production of data did not correspond genuine research efforts into the fundamental aspects of partitioning processes and their significance to drug research.

To conclude this section on parametrization, let us briefly mention the problem posed by colinearity of structural descriptors. Often parameters have overlapping informational contents which preclude an adequate exploration of propriety spaces in correlation equations. It is therefore of considerable interest for the proper design of test series of potential drugs that rational substituent sets are proposed which allow high data variance and low colinearity (e.g. Streich *et al.*, 1980; Wooldridge, 1980).

2.3 DRUG INTERACTIONS WITH A BIOLOGICAL ENVIRONMENT

Having focused our attention first on biological systems and then on drug molecules, let us now discuss some general aspects of their interactions. As schematized in Fig. 2, the situations encountered are: (a) pharmacodynamic effects of a drug on a biological system; (b) metabolism undergone by a chemical compound; and (c) "silent" interactions. The latter imply that both the biological and the chemical partner will return to their prior state as soon as the interaction is over. This is exemplified by the binding of a drug to a plasma protein, where the partners (or at least the smaller one) should exhibit modified properties only as long as the complex lasts. At the molecular level, consider how spectral properties of both the protein and the ligand can vary. At high levels of biological organization, focus on the profound influence which protein binding exerts on a drug's disposition and pharmacokinetics. This topic is aptly presented by Tillement and collaborators in the present volume.

For the sake of the following discussion, let us briefly consider a point of definition. A compound interacting with any binding site (receptor, enzymatic active site, "silent" acceptor . . .) is termed a *ligand*. If biotransformation of this compound occurs following its binding to an enzyme, it is called a *substrate*. Thus, and strictly applying the definition, a substrate is a particular case of a ligand. Such a view may not be to the liking of biochemists, who apply the either/or classification to ligands and substrates of cytochrome P-450 (see section 2.3.3.). Agonists and antagonists are also particular cases of ligands when receptors are involved (section 2.3.2).

2.3.1 Biological events and types of selectivity

From a general viewpoint, the interactions of a drug with a biological environment can be broken down into three steps, as illustrated in Fig. 4. Step 1 is the penetration, which includes the pharmaceutical phase and part of the pharmacokinetic phase: absorption, distribution, entry into the compartment of receptor, enzyme, etc. In step 2, the drug molecule is recognized by the receptor, enzymatic active site, etc., to which it binds. And then, the activation occurs (Weinstein *et al.*, 1981), which is measurable as a pharmacodynamic response (pharmacological, toxicological) or as metabolite formation. Note that activation does not need to involve a specific receptor or enzyme. Indeed, alterations in membrane fluidity which modify the state of wakefulness result from non-specific interactions. Similarly, metabolite formation can also occur non-enzymatically (see section 2.3.3.).

Drug researchers are well aware that situations exist which involve only two out of the three steps in Fig. 4. Penetration is obviously bypassed when working with isolated enzymes or macromolecules. Recognition does not occur, or only to a small extent, in non-enzymatic biotransformation reactions and in non-specific receptor-independent mechanisms of action (e.g. Seeman, 1972). And there is no activation when "silent" binding occurs.

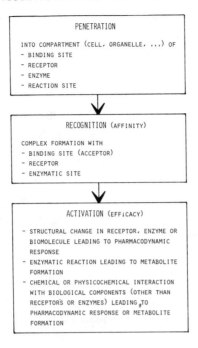

FIG. 4. A scheme of biological events in drug action.

Of course the biological events do not end with activation. Rather, in the simplest of cases, the road is traced backwards, first by dissociation of the complex, then by elimination of the drug and its metabolites.

To three types of biological events discussed above correspond in a complex manner three types of selectivity encountered in pharmacology, biochemistry, drug metabolism, etc. (Fig. 5). Depending on differences in penetration and recognition, a given compound will interact preferentially with one type of receptor among several, or with one enzyme or isozyme among several. This is expressed as *"discrimination" of receptors, acceptors or enzymes* by a given drug. We may note that when the determinants of such a discrimination are investigated, the penetration component is often neglected. This may lead to unsatisfactory rationalizations, in particular when assessing discrimination of receptor subtypes by *in vivo* studies (see section 2.3.2.). Thus, Landau *et al.* (1979) in an enlightening study showed that differential solubilities in membrane subregions afford a non-steric (i.e. receptor-independent) mechanism of drug selectivity. Similarly, Bergman *et al.* (1981) showed that for completely unknown reasons, some chlorinated xenobiotics accumulate selectively in a few brain structures, while analogous compounds distribute evenly in the brain. These penetration-related aspects of selectivity are essentially unexplored, and unfortunately are sometimes ignored.

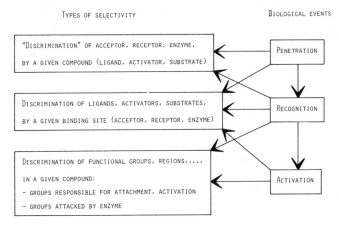

FIG. 5. Types of selectivity resulting from biological events in drug action.

The second type of selectivity is certainly the best-known one, namely the *discrimination of ligands* by a given binding site. The main determinant of this selectivity is the recognition process (e.g. Chapeville and Haenni, 1980; Dean, 1981; Pincus and Scheraga, 1981), but the role of penetration again should not be underestimated. The process of activation may also contribute to this selectivity, for example in molecular pharmacology when two drugs with identical receptor affinities have different efficacies; another example is found in biotransformation processes, when two substrates with identical affinities may be discriminated according to the energy of the transition state leading to the formation of the metabolite.

According to the structural relationships between the compounds investigated as ligands, three subtypes of selectivity can be characterized (Fig. 6). Indeed, the discrimination can be between congeners or analogs, between regioisomers, or between stereoisomers. If two enantiomers are examined, enantioselectivity may be found to occur (Lehmann, 1982), a particular case of stereoselectivity. The general case of ligand selectivity shows a close analogy with the more particular case of substrate selectivity as documented in drug metabolism. This analogy is illustrated in Fig. 6.

The third type of selectivity in Fig. 5 involves the *discrimination of functional groups, regions*, etc., in a given molecule. Such a discrimination is a robust one in drug metabolism, where the enzymatic attack at different groups or regions leads to different products and hence is easily characterized. This discrimination is recognized in drug metabolism as product selectivity, which can be subdivided as shown in Fig. 7, in analogy with Fig. 6.

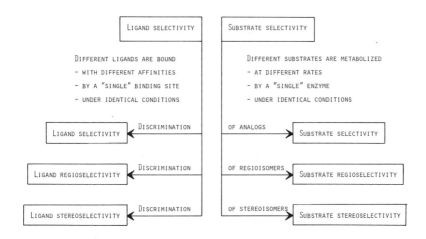

FIG. 6.   The discrimination of ligands or substrates by a given binding site or enzyme.

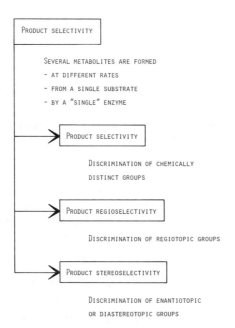

FIG. 7.   A schematic definition of product selectivities.

In ligands on the other hand, the third type of discrimination in Fig. 5 is a rather soft one because it is difficult to assign to each group an accurate contribution to the overall attachment or activation process. Certainly some groups contribute more than others, constituting the haptophore, and hence they are indeed discriminated by the binding site. Similarly, some groups in activator molecules play a privileged role in eliciting a pharmacodynamic response, e.g. groups believed to account for an antagonistic type of response at a receptor, or deceptor groups in inhibitors of enzymatic pathways. Quantitatively assessing these contributions is an important and as yet poorly met challenge to drug designers, but promising approaches have recently been developed (e.g. Crippen, 1979, 1982).

In drug metabolism, the products one obtains are chemical compounds which allow a reliable assessment of product selectivity. In contrast, the products of ligand binding are usually biochemical, pharmacological or toxicological responses to which the concept of product selectivity is not applicable as such, in agreement with the discussion of the previous paragraph. Thus drug metabolism and pharmacodynamics only partly mirror each other, as opposed to the first approximation schematized in Fig. 2.

2.3.2 Drug receptors: A meeting ground for pharmacologists and medicinal chemists

The receptor theory, which we owe to the fertile minds of Langley and Ehrlich (see the very readable historical mini-review of Parascandola, 1980) stands as one of the most prominent milestones in drug research. Although the emergence of this theory is to be traced back to the end of the nineteenth century and to the beginnning of the twentieth century, c. five decades passed before it gained general acceptance. Since then, receptor research has led to an impressive number of minor findings and major discoveries.

Until the first successful attempts at isolating receptors and the use of labeled ligands (see later), pharmacologists were dealing with "happenings in a garbage can" (Mautner, 1980), these "happenings" being expressed primarily as dose–response curves. Their interpretations have necessitated many theoretical efforts which have generated the fundamental concepts of agonism, antagonism, and partial agonism, as well as two major theories to model dose–response curves. The first theory is the "occupation theory" which states that drug effect is related to receptor occupation (e.g. Ariëns, 1966; Ariëns and Simonis, 1964; van Rossum, 1966). The second theory is the "rate theory" which proposes that a drug's response is related to the rate of formation of the drug–receptor complex (e.g. Paton and Rang, 1966). While the latter theory is useful in explaining some phenomena, there is much evidence to support the occupation theory. Thus, Paul et al. (1979) have found an excellent linear correlation between the anticonvulsant effect of diazepam and the percentage of occupied benzodiazepine receptors. Much information on the state of receptor research during the sixties can be found in two well-known reviews (Mautner, 1967; Waud, 1968).

Recent years have witnessed unprecedented developments which have literaly revolutionized receptor research. Three review articles among many are particularly recommended for their clarity and lucidity (Ariëns, 1979; Ariëns and Rodrigues de Miranda, 1979; Mautner, 1980). Perhaps the most significant advance has been the study of the binding of *labeled ligands*, as reviewed for example by Hamblin and Creese (1981). This technique allows one to conveniently determine the affinity of series of compounds for a given population of receptors and/or for different receptor types. It has thus proved to be an invaluable if obviously incomplete tool in drug screening and drug profiling.

Another domain of technical advances in receptor research is that of receptor purification and isolation (Moran and Triggle, 1970; Mautner, 1980). Much significant progress has already been made, but much more remains to be done before we can claim to have acquired some understanding of the fundamental nature and function of receptors.

The concept of *receptor mapping* has been an important contribution of medicinal chemists to receptor research. At the most elementary chemical level, drug receptors are thus viewed as a complementary pattern to pharma-cophores (see section 2.2.2), with additional regions responsible for steric hindrance or binding of non-pharmacophoric groups in the drug molecule (e.g. non-essential binding groups, moieties responsible for antagonistic properties). Rationalization of structure–activity relationships in terms of receptor mapping has thus evolved into a valuable tool in drug design (see for example Ariëns, 1966; Kuntz, 1980), and it is now greatly benefiting from such recent advances as distance geometry analysis (section 2.2.4) and computer graphics (section 2.2.3). Numerous examples of receptor mapping have been published, as exemplified by the currently hot field of dopamine agonists and antagonists. A most elaborate topographical model of the dopamine receptor is that of Humber and colleagues (Philipp *et al.*, 1979) which we have been able to tentatively enlarge (van de Waterbeemd and Testa, 1983a). Note however that receptor mapping does not need to be restricted to purely topographical considerations. Indeed, from the latter and from chemical arguments, molecular models of receptors can sometimes be conceived and offered as working hypotheses to the scrutiny of colleagues at large. This is nicely illustrated by the model of the H_1-receptor presented some years ago by Rekker *et al.* (1971). Obviously such studies lose some or much of their speculative nature when independent approaches yield information on the chemical nature of the receptor, e.g. evidence for the presence of a reactive group. In ideal cases where the site of action of a drug can be examined by X-ray crystallography (as is the case for some enzymes and macromolecules), receptor topography and chemical characterization merge to yield a powerful understanding of structure-binding relationships, but this brings us back to some of the arguments developed in section 2.2.3.

The concepts of pharmacophores and receptor topography tend to suggest a lock-and-key image of the drug–receptor complex, but this model is too limited in that it neglects an inherent *flexibility* which may be found in the drug and its receptor alike. The preferred conformation of a drug may not be its pharmacophoric conformation (see section 2.2.2.). In general, such a drug would be considered to be of relative low activity, since a greater activity is expected *a priori* for molecules which exist exclusively or predominantly in the correct pharmacophoric pattern, be they rigid or flexible compounds. However, there are cases in which flexibility itself is believed to be beneficial in terms of activity. From an impressive collection of conformational data and energies, Delettré *et al.* (1980) were able to demonstrate that when steroids interact with their receptors, the kinetics of complex formation and the responses are determined to a notable extent by ligand flexibility. These facts can gainfully be compared with the model of Portoghese (1971) postulating translocation of ligand conformational free energy in receptor activation; in other words, a ligand binding in a non-preferred conformation may, once bound, return to a low-energy conformation, the free energy thus liberated contributing to receptor activation. This model postulates the flexibility of the drug–receptor complex as being a condition for receptor activation. In fact, a conformational change in the receptor following ligand binding is often recognized as important in the sequence of events leading to the pharmacological response. Belleau (e.g. 1965) was one of the first to relate conformational perturbation to the regulation of receptor as well as enzyme behaviour. More recently, Burgen (1981) has also examined how the initial transduction of binding energy into action could be accomplished through a conformational change in the drug–receptor complex. This entire topic of the transduction of a molecular binding process into a macroscopic event is one of the major challenges faced by pharmacological sciences. In contrast, some *seconday events* in this sequence are already reasonably well understood, e.g. the drug–receptor complex may trigger an enzymatic transducer, resulting in the liberation of a messenger such as cAMP or Ca^{2+}; effectors or amplifiers systems are thus involved (Berridge, 1980). The understanding of these mechanisms is important not only at the fundamental level, but also in suggesting new target systems for drug research, with particularly fruitful results being reported in recent years—witness the calcium antagonistic drugs (Rahwan *et al.*, 1979).

Drug–receptor interactions have also allowed some insights into the different behaviours of agonists and antagonists, and this brings us back to the primary events of drug action. Thus, Weiland et al. (1979) have shown that, at least for the β-adrenergic receptor, the binding of antagonists is essentially entropy-driven with little change in enthalpy. In contrast, agonist binding is accompanied by a large decrease in enthalpy permitting an unfavourable decrease in entropy; these changes occur mainly in the second stage of the binding, when the complex undergoes a conformational change triggering the action. Such thermodynamic studies should certainly become more prevalent because they address precisely those upstream events in drug action where much obscurity remains (see Page, 1983).

A major issue of molecular pharmacology has been, and still remains, *receptor multiplicity*. This multiplicity is documented for a number of receptor types, with much controversy often attached to it. Indeed, a neutral observer (if such exists) sometimes gets the impression of a highly competitive field where alternate classifications are proposed prematurely, and where similar evidence may be interpreted differently to support or to dispute receptor multiplicity. The dopamine receptor is exemplary in this respect, and the interested reader is referred to the careful and balanced review of Horn and colleagues (1981). These authors give attention not only to pre- and postsynaptic dopamine receptors and to the various classifications proposed, but also to the obviously critical aspect of their clinical significance (concerning the latter, see also Calne, 1980). An important classification is that of Kebabian and Calne (1979) who distinguish between two populations of dopamine receptors, namely those linked to adenylate cyclase (D-1), and those which are not (D-2). Based on various binding behaviours, this classification has been expanded to D-3 and D-4 receptors (Sokoloff et al., 1980; Seeman, 1982), but the existence of the D-4 receptors is challenged (Creese and Sibley, 1982). For Laduron (1983), only the D-2 site meets the criteria of a genuine pharmacological receptor, whereas the D-3 and D-4 sites must be considered as binding sites devoid of any physiological meaning.

While the existence of multiple dopamine receptors is supported by generally strong evidence, the contrasting unitary dopamine receptor model (e.g. Van Gompel et al., 1982) is also coherent in explaining many findings. The latter model involves various specific binding sites differentially exposed. In most people's mind, the two models are perceived as incompatible, making it difficult to avoid dogmatic attitudes. But are these two models really incompatible? Can they not be perceived as different and partial representations of a single reality? Furthermore, how much do differences in membranes and membrane uptake, differential distribution into different organ areas or into different organs, account for receptor selectivity and multiplicity? We have already stressed (see section 2.3.1) that uneven distribution into such organs as the brain does occur. On a broader scale, organ selectivity of drugs has been proposed as an alternative to receptor selectivity (Kenakin, 1982).

But whether receptor multiplicity is due to differences in the receptor core, in accessory sites, in the microenvironment, or in the membrane, and whatever the physiological differences between binding sites, the fact remains that this multiplicity is an operational reality and even a truism as far as structure–activity relationships are concerned. Just consider the histamine H_1 and H_2 receptors, the existence of which is undisputed because they are so clearly discriminated pharmacologically or by structurally distinct ligands.

The concept of multiple receptor sites, which has been analyzed from a theoretical viewpoint by De Lean et al. (1979), is of interest not only as far as receptor multiplicity is concerned, but also with respect to *complex receptor systems*. This again leads us back to the cascade of events following receptor binding. Indeed, the nature and coupling of binding sites within a receptor complex partly reveals its mechanism of action. The best example of such a complex is the oligomeric GABA receptor (e.g. De Feudis, 1981) which is now viewed as comprising the GABA, benzodiazepine, and picrotoxin/ barbiturate recognition sites, which are interrelated in controlling anion (chloride) and cation ionophores (Squires and Saederup, 1982). Less well understood, but equally fascinating, is the opiate receptor, for which an allosteric coupling of yet unknown function has been documented between the morphine and enkephalin receptors (Rothman and Westfall, 1982).

The concept of receptors is an eminently reductionistic one as far as pharmacology is concerned. However, the value of this concept derives not only from it being a pillar of molecular pharmacology, but also from its utility in general pharmacology. In other words, the receptor concept is compatible and integral with global pharmacological approaches.

Over the years, it has been increasingly recognized that drug–receptor interactions not only produce "immediate" effects, but may also affect the receptors themselves in their number and/or properties. This of course suggests that the artificial (drug-induced) activation or blockade of receptors stimulates some regulatory mechanisms. Extensive data on *receptor adaptations* to neuropharmacological agents have been compiled by Creese and Sibley (1981). Thus, chronic administration of neuroleptics, which act primarily through dopamine receptor blockade, renders these receptors supersensitive (Clow et al., 1979; Costa, 1980). In this context, it is worth remembering that as early as 1966, Collier (1966) proposed that tolerance and physical dependence might be due to drug-induced changes in the number of receptors.

In addition to these external influences, receptors must also be under the control of endocrine influences. However, this topic has not as yet been sufficiently investigated in its own right. Interesting studies report endocrine influences on the actions of some drugs, e.g. morphine (Kasson *et al.*, 1983), but how much receptors themselves are affected remains to be better understood. Hopefully future research will place receptors in a more holistic perspective (see Table 2).

In conclusion, there is much more in discussing drug interactions with a biological environment than merely deriving various types of selectivity (see Fig. 5) or assessing the influence of chemico-structural factors (sections 2.2 and 3.1). Indeed, due acknowledgement must be given to the hierarchical levels of biological organizations of relevance to the studies or results under consideration, bearing in mind that the extrapolation from one level to the other is not straightforward (see section 2.1.). Furthermore, any biological response is under the influence of a number of physiological factors, both endocrine or caused by external influences, which can vary from one individual to the other at a given time, or for a given individual at different times. Figure 5 can thus be completed as shown in Fig. 8 which schematizes various ways of approaching biological responses of any kind.

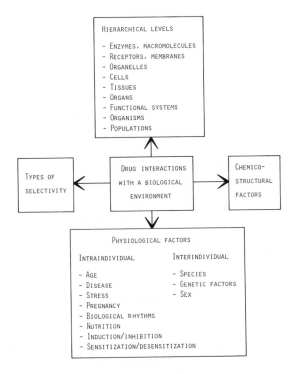

FIG. 8. Approaches to the study of biological events in drug action.

2.3.3 Drug metabolism: A meeting ground for medicinal chemists, pharmacologists, and biochemists

Figure 6 is relevant not only to pharmacodynamic effects, but also to drug metabolism which we have viewed as reverse of the former (see Fig. 2). As such, it offers a convenient transition between the previous and the present section.

When compared to "classical" sciences such as pharmacology, toxicology and chemistry, drug metabolism (for a definition, see Di Carlo, 1982) is a "young" science (Testa, 1976). However, its maturation to a "full" science has been exceptionally swift. This took place over the last two or three decades, once it had been universally recognized that the pharmacodynamic properties of any xenobiotic are influenced by its metabolism quantitatively and kinetically (intensity and time course of effects) as well as qualitatively (pharmacologically active or chemically reactive metabolites). Some qualitative aspects of xenobiotic metabolism of particular interest in drug research will be discussed here.

The *process of drug absorption* has been taken for granted for a long time. But things have changed, and for the better. The various modes of absorption are now being systematically investigated for all factors influencing them (e.g. Houston and Wood, 1980), and new routes of absorption are being used therapeutically for systemic administration. The dermal route now enjoys a marked interest, witness the novel device known as the transdermal therapeutic system. Obviously pharmaceutical technology and biopharmacy have much to contribute to drug research.

Distribution and *excretion* are two processes which have much in common, since elimination can be considered as the distribution (active or passive) to a "flush-out" compartment such as bile or urine. Distribution to the brain is of particular importance not only because it is the target organ of an impressive number of drugs, but also because a number of side-effects of drugs result from their crossing of the blood–brain barrier. A better understanding of all those factors (physiological and chemical) influencing distribution to the brain is thus an explicit goal of drug research. It is well known for many QSAR studies (e.g. Kubinyi, 1979) that the optimal $\log P$ for brain penetration is c. 2. Nevertheless, highly lipophilic neuroleptics readily enter the brain, whereas a new generation of very potent and lipophilic antihistamines, e.g. terfenadine (Cheng and Woodward, 1982), are devoid of central side-effects. Obviously many questions remain to be answered.

In relation with the safety of unborn and newborn children, xenobiotic *distribution to the fetus* and *excretion in milk* are now receiving intensive attention which was long overdue. Placental transfer, disposition in the fetus, and species differences in milk excretion, are now reasonably well understood even if the data available are relatively limited. A number of useful reviews are available (e.g. Green *et al.*, 1979; Wilson *et al.*, 1980; Welch and Findlay, 1981).

Reversible *binding to proteins* and other macromolecules is a major determinant of drug distribution. Binding to serum albumin is a well-documented phenomenon, although obviously there is still much to be discovered in this field. However, albumin is not, and by far, the only plasmatic macromolecule, and the significance of drug binding to several other plasmatic macromolecules is only now being uncovered. This topic, which has important pharmacological and therapeutic implications, is an active research front reviewed by Tillement and colleagues in the present volume.

Recent findings suggest that binding to blood constituents such as erythrocytes and leucocytes, as well as to tissue macromolecules, may have a marked influence on the pharmacokinetic behaviour of a given xenobiotic (e.g. Curry, 1970). These binding processes are conceptually quite distinct from storage into lipidic tissues, although experimentally the discrimination is a delicate one. In addition, the study of binding to macromolecules in some tissues is difficult to perform without interference from biotransformation processes. For the above and other reasons, this entire topic is still in its infancy, and relatively few research papers have been published (e.g. Bickel and Steele, 1974; Fichtl *et al.*, 1980). Improved experimental approaches and a greater interest in this topic are expected to permit a better understanding of these processes and of their contribution to drug–drug interactions and pharmacokinetic variations.

Before turning to biotransformation, let us briefly mention that scientists and the educated public are now aware that the concept of disposition applies to organisms as well as to ecological systems. A topic of particular worry is the *ecodisposition* of persistent polyhalogenated compounds and its relationship with toxicokinetics (Bickel and Muehlebach, 1980; Jondorf, 1981a).

Xenobiotic biotransformation (or metabolism, in a narrow sense) is a field which has developed at a surprising rate when considered in proper perspective. At the chemical level, the ever increasing number and structural complexity of drugs, the constant improvement of instrumentation and techniques, as well as regulatory requirements for metabolic data, have resulted in many novel pathways being discovered. For a number of years, many findings belonged to functionalization reactions (phase I reactions), improving our understanding of enzymatic reaction mechanisms, and bringing evidence for the involvement of enzymes previously believed to react exclusively with endogenous substrates (Jenner and Testa, 1978; Testa and Jenner, 1978). Several newly discovered *conjugation reactions* have regularly enriched our knowledge in the past but it appears that the recent years have been particularly fruitful in this respect. For example, and in contrast to the obsolete belief that conjugates must be hydrosoluble, highly lipophilic conjugates of xenobiotics have now been characterized. Thus, various compounds are conjugated with fatty acids (e.g. Leigthy *et al.*, 1976; Lange *et al.*, 1981); the structural variety of the substrates tends to indicate that the reaction may be the rule rather than the exception for hydroxylated compounds. Other fascinating discoveries involve cholesterol (Fears *et al.*, 1982) and biliary acids (Quistad *et al.*, 1982) as the endogenous conjugating moiety for exogenous acids. An entire new field of research is opened by these novel metabolites; their physicochemical properties, their peculiar pharmacokinetics (high potential for tissue accumulation), and the consequences thereof at the cellular level, will certainly attract a number of investigators, and we can look forward to many findings.

Functionalization and conjugation reactions are typically high-energy processes, i.e. involving the cleavage and creation of covalent bonds. This contrasts with reversible binding to proteins and other macromolecules, as discussed previously. From a conceptual viewpoint, it is of interest to note that intermediate cases do exist, even if they are not always recognized as such. Indeed, *drug–macromolecule conjugates* are quite common (Caldwell, 1982). One case involves the oxidative formation of a disulfide bond between a cysteinyl residue and a thiol-containing drug (e.g. captopril, see Soudijn, 1982). Other quite common cases involve the covalent binding of reactive metabolic intermediates to various enzymes (suicide substrates) or macromolecules (post-enzymatic reactions, see later). The toxicological consequences of these macromolecular conjugates are being actively investigated (see later), in contrast to their pharmacokinetic behaviour and subsequent fate, which are essentially unexplored. Figure 9 summarizes the above discussion.

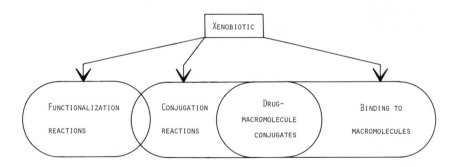

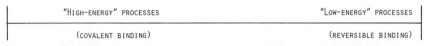

FIG. 9. Chemical processes in xenobiotic metabolism.

Enzymological aspects are perhaps that field of drug metabolism where advances occur at the fastest pace. Some years ago, it was possible to consider endogenous and exogenous molecules as substrates for distinct enzymes; such a distinction can no longer be accepted today (see Jenner *et al.*, 1981; Testa *et al.*, 1981). Enzymes which were once believed to metabolize exclusively endogenous molecule, e.g. prostaglandin endoperoxide synthetase, are now known to metabolize xenobiotics as well; a number of relevant examples can be found in the chapter by Mesnil *et al.* (this volume, p. 95). Furthermore, enzyme systems originally believed to be xenobiotic metabolizers have since revealed endogenous functions. The best-known example is certainly cytochrome P-450, which plays progressively discovered key roles in the metabolism of such endogenous compounds as hormonal steroids, vitamin D, fatty acids and prostaglandins (e.g., Kupfer, 1980; Jenner *et al.*, 1981). As a consequence of the above, the discrimination between xenobiotic- and endobiotic-metabolizing enzymes, if intellectually pleasing in its dualistic simplicity, is in fact a dangerously misleading oversimplification. The metabolism of endogenous compounds and that of xenobiotics are intimately intertwined, with consequences that may be dramatic (induction, competitive or irreversible inhibition, disregulation), and cannot be ignored (Parke, 1981). A number of toxic effects of environmental chemicals and drugs at the molecular, cellular and organ level result precisely from such interconnections (see also later).

Today, the question of distinct xenobiotic- and endobiotic-metabolizing enzymes is still being debated, but at the level of isozymes. Indeed, the concept of *enzyme multiplicity* (e.g. Lu, 1979) offers fascinating perspectives and developments. The problem discussed above can thus be reworded: considering enzymes which metabolize xenobiotics and their usually broad substrate selectivity, does the latter result from the superimposed rather broad substrate selectivities of a few isozymes, or from the superimposed very narrow substrate selectivities of a considerable number of isozymes? The answer to such a question awaits a definitive knowledge of the real number of isozymes of a given enzyme, if such a datum has any meaning at all and can be obtained.

The enzyme most actively investigated at present for its multiplicity is *cytochrome P-450*, with speculations for the number of its multiple forms ranging from ten or twenty to thousands (see the remarkable commentary by Nebert and Negishi, 1982). There are now numerous publications showing that the cytochrome P-450 multiple forms so far isolated have distinct substrate and product selectivities which overlap only partly. In this context, an important finding is that regioselective hydroxylation by cytochrome P-450 isozymes is at least in part accounted for by distinct modes of binding of the substrate (Novak and Vatsis, 1982), whereas earlier studies had implicated electronic factors (Testa and Mihailova, 1978). In connection with these approaches, studies are now in progress to determine amino acid sequences (e.g. Gotoh *et al.*, 1983) of apocytochromes P-450, with the goal of explaining immunochemical differences and also mapping the substrate-binding site(s). Results of such investigations at the molecular level, when replaced in higher context, will do much to enrich our fundamental understanding of metabolic phenomena.

Enzyme multiplicity cannot be dissociated from the well-known phenomena of *induction* and *inhibition*. Cytochrome P-450 again is exemplary in this respect, the isozyme selectivity displayed by inhibitors (e.g. Testa and Jenner, 1981) and even more by inducers (e.g. Sharma *et al.*, 1979) being a precious experimental tool. These studies recently gained a new dimension when it was shown that *genetic mechanisms* control the induction of at least some monooxygenase activities (e.g. Nebert, 1979; Nebert *et al.*, 1981). The relationships between carcinogenesis and bioactivation by some cytochrome P-450 isozymes (see later) have created immense interest in the induction of cytochrome P_1-450, its regulation via a cytosolic receptor, and its control by a cluster of genes called the Ah locus (Nebert, 1980; Nebert and Jensen, 1979). These points aptly illustrate how drug metabolism, once the "poor relative" of pharmacology, has evolved from the factual to the fundamental level and is now growing at an explosive rate in many directions.

Tissue and organ differences is one field of xenobiotic metabolism still dominated by facts and data more than by concepts and fundamental differences. That the body of a higher organism should be "anisotropic" with respect to biotransformation has been common sense for a long time. However, the former assumption was more of a yes–no type—yes in the liver, very little elsewhere. Today's assessment can be summarized as follows: (a) non-hepatic tissues play a significant role in xenobiotic metabolism, and (b) the differences between tissues or organs are very large, both quantitatively and qualitatively. These differences and their consequences in terms of *in vivo* metabolism are now being actively studied by a considerable number of investigators (e.g. Vainio and Hietanen, 1980; Connelly and Bridges, 1980). For a number of reasons related to drug action and xenobiotic toxicity, some organs and tissues are of particular interest, e.g. gut wall, blood, bone marrow, lung, placenta, brain (see an extensive chapter in this volume), as well as the gut microflora, which in this context can be regarded as an organ.

A particular and very important case is the *fetus*, which in terms of xenobiotic metabolism is simultaneously an "organ", and an organism in a peculiar environment. The fetus globally displays a relatively large potential for biotransformation (Pelkonen, 1980a, 1980b), the consequences of which are far from being sufficiently understood. Many fragmentary results have been published, as well as some generalizations. But a global understanding of xenobiotic disposition and metabolism is urgently needed at the level of the mother–placenta–fetus triad.

Xenobiotic metabolism is affected by a number of *physiological factors* (Fig. 8) which are all being investigated, though to varying extents. Species differences have always been of considerable concern to biologists, pharmacologists and toxicologists, and the enormous amount of information available (e.g. Kato, 1979; Walker, 1980) is progressively making sense. The interested reader is referred to a concise and striking review by Caldwell (1981), as well as two stimulating and masterly reviews by Jondorf (1981a, 1981b) where xenobiotic metabolism is examined from an evolutionary viewpoint. Genetic factors have in recent years become a major issue in drug metabolism. Besides the previously mentioned genetic control of induction, it is now well established that genetic differences between individuals of a given species may account for large differences in some xenobiotic-metabolizing activities. For obvious reasons, genetic differences in humans are of particular significance as far as drug research is concerned. Classical examples of genetically controlled enzymes include acetyltransferase and alcohol dehydrogenase (Kalow, 1980). More recently, the cytochrome P-450 oxidation of several drugs has also been shown to be genetically controlled, with important therapeutic consequences actively investigated by clinical pharmacologists (e.g. Eichelbaum, 1982). To make sense, these genetic differences must be assessed in relatively large human populations, and the ethnic differences thus detected are opening a new biological level at which to study drug metabolism (Kalow, 1982).

Sex differences in drug metabolism occur primarily in the rat and also in the mouse, and seemingly much less in other species. These variations raise a number of question as to their origin; they may be due to multiple enzymatic forms, to hormonal regulation, or more likely to both since these factors should be interrelated. And why should sex differences be species-dependent? As regards humans, a few cases are documented, for example the longer half-life of oxazepam in women than in men, a difference which varies with age (Greenblatt *et al.*, 1980). However, the therapeutic consequences of these few cases may be rather modest.

In contrast, age-related differences in drug metabolism are supported by numerous publications and are gaining a long overdue recognition as non-negligible determinants of drug kinetics. Two fractions of the population are particularly concerned, namely the newborns and very young children on one side, and the elderly on the other. The fetus is a particular case which we have considered earlier.

Besides age, other factors can operate to produce intraindividual variations (Fig. 8) in drug metabolism. This is true for circadian and other biological rhythms (Reinberg and Smolensky, 1982) which should be taken into account to optimize administration schedules. Disease states, at least a number of them, may profoundly affect drug kinetics (Jenner and Testa, 1981). Many findings have been made, several of them in animal models which do not always show enough relevance to clinical situations.

Environmental factors such as food constituents and pollutants, as well as other drugs, can also modify xenobiotic metabolism by influencing physiological conditions and modifying enzymatic activities (activation, induction, or inhibition) (Alvares *et al.*, 1980; Park and Beckenridge, 1981). Ethanol affords a particularly illustrative example due to the complexity of its effects, acute, chronic, and pathological; in fact, drug metabolism shows a number of alterations in alcoholics (Pelkonen and Sotaniemi, 1982) which have marked therapeutic consequences. However, clinical pharmacologists know that physiological factors influencing drug kinetics cannot always be examined individually, and that many combinations of modifying factors are encountered in clinical situations. Assessing and understanding such combined influences while also taking drug–drug interactions into account is a major prerequisite for optimizing the therapeutic use of known and future drugs.

One of the reasons which provides so much incentive to the fast development of xenobiotic metabolism studies is the fact that many metabolites are pharmacodynamically active (Drayer, 1982). Pharmacologically active metabolites will not be discussed here, as opposed to *toxic metabolites*, be they metabolic intermediates or stable compounds.

A xenobiotic may be transformed by enzymatic or non-enzymatic reactions, or even by reactions which are difficult to categorize (for more details, see Testa, 1982b). The metabolite(s) thus generated may be stable, or may be reactive and spontaneously undergo post-enzymatic reactions (Fig. 10). When the primary metabolites are electrophiles (e.g., diol-epoxides) or radicals (e.g. semiquinone radicals) which covalently bind to some critical biomolecules, the initial conditions which may lead to such phenomena as mutagenesis, carcinogenesis, or teratogenesis are met (e.g. Nelson, 1982). Oxidative stress, namely the generation of activated oxygen species and the biological consequences thereof, is now recognized as an important determinant of toxicity (Holtzman, 1982). Conjugation reactions, which until some years ago were believed to be exclusively detoxication processes, have been shown in a number of cases to generate reactive and/or toxic metabolites (Reichert, 1981). For example, macromolecular conjugates are potential haptens which may lead to allergic responses or immunological disorders.

The present section has considered some aspects of xenobiotic metabolism as viewed from a qualitative and general viewpoint. Another major aspect is the mathematical description of metabolic processes as a function of time (pharmacokinetics and toxicokinetics, see Di Carlo, 1982). These *kinetic aspects* have been and are an important field of drug research to which innumerable papers, many review articles and an impressive number of books have been devoted. The time is now over when progress meant longer pharmacokinetic equations. Clinical relevance and applicability has become the major goal of research in pharmacokinetics (e.g. Wagner, 1975; Rowland and Tozer, 1980), with the description of time-dependent phenomena becoming a major issue (Lévy, 1982).

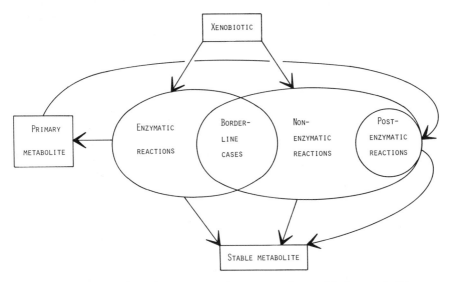

FIG. 10. Enzymatic and non-enzymatic processes in xenobiotic metabolism.

In conclusion, drug metabolism has now established itself as the counterpart of pharmacodynamics. These two aspects of drug research are complementary and of equal importance, and a lack of balance in future progresses does not appear desirable.

2.3.4 Overview

In Fig. 5 we have stressed that drug-related biological events can be broken down into various types of selectivity. Furthermore, these events are influenced both qualitatively and quantitatively by the chemico-structural features of the drugs, and assessing these influences implies the reduction of drug molecules to a number of properties (see section 2.2). In short, the horizontal axis in Fig. 8, which displays these two analytical approaches, may be labeled a reductionistic axis where complex phenomena are viewed as a summation of simpler ones.

In section 2.3.2 and 2.3.3, the importance of hierarchical levels in biological studies has been repeatedly mentioned, as resulting from uninterrupted increases in complexity/organization (section 2.1.1) as we climb the biological ladder. Similarly, the role of physiological factors becomes overwhelming as higher hierarchial levels are reached. These two approaches, displayed on the vertical axis in Fig. 8, thus aim at taking biological complexity into account and viewing drug-related events in the global context of living systems. This axis can therefore be labeled a holistic one since it symbolizes attempts to view phenomena in their totality as an integrated whole, and not as a collection of dissected parts.

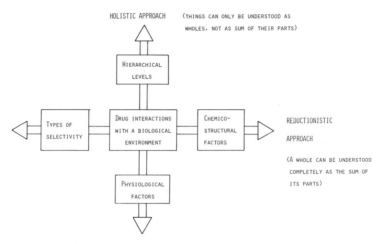

FIG. 11. The two axes of scientific research as applied to the study of biological events in drug action.

To summarize the above, Fig. 8 is transformed into Fig. 11 which defines the reductionistic and the holistic approaches. To avoid all misunderstanding, let me clearly state that no value judgement is implied here. Philosophers, epistemologists and scientists have fought over one or the other approach when in fact they are complementary. The conclusion offered here is therefore that advances in drug research, to be of any real significance, must result from coordinated efforts at both the molecular and the biological levels.

3 Advances in drug research?

Drug research progresses through the study of biological systems, of drug molecules, and of their interactions (section 2). Taken together and integrated, these three fields of research yield the broad discipline of structure–activity relationships, the current spearhead in the search for new drugs, and the central paradigm of medicinal chemistry. Structure–activity relationships, as will be discussed below, are central not only for the optimization of lead compounds, but may also contribute to, and help understand, lead finding. A number of stimulating reviews have appeared, e.g. Albert (1971, 1982), Burger (1979), and Hathway (1982).

3.1 DRUG DESIGN

In a series of compounds, the biological activity can vary in two ways:

1. *qualitatively*, when different pharmacophores (section 2.2.2) are present, resulting in interactions with different receptors or other sites and hence in different mechanisms of action;
2. *quantitatively*, when the same pharmacophore is present in all compounds, resulting in a single mechanism of action, while differences in substitution produce differences in the intensity of the biological response.

Such a view is quite a schematic one, and hence often misleading, especially when the therapeutic effect results from actions at several sites as is often the case with neuropharmacological drugs. Nevertheless, the above discrimination has its interest as a first approximation, since qualitative and quantitative differences in activity are related respectively to the concepts of lead finding and lead optimization which are central to drug design (Austel and Kutter, 1980; Craig, 1980).

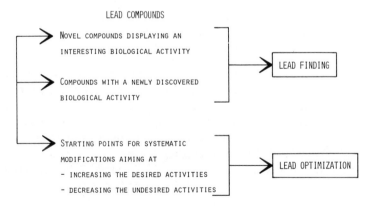

FIG. 12. The concept of lead compounds in drug design.

Defining *lead compounds* may not be as easy as intuitively believed, and an attempt at definition is presented in Fig. 12. The underlying idea of novelty is evident, either in novel compounds, or in new activities displayed by known compounds. Discovering either of these novelties is the aim of lead finding. But lead compounds are also starting points for lead optimization, as discussed later.

Lead finding can be accomplished in a number of ways. The most important origins of lead compounds are listed in Table 4. Regarding biological hypotheses, mention can be made of enzyme-directed research. Understanding of enzyme function, mechanism and structure can indeed be the starting point for the design of enzyme inhibitors, a promising approach in lead finding (e.g. Hansch, 1979; Krenitsky and Elion, 1982). Note as regards Table 4 that the various origins of lead compounds are not mutually exclusive, and that several combinations have been observed.

TABLE 4

Lead compounds

Origin of leads	Definition and/or relevant disciplines
Mass (random) screening	Systematic synthesis and evaluation
Rational approach (based on correct or incorrect hypothesis)	Biological hypotheses
	Artificial intelligence (pharmacophore recognition, molecular graphics)
Natural products	Pharmacognosy
	Ethnopharmacology
	Marine biology
Drug metabolites	Systematic synthesis and evaluation of metabolites
Side-effects of drugs	Recognition of unexpected effects in (clinical) pharmacology
Serendipity[a]	Discovery by accident and sagacity

[a]"The three princes of Serendip . . . were always making discoveries, by accident and sagacity, of things they were not in quest of." Horace Walpole, 1794 (see Clarke, 1979).

Lead optimization can be pursued using a number of approaches, be they intuitive, at random, or rational (qualitatively or quantitatively), these three categories overlapping to some extent. In these pages, we shall restrict ourselves to two important rational approaches, namely an essentially qualitative one based on biotransformation considerations, and quantitative structure–activity relationships. Other important approaches obviously also exist, e.g. the concept of bioisosteric which can provide many ideas of molecular modification and is complementary to the methods discussed below (Thornber, 1979).

From a therapeutic viewpoint, drug metabolism can be beneficial (e.g. if active metabolites are produced, or if their formation corresponds to a detoxication), or it can be detrimental (e.g. if the drug is eliminated too rapidly, or if toxic metabolites are produced). According to these circumstances, several approaches are useful in drug design, the extremes of which are "hard" drugs and prodrugs. Ariëns (e.g. Ariëns and Simonis, 1982) has advocated the design of unmetabolizable drugs called *"hard" drugs*, by "metabolic stabilization". Such drugs should display a number of advantages, for example longer half-lives, decreased intra- and interpatient variability, decreased species differences, and decreased number and significance of active metabolites. A less extreme approach is "metabolic switching", which aims at increasing the generation of therapeutic active metabolites, and decreasing the generation of toxic metabolites. *Metabolic switching* is achieved by molecular modifications which block metabolic attack at some groups, or promote it at other groups.

Promotion and control of biotransformation underlie the concepts of "soft" drugs and prodrugs. In both classes of drugs, extensive and relatively rapid metabolism occurs as a *sine qua non* condition due to the incorporation of labile groups. *"Soft" drugs*, a concept pioneered by Bodor (e.g. 1982a, 1982b), are "biologically active compounds characterized by a predictable *in vivo* metabolism to nontoxic moieties". In contrast, the well-known class of *prodrugs* consists of compounds with little or no activity undergoing metabolic transformation to a therapeutically active compound (e.g. Albert, 1958; Roche, 1977; Notari, 1981; Pitman, 1981; Wermuth, 1984). In many prodrugs, the metabolic activation occurs by hydrolytic cleavage which liberates the active moiety. However, activation by other reactions, e.g. oxidation, is also documented, and the designation of "bioprecursors" is sometimes used in such cases.

Prodrugs have contributed significantly to drug design, and many of them are in wide therapeutic use. Reasons for their creation are numerous, aiming for example at improved pharmaceutical properties, improved compliance, improved pharmacokinetics, improved organ selectivity, or decreased side effects; marketing considerations sometimes also play a role. From the point of view of a rational therapy, the design of prodrugs as site-specific delivery systems (Stella and Himmelstein, 1980; Bundgaard *et al.*, 1982) appears a particularly interesting and promising topic of research, and we can certainly look forward to noteworthy advances (see also Bodor's chapter in this volume).

To summarize the above discussion, Fig. 13 schematically presents prodrugs, soft drugs and hard drugs categorized according to their metabolic stability and their activity prior to metabolism. These three classes should not hide the forest of innumerable "plain" drugs, which are active as such, which undergo metabolism to various degrees, and which may or may not yield active metabolites contributing to their therapeutic effects. Note that inactive unmetabolizable compounds do not usually qualify as drugs.

Quantitative structure–activity relationships (QSAR) are the application to pharmacology and medicinal chemistry of Mach's Principle ("Every statement in physics has to state relations between observable quantities"). In a classical paper, Hansch and Fujita (1964) presented the first quasi-general mathematical approach to structure–activity relationships Since then, the *"Hansch approach"* has undergone an explosive development (Tute, 1971, 1980; Hansch, 1981). In particular, the relationship between partition coefficient and biological response has been extensively analyzed using a number of models (e.g. Kubinyi, 1979; Cooper *et al.*, 1981). Biological activity is often found to be heavily dependent on lipophilicity, hence the capital importance of gaining an in-depth understanding of this relationship.

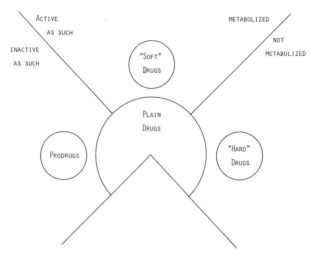

FIG. 13. A metabolic basis for qualitative drug design.

The parametric approach of Hansch is in its essence an application to biology of linear free-energy relationships (LFER). As such, it is often contrasted with the *de novo, non-parametric method* first proposed by Free and Wilson (1964), although both methods are closely related. These two regression analysis methods are categorized by Lewi (1976) as strongly predictive. To this group also belongs the highly sophisticated DARC/PELCO method of Dubois (e.g. Mercier *et al.*, 1981), the full potential of which does not appear to be recognized everywhere.

The classification of compounds into two or few classes (e.g. active versus inactive) is performed by the so-called weak predictive methods, most of which belong to the domain of *multivariate statistics* (Lewi, 1980). These methods, which have progressed considerably in recent years, include discriminant analysis, pattern recognition, factor analysis and principal component analysis, spectral mapping, and cluster analysis (Lewi, 1976, 1978; Kirschner and Kowalski, 1979).

In addition to the above methods, the drug designer also has at his disposal a number of *manual methods* (Purcell *et al.*, 1973; Chu, 1980) which despite their relative simplicity can prove quite useful. Recently, the theory of sets has been applied as a promising tool in drug design (Austel and Kutter, 1981). For a general, and indeed critical, review of several methods used in QSAR, the interested reader is referred to the useful book by Martin (1978); some methodological advances are extensively treated in a review chapter (Martin, 1979).

Despite being only 20 years old, the QSAR methodology has come of age a number of years ago, and is still developing at an impressive pace. The mathematical and statistical foundations of QSAR are receiving some (e.g. Martin and Panas, 1979; Topliss and Edwards, 1979), but perhaps not sufficient, attention. The various methods themselves, be they manual or statistical, parametric or not, are a very active field of research, as outlined above. In this context, the entirely novel methods of *computer graphics* (see section 2.2.3) must be considered as a major development, if not a break-through, in quantitative drug design, the potential of which they expand considerably. In some circles one can hear experts serenely voicing the opinion that molecular graphics will supersede QSAR. Such a belief is unwarranted and will not come true, any more than QSAR could have prevented medicinal chemists from continuing to use their intelligence, creativity and intuition when designing drugs. In fact, QSAR and molecular graphics are remarkably complementary tools at the command of the medicinal chemist, and their combined use should prove very fruitful.

In an inspired article, Cavalla (1980) wrote:

One area that does excite a growing academic interest is the study of Quantitative Structure–Activity Relationships and the hope is always there that one day even this Christmas cactus will bloom.

Indeed, the interest is still growing; but does this growth occur in academic circles only? Certainly the interest is just as great, if not greater, in industrial research. And to admire the cactus' bloom, no need to look in a crystal ball—the scientific literature contains relatively few examples of QSAR success, but they are genuine. For example, a successful improvement of antiallergic pyranenamines has been reported (Cramer *et al.*, 1979; Cramer, 1980b). Martin (1981), in a review of rare clarity and lucidity, has discussed the accomplishments and limitations of QSAR as judged from her own extensive experience.

To the above, we may also add that the few QSAR predictive successes appearing in the literature are certainly far outnumbered by undisclosed ones. Furthermore, as shown in Fig. 2, QSAR not only aims at predictions and drug design, but also at a better understanding of mechanisms of action.

The contributions of QSAR to this second goal are innumerable, and they concern not only pharmacodynamic actions, but also metabolism and pharmacokinetics (e.g. Hansch, 1972; Seydel and Schaper, 1982; Seydel, 1983). And even if QSAR had not met with tangible success, it could at least be claimed that they have completely transformed the way medicinal chemists and pharmacologists comprehend molecular structure and structure–activity relationships. If only for this intellectual evolution, the contribution of Hansch deserves the highest recognition.

3.2 CONCLUDING AN INTRODUCTION

Drug research today is faced with a number of specific changes, problems, and opportunities which have been stimulatingly discussed by Konig (1980). In addition, problems exist which are of a more general nature, rather than specific to drug research. Such is the case of two alternatives, namely human versus artificial intelligence, and research versus development, which are encountered in many if not all areas of science.

In previous pages, we have stressed the ever-increasing role of *artificial intelligence* (AI) in drug research. Does this imply a proportionally decreasing role of human intelligence? The danger certainly exists, because some scientists and managers are tempted to rely too much on AI. One marvels at the apparently unlimited opportunities which AI now opens to scientific research in general and drug research in particular. Assessing structure–activity relationships, understanding in detail and globally the mechanisms of interactions between drugs and biological systems, and predicting biological activities, are tasks for which human intelligence benefits considerably from AI (see sections 2.2 and 2.1). But AI cannot and must not be anything else than a subordinate extension of human intelligence. How can the latter be and remain dominant? The answer can be found in irreducible differences implicit in a citation offered as our first conclusion:

> Not to be absolutely certain is, I think, one of the essential things of rationality.
> Bertrand Russell

In scientific endeavours, it is customary to discriminate between *research and development* (R and D), although the two overlap considerably. Schematically, research is a long-range task with the potential for considerable scientific benefits and a high risk of failure. Development is a short-range task with the potential for considerable material profits and a lower risk of failure. Drug research is composed of both R and D. But an equilibrium must exist in science. Research could be maintained without development, but who would benefit from it? Without research, development cannot survive for long.

The series "Advances in Drug Research" is obviously oriented towards the long-range perspective, towards offering to drug researchers ample matter for thought. Our final conclusion will therefore take the form of a well-known citation:

> The important thing in science is not so much to obtain new facts as to discover new ways of thinking about them.
>
> William L. Bragg

References

The titles of the articles are given here because they often complement the text.

Albert, A. (1958). Chemical aspects of selective toxicity. *Nature* **182**, 421–423.

Albert, A. (1971). Relations between molecular structure and biological activity: stages in the evolution of current concepts. *Ann. Rev. Pharmacol.* **11**, 13–36.

Albert, A. (1973). "Selective Toxicity. The Physico-chemical Basis of Therapy", 5th Edition. Chapman and Hall, London.

Albert, A. (1982). The long search for valid structure–action relationships in drugs. *J. Med. Chem.* **25**, 1–5.

Alvares, A. P., Pantuck, E. J., Anderson, K. E., Kappas, A. and Conney, A. H. (1980). Regulation of drug metabolism in man by environmental factors. *Drug Metab. Rev.* **9**, 185–205.

Andrews, P. R. and Lloyd, E. J. (1982). Molecular conformation and biological activity of central nervous system active drugs. *Med. Res. Rev.* **2**, 355–393.

Arenas, C. A., Lacourly, N., Sepúlveda, A. and Tohá, J. C. (1981). Biological molecular information and its representation. *J. Theor. Biol.* **89**, 335–339.

Ariëns, E. J. (1966). Receptor theory and structure–action relationships. *In* "Advances in Drug Research" (N. J. Harper and A. B. Simmonds, eds), vol. 3, pp. 235–285. Academic Press, London, Orlando and New York.

Ariëns, E. J. (1979). Receptors: from fiction to fact. *Trends Pharmacol. Sci.* **1**, 11–15.

Ariëns, E. J. and Rodrigues de Miranda, J. F. (1979). The receptor concept: recent experimental and theoretical developments. *In* "Recent Advances in Receptor Chemistry" (F. Gualtieri, M. Giannella and C. Melchiorre, eds), pp. 1–36. Elsevier, Amsterdam.

Ariëns, E. J. and Simonis, A. M. (1964). A molecular basis for drug action. *J. Pharm. Pharmacol.* **16**, 137–157, 289–312.

Ariëns, E. J. and Simonis, A. M. (1982). Optimalization of pharmacokinetics—an essential aspect of drug development—by "metabolic stabilization". *In* "Strategy in Drug Research" (J. A. Keverling Buisman, ed.), vol. 4, pp. 165–178. Elsevier, Amsterdam.

Austel, V. and Kutter, E. (1980). Practical procedures in drug design. *In* "Drug Design" (E. J. Ariens, ed.), vol. X, pp. 1–69. Academic Press, Orlando, New York and London.

Austel, V. and Kutter, E. (1981). The theory of sets as a tool in systematic drug design, *Arzneim.-Forsch.* **31**, 130–135.

Bader, R. F. W., Tal. Y., Anderson, S. G. and Nguyen-Dang, T. T. (1980). Quantum topology: theory of molecular structure and its change. *Isr. J. Chem.* **19**, 8–29.

Barton, D. H. R. (1950). The conformation of the steroid nucleus. *Experientia* **6**, 316–320.

Belleau, B. (1965). Conformational perturbation in relation to the regulation of enzyme and receptor behaviour. *In* "Advances in Drug Research" (N. J. Harper and A. B. Simmonds, eds), vol. 2, pp. 89–126. Academic Press, London, Orlando and New York.

Bergman, K., Brandt, I., Appelgren, L. E. and Slanina, P. (1981). Structure-dependent, selective localization of chlorinated xenobiotics in the cerebellum and other brain structures. *Experientia* **37**, 1184–1185.

Berridge, M. J. (1980). Receptors and calcium signalling. *Trends Pharmacol. Sci.* **1**, 419–424.

Beveridge, D. L., Mezei, M., Mehrotra, P. K., Marchese, F. T., Thirumalai, V. and Ravi-Shanker, G. (1981). Liquid state computer simulations of biomolecular solvation problems. *In* "Quantum Chemistry in Biomedical Sciences" (H. Weinstein and J. P. Green, eds), vol. 367, pp. 108–131. *Annals N.Y. Acad. Sci.*, New York.

Bickel, M. H. and Muehlebach, S. (1980). Pharmacokinetics and ecodisposition of polyhalogenated hydrocarbons: aspects and concepts. *Drug Metab. Rev.* **11**, 149–190.

Bickel, M. H. and Steele, J. W. (1974). Binding of basic and acidic drugs to rat tissue subcellular fractions. *Chem.-Biol. Interact.* **8**, 151–162.

Bodor, N. (1982a). Designing safer drugs based on the soft drug approach. *Trends Pharmacol. Sci.* **3**, 53–56.

Bodor, N. (1982b). Soft drugs: strategies for design of safer drugs. *In* "Strategy in Drug Research" (J. A. Keverling Buisman, ed.), vol. 4, pp. 137–164. Elsevier, Amsterdam.

Bolender, R. P. (1981). Stereology: applications to pharmacology. *Ann. Rev. Pharmacol. Toxicol.* **21**, 549–573.

Bundgaard, H., Hansen, A. B. and Kofod, H. (eds) (1982). "Optimization of Drug Delivery." Munksgaard, Copenhagen.

Burgen, A. S. V. (1981). Conformational changes and drug action. *Fed. Proc.* **40**, 2723–2728.

Burger, A. (1979). Relationships of chemical structure and biological activity in drug design. *Trends Pharmacol. Sci.* **1**, 62–64.

Caldwell, J. (1981). The current status of attempts to predict species differences in drug metabolism. *Drug. Metab. Rev.* **12**, 231–237.

Caldwell, J. (1982). Conjugation reactions in foreign-compound metabolism: definition, consequences, and species variations. *Drug Metab. Rev.* **13**, 745–777.

Calne, D. B. (1980). Clinical relevance of dopamine receptor classification. *Trends Pharmacol. Sci.* **1**, 412–414.

Cavalla, J. (1980). The team approach or doing without genius. *Trends Pharmacol. Sci.* **1**, 225–227.

Chapeville, F. and Haenni, A.-L. (eds) (1980). "Chemical Recognition in Biology." Springer-Verlag, Berlin.

Cheng, H. C. and Woodward, J. K. (1982). Antihistaminic effect of terfenadine: a new piperidine-type antihistamine. *Drug Dev. Res.* **2**, 181–196.

Christoffersen, R. E. (1976). Molecules of pharmacological interest. *In* "Quantum Mechanics of Molecular Conformations" (B. Pullman, ed.), pp. 193–293. Wiley, London.

Chu, K. C. (1980). The quantitative analysis of structure–activity relationships. *In* "Burger's Medicinal Chemistry," 4th Edition, Part I, "The Basis of Medicinal Chemistry" (M. E. Wolff, ed.), pp. 393–418. Wiley, New York.

Clarke, A. (1979). "The View from Serendip", pp. 9–13. Pan Books, London.

Clow, A., Jenner, P. and Marsden, C. D. (1979). Changes in dopamine-mediated behaviour during one year's neuroleptic administration. *Eur. J. Pharmacol.* **57**, 365–375.

Cohen, N. C. (1971). GEMO, a computer program for the calculation of the preferred conformations of organic molecules. *Tetrahedron* **27**, 789–797.

Cohen, N. C. (1979). Beyond the 2-D chemical structure. *In* "Computer-Assisted Drug Design", (E. C. Olson and R. E. Christoffersen, eds), pp. 371–381. *Am. Chem. Soc.*, Washington DC.

Collier, H. O. J. (1966). Tolerance, physical dependence and receptors. A theory of the genesis of tolerance and physical dependence through drug-induced changes in the number of receptors. *In* "Advances in Drug Research" (N. J. Harper and A. B. Simmonds, eds), vol. 3, pp. 171–188. Academic Press, London, Orlando and New York.

Connelly, J. C. and Bridges, J. W. (1980). The distribution and role of cytochrome P-450 in extrahepatic organs. *In* "Progress in Drug Metabolism" (J. W. Bridges and L. F. Chasseaud, eds), vol. 5, pp. 1–111. Wiley, Chichester.

Conrad, M. (1979). Unstable electron pairing and the energy loan model of enzyme catalysis. *J. Theor. Biol.* **79**, 137–156.

Cooper, E. R., Berner, B. and Bruce, R. D. (1981). Kinetic analysis of relationship between partition coefficient and biological response. *J. Pharm. Sci.* **70**, 57–59.

Costa, E. (1980). Receptor plasticity: biochemical correlates and pharmacological significance. *Adv. Biochem. Psychopharmacol.* **24**, 363–377.

Craig, P. N. (1980). Guidelines for drug and analog design. *In* "Burger's Medicinal Chemistry," 4th Edition, Part I, "The Basis of Medicinal Chemistry" (M. E. Wolff, ed.), pp. 331–348. Wiley, New York.

Cramer, F. (1979). Fundamental complexity: a concept in biological sciences and beyond. *Interdisciplin. Sci. Rev.* **4**, 132–139.

Cramer, R. D. III. (1980a). BC(DEF) parameters. *J. Am. Chem. Soc.* **102**, 1837–1849, 1849–1859.

Cramer, R. D. III. (1980b). A QSAR success story. *Chemtech.* 744–747.

Cramer, R. D. III, Snader, K. M., Willis, C. R., Chakrin, L. W., Thomas, J. and Sutton, B. M. (1979). Application of quantitative structure–activity relationships in the development of the antiallergic pyranenamines. *J. Med. Chem.* **22**, 714–725.

Creese, I. and Sibley, D. R. (1981). Receptor adaptations to centrally acting drugs. *Ann. Rev. Pharmacol. Toxicol.* **21**, 357–391.

Creese, I. and Sibley, D. R. (1982). Comments on the commentary by Dr. Seeman (see Seeman, 1982). *Biochem. Pharmacol.* **31**, 2568–2569.

Crippen, G. M. (1979). Distance geometry approach to rationalizating binding data. *J. Med. Chem.* **22**, 988–997.

Crippen, G. M. (1982). Distance geometry analysis of the benzodiazepine binding site. *Molec. Pharmacol.* **22**, 11–19.

Curry, S. H. (1970). Theoretical changes in drug distribution resulting from changes in binding to plasma proteins and to tissues. *J. Pharm. Pharmacol.* **22**, 753–757.

Cushny, A. (1926). "Biological Relations of Optical Isomeric Substances". Williams and Wilkins, Baltimore.

Dean, P. M. (1981). Drug-receptor recognition: elestrostatic field lines at the receptor and dielectric effects. *Brit. J. Pharmacol.* **74**, 39–46.

Dean, P. M. and Wakelin, L. P. G. (1979). The docking manoeuvre at a drug receptor: a quantum mechanical study of intercalative attack of ethidium and its carboxylated derivative on a DNA fragment. *Phil. Trans. R. Soc. Lond., Series B* **287**, 571–607.

Dearden, J. C. and Bresnen, G. M. (1982). Thermodynamics of partitioning—Absence of constant hydrophobic effect of intramolecular hydrogen bonding. *J. Pharm. Pharmacol.* **34** (supplement), 82P.

De Feudis, F. V. (1981). Recent studies on the pharmacology of GABA: therapeutic perspectives. *Trends Pharmacol. Sci.* **2**, VI–IX.

De Lean, A., Munson, P. J. and Rodbard, D. (1979). Multi-subsite receptors for multivalent ligands. Application to drugs, hormones and neurotransmitters. *Molec. Pharmacol.* **15**, 60–70.

Delettré, J., Mornon, J. P., Lepicard, G., Ojasoo, T. and Raynaud, J. P. (1980). Steroid flexibility and receptor specificity. *J. Steroid Biochem.* **13**, 45–59.

Di Carlo, F. J. (1982). Metabolism, pharmacokinetics, and toxicokinetics defined. *Drug Metab. Rev.* **13**, 1–4.

Drayer, D. E. (1982). Pharmacologically active metabolites of drugs and other foreign compounds: clinical, pharmacological, therapeutic and toxicological considerations. *Drugs* **24**, 519–542.

Drost-Hansen, W. (1971). Role of water structure in cell-wall interactions. *Fed. Proc.* **30**, 1939–1948.

Edmonds, D. T. (1980). Membrane ion channels and ionic hydration energies. *Proc. R. Soc. Lond., Series B* **211**, 51–62.

Eichelbaum, M. (1982). Defective oxidation of drugs: pharmacokinetic and therapeutic implications. *Clin. Pharmacokinet.* **7**, 1–22.

Eigen, M. and Schuster, P. (1979). "The Hypercycle. A Principle of Natural Self-Organization." Springer-Verlag, Berlin.

Esaki, T. (1982). Quantitative drug design studies. V. Approach to lead generation by pharmacophoric pattern searching. *Chem. Pharm. Bull.* **30**, 3657–3661.

Fadhil, G. F. and Godfrey, M. (1982). The interpretation of quantitative linear correlations. Studies on the substituent shell concept. *J. Chem. Soc. Perkin Trans.* **II**, 933–941.

Fears, R., Baggaley, K. H., Walker, P. and Hindley, R. M. (1982). Xenobiotic cholesteryl ester formation. *Xenobiotica* **12**, 427–433.

Fichtl, B., Bondy, B. and Kurz, H. (1980). Binding of drugs to muscle tissue: dependence on drug concentration and lipid content of tissue. *J. Pharmacol. Exp. Ther.* **215**, 248–253.

Free, S. M. Jr. and Wilson, J. W. (1964). A mathematical contribution to structure–activity studies. *J. Med. Chem.* **7**, 395–399.

Ganellin, C. R. (1977). Chemical constitution and prototropic equilibria in structure–activity analysis. *In* "Drug Action at the Molecular Level" (G. C. K. Roberts, ed.), pp. 1–39. Macmillan Press, London.

Garfinkel, D. (1982). How can we effectively handle the large information content and complexity of biology? *J. Theor. Biol.* **96**, 3–8.

Gotoh, O., Tagashira, Y., Iizuka, T. and Fujii-Kiriyama, Y. (1983). Structural characteristics of cytochrome P-450. Possible location of the heme-binding cysteine in determined amino-acid sequences. *J. Biochem.* **93**, 807–818.

Green, T. P., O'Dea, R. F. and Mirkin, B. L. (1979). Determinants of drug disposition and effect in the fetus. *Ann. Rev. Pharmacol. Toxicol.* **19**, 285–322.

Greenblatt, D. J., Divoll, M., Harmatz, J. S. and Shader, R. I. (1980). Oxazepam kinetics: effects of age and sex. *J. Pharmacol. Exp. Ther.* **215**, 86–91.

Grieco, C., Silipo, C. and Vittoria, A. (1979). Physicochemical parameters in biological correlation analysis: meaning and limits. *Farmaco Ed. Sci.* **34**, 433–464.

Gund, P. (1979). Pharmacophoric pattern searching and receptor mapping. *In* "Annual Reports in Medicinal Chemistry" (H.-J. Hess, ed.), vol. 14, pp. 299–308. Academic Press, Orlando, New York and London.

Gund, P. (1982). Molecular geometry as an indicator of drug activity. *Trends Pharmacol. Sci.* **3**, 56–58.

Haken, H. (1980). Synergetics: are cooperative phenomena governed by universal principles? *Naturwissenschaften* **67**, 121–128.

Hamblin, M. and Creese, I. (1981). Receptor binding and the discovery of psychotherapeutic drugs. *Drug Dev. Res.* **1**, 343–372.

Hansch, C. (1972). Quantitative relationships between lipophilic character and drug metabolism. *Drug Metab. Rev.* **1**, 1–14.

Hansch, C. (1979). The interaction of ligands with enzymes. A starting point in drug design. *Farmaco Ed. Sci.* **34**, 729–742.

Hansch, C. (1981). The physicochemical approach to drug design and discovery (QSAR). *Drug Dev. Res.* **1**, 267–309.

Hansch, C. and Fujita, T. (1964). ρ-σ-π analysis. A method for the correlation of biological activity and chemical structure. *J. Am. Chem. Soc.* **86**, 1616–1626.

Hansch, C. and Leo, A. (1979). "Substituent Constants for Correlation Analysis in Chemistry and Biology." Wiley, New York.

Hansch, C., Muir, R. M., Fujita, T., Maloney, P. P., Geiger, F. and Streich, M. (1963). The correlation of biological activity in plant growth regulators and chloromycetin derivatives with Hammett constants and partition coefficients. *J. Am. Chem. Soc.* **85**, 2817–2824.

Hartley, B. S. (1979). Evolution of enzyme structure. *Proc. R. Soc. Lond. Series B* **205**, 443–452.

Hassel, O. (1943). The cyclohexane problem. *Tidsskr. Kjemi Bergvesen Metal.* **3**, 32.

Hathway, D. E. (1982). Structure–activity considerations: a synthesis of ideas. *Chem.-Biol. Inter.* **42**, 1–26.

Hazlewood, C. F. (1977). Bound water in biology. *Acta Biochim. Biophys.* **12**, 263–274.

Holtzman, J. L. (1982). Role of reactive oxygen and metabolite binding in drug toxicity. *Life Sci.* **30**, 1–9.

Hopfinger, A. J. (1981). A general QSAR for dihydrofolate reductase inhibition by 2,4-diaminotriazines based upon molecular shape analysis. *Arch. Biochem. Biophys.* **206**, 153–163.

Horn, A. S., Feenstra, M. G. P., Grol, C. J., Rollema, H., van Oene, J. C. and Westerink, B. H. C. (1981). Multiple dopamine receptors: fact, fiction or confusion? *Pharm. Weekblad Sci. Ed.* **3**, 145–165.

Houston, J. B. and Wood, S. G. (1980). Gastrointestinal absorption of drugs and other xenobiotics. *In* "Progress in Drug Metabolism" (J. W. Bridges and L. F. Chasseaud, eds), vol. 4, pp. 57–129. Wiley, Chichester.

Huber, R. and Bennett, W. S. Jr. (1983). Functional significance of flexibility in proteins. *Biopolymers* **22**, 261–279.

B. TESTA

Humblet, C. and Marshall, G. R. (1980). Pharmacophore identification and receptor mapping. In "Annual Reports in Medicinal Chemistry" (H.-J. Hess, ed.), vol. 15, pp. 267–276. Academic Press, Orlando, New York and London.

Humblet, C. and Marshall, G. R. (1981). Three-dimensional computer modelling as an aid to drug design. Drug Dev. Res. 1, 409–434.

Isogai, Y., Némethy, T., Rackovsky, S., Leach, S. J. and Scheraga, H. A. (1980). Characterization of multiple bends in proteins. Biopolymers 19, 1183–1210.

Jenner, P. and Testa, B. (1978). Novel pathways of drug metabolism. Xenobiotica 8, 1–25.

Jenner, P. and Testa, B. (1981). Altered drug disposition in disease states: the first pieces of the jigsaw. In "Concepts in Drug Metabolism" (P. Jenner and B. Testa, eds), part B, pp. 423–513. Dekker, New York.

Jenner, P., Testa, B. and Di Carlo, F. J. (1981). Xenobiotic and endobiotic metabolizing enzymes: an overstretched discrimination? Trends Pharmacol. Sci. 2, 135–137.

Jondorf, W. R. (1981a). Drug metabolism and drug toxicity: some evolutionary considerations. In "Concepts in Drug Metabolism" (P. Jenner and B. Testa, eds), part B, pp. 307–376. Dekker, New York.

Jondorf, W. R. (1981b). Drug-metabolizing enzymes as evolutionary probes. Drug Metab. Rev. 12, 379–430.

Kalow, W. (1980). Pharmacogenetics of drug metabolism. Trends Pharmacol. Sci. 1, 403–405.

Kalow, W. (1982). Ethnic differences in drug metabolism. Clin. Pharmacokinet. 7, 373–400.

Kasson, B. G., Carlson, H. E. and George, R. (1983). Endocrine influences on the actions of morphine. II. Responses to pituitary hormones. J. Pharmacol. Exp. Ther. 224, 282–288.

Kato, R. (1979). Characteristics and differences in the hepatic mixed function oxidases of different species. Pharmacol. Ther. 6, 41–98.

Kaufman, J. J., Hariharan, P. C., Popkie, H. E. and Petrongolo, C. (1981). Ab-initio MODPOT/VRDDO/MERGE calculations on large biomedical molecules and electrostatic molecular potential contour maps. In "Quantum Chemistry in Biomedical Sciences" (H. Weinstein and J. P. Green, eds), vol. 367, pp. 452–477. Annals N.Y. Acad. Sci., New York.

Kebabian, J. W. and Calne, D. B. (1979). Multiple receptors for dopamine. Nature 277, 93–96.

Kenakin, T. P. (1982). Organ selectivity of drugs. Alternatives to receptor selectivity. Trends Pharmacol. Sci. 3, 153–156.

Kier, L. B. (1980). Molecular connectivity as a description of structure for SAR analyses. In "Physical Chemical Properties of Drugs" (S. H. Yalkowsky, A. A. Sinkula and S. C. Valvani, eds), pp. 277–319. Dekker, New York.

Kier, L. B. and Hall, L. H. (1976). "Molecular Connectivity in Chemistry and Drug Research." Academic Press, New York.

Kier, L. B. and Hall, L. H. (1977). The nature of structure–activity relationships and their relation to molecular connectivity. Eur. J. Med. Chem. 12, 307–312.

Kier, L. B. and Hall, L. H. (1981). Derivation and significance of valence molecular connectivity. J. Pharm. Sci. 70, 583–589.

Kirschner, G. L. and Kowalski, B. R. (1979). The application of pattern recognition to drug design. In "Drug Design" (E. J. Ariëns, ed.), vol. VIII, pp. 73–131. Academic Press, Orlando, New York and London.

Konig, H. (1980). Pharmaceutical chemistry today—Changes, problems, and opportunities. Angew. Chem. Inter. Ed. 19, 749–761.

Krenitsky, T. A. and Elion, G. B. (1982). Enzymes as tools and targets in drug research. *In* "Strategy in Drug Research" (J. A. Keverling Buisman, ed.), pp. 65–87. Elsevier, Amsterdam.

Kubinyi, H. (1979). Lipophilicity and drug activity. *In* "Progress in Drug Research" (E. Jucker, ed.), vol. 23, pp. 97–198. Birkhäuser Verlag, Basel.

Kuntz, I. D. Jr. (1980). Drug-receptor geometry. *In* "Burger's Medicinal Chemistry," 4th Edition, Part I, "The Basis of Medicinal Chemistry" (M. E. Wolff, ed.), pp. 285–312. Wiley, New York.

Kupfer, D. (1980). Endogenous substrates of monooxygenases: fatty acids and prostaglandins. *Pharmacol. Ther.* **11**, 469–496.

Laduron, P. (1983). More binding, more fancy. *Trends Pharmacol. Sci.* **4**, 333–335.

Landau, E. M., Richter, J. and Cohen, S. (1979). Differential solubilities in subregions of the membrane: a nonsteric mechanism of drug specificity. *J. Med. Chem.* **22**, 325–327.

Lang, E. W. and Lüdermann, H.-D. (1982). Anomalies of liquid water. *Angew. Chem. Int. Ed.* **21**, 315–329.

Lange, L. G., Bergmann, S. R. and Sobel, B. E. (1981). Identification of fatty acid ethyl esters as products of rabbit myocardial ethanol metabolism. *J. Biol. Chem.* **256**, 12968–12973.

Langridge, R., Ferrin, T. E., Kuntz, I. D. and Connolly, M. L. (1981). Real-time color graphics in studies of molecular interactions. *Science* **211**, 661–666.

Lehmann F., P. A. (1982). Quantifying stereoselectivity or how to choose a pair of shoes when you have two left feet. *Trends Pharmacol. Sci.* **3**, 103–106.

Leighty, E. G., Fentiman, A. F. Jr. and Foltz, R. L. (1976). Long-retained metabolites of delta-9- and delta-8-tetrahydrocannabinols identified as novel fatty acid conjugates. *Res. Commun. Chem. Pathol. Pharmacol.* **14**, 13–28.

Leo, A., Hansch, C. and Elkins, D. (1971). Partition coefficients and their uses. *Chem. Rev.* **71**, 526–616.

Lévy, R. H. (1982). Time-dependent pharmacokinetics. *Pharmacol. Ther.* **17**, 383–397.

Lewi, P. J. (1976). Computer technology in drug design. *In* "Drug Design" (E. J. Ariëns, ed.), vol. VII, pp. 209–278. Academic Press, Orlando, New York and London.

Lewi, P. J. (1978). The use of multivariate statistics in industrial pharmacology *Pharmacol. Ther.* Part B **3**, 481–537.

Lewi, P. J. (1980). Multivariate data analysis in structure-activity relationships *In* "Drug Design" (E. J. Ariëns, ed.), vol. X, pp. 307–342. Academic Press, Orlando, New York and London.

Lewin, S. (1974). "Displacements of Water and its Control of Biochemical Reactions." Academic Press, London, Orlando and New York.

Lu, A. Y. H. (1979). Multiplicity of liver drug metabolizing enzymes. *Drug Metab. Rev.* **10**, 187–208.

Luisi, P. L. (1979). Why are enzymes macromolecules? *Naturwissenschaften* **66**, 498–504.

Lyle, G. G. (1976). The chiroptical properties of bistetrahydroisoquinolines and polycyclic biaryl derivatives. *J. Org. Chem.* **41**, 850–855.

Marshall, G. R., Barry, C. D., Bosshard, H. E., Dammkoehler, R. A. and Dunn, D. A. (1979). The conformational parameter in drug design: the active analog approach. *In* "Computer-Assisted Drug Design" (E. C. Olson and R. E. Christoffersen, eds), pp. 205–226. *Am. Chem. Soc.*, Washington DC.

Martin, Y. C. (1978). "Quantitative Drug Design. A Critical Introduction." Dekker, New York.

Martin, Y. C. (1979). Advances in the methodology of quantitative drug design. *In* "Drug Design" (E. J. Ariëns, ed.), vol. VIII, pp. 1–72. Academic Press, Orlando, New York and London.

Martin, Y. C. (1981). A practitioner's perspective of the role of quantitative structure-activity analysis in medicinal chemistry. *J. Med. Chem.* **24**, 229–237.

Martin, Y. C. and Panas, H. N. (1979). Mathematical considerations in series design. *J. Med. Chem.* **22**, 784–791.

Mautner, H. G. (1967). The molecular basis of drug action. *Pharmacol. Rev.* **19**, 107–144.

Mautner, H. G. (1980). Receptor theories and dose-response relationships. *In* "Burger's Medicinal Chemistry," 4th Edition, Part I, "The Basis of Medicinal Chemistry" (M. E. Wolff, ed.), pp. 271–284. Wiley, New York.

Mayer, J. M., van de Waterbeemd, H. and Testa, B. (1982). A comparison between the hydrophobic fragmental methods of Rekker and Leo. *Eur. J. Med. Chem.* **17**, 17–25.

Mehrotra, P. K., Marchese, F. T. and Beveridge, D. L. (1981). Statistical state solvation sites. *J. Am. Chem. Soc.* **103**, 672–673.

Mercier, C., Sobel, Y. and Dubois, J.-E. (1981). Méthode DARC/PELCO: QSAR unique de phénylalkylamines inhibitrices de la PNMT. *Eur. J. Med. Chem.* **16**, 473–476.

Merrifield, R. E. and Simmons, H. E. (1980). The structures of molecular topological spaces. *Theoret. Chim. Acta* **55**, 55–75.

Milner-White, E. J. (1980). Description of the quaternary structure of tetrameric proteins. Forms that show either right-handed or left-handed symmetry at the subunit level. *Biochem. J.* **187**, 297–302.

Mitchell, P. (1979). Compartmentation and communication in living systems. Ligand conduction: a general catalytic principle in chemical, osmotic and chemiosmotic reaction systems. *Eur. J. Biochem.* **95**, 1–20.

Moran, J. F. and Triggle, D. J. (1970). Approaches to the quantitation and isolation of pharmacological receptors. *In* "Fundamental Concepts in Drug-Receptor Interactions" (J. F. Danielli, J. F. Moran and D. J. Triggle, eds), pp. 133–176. Academic Press, Orlando, New York and London.

Murdoch, J. R. and Magnoli, D. E. (1982). The relationship between energy additivity and the equivalent group. *J. Am. Chem. Soc.* **104**, 2782–2789.

Nebert, D. W. (1979). Genetic aspects of enzyme induction by drugs and chemical carcinogens. *In* "The Induction of Drug Metabolism" (R. W. Estabrook and E. Lindenlaub, eds), pp. 419–452. Schattauer Verlag, Stuttgart.

Nebert, D. W. (1980). The Ah locus. A gene with possible importance in cancer predictability. *Arch. Toxicol. Suppl.* **3**, 195–207.

Nebert, D. W. and Jensen, N. M. (1979). The Ah locus: genetic regulation of the metabolism of carcinogens, drugs, and other environmental chemicals by cytochrome P-450-mediated monooxygenases. *CRC Crit. Rev. Biochem.* **6**, 401–438.

Nebert, D. W. and Negishi, M. (1982). Multiple forms of cytochrome P-450 and the importance of molecular biology and evolution. *Biochem. Pharmacol.* **31**, 2311–2317.

Nebert, D. W., Eisen, H. J., Negishi, M., Lang, M. A., Hjelmeland, L. M. and Okey, A. B. (1981). Genetic mechanisms controlling the induction of polysubstrate monooxygenase (P-450) activities. *Ann. Rev. Pharmacol. Toxicol.* **21**, 431–462.

Nelson, S. D. (1982). Metabolic activation and drug toxicity. *J. Med. Chem.* **25**, 753–765.

Némethy, G. and Scheraga, H. A. (1980). Stereochemical requirements for the existence of hydrogen bonds in β-bends. *Biochem. Biophys. Res. Commun.* **95**, 320–327.

Notari, R. E. (1981). Prodrug design. *Pharmacol. Ther.* **14**, 25–53.

Novak, R. F. and Vatsis, K. P. (1982). ^{1}H Fourier transform nuclear magnetic resonance relaxation rate studies on the interaction of acetanilide with purified isozymes of rabbit liver microsomal cytochrome P-450 and with cytochrome b_5. *Molec. Pharmacol.* **21**, 701–709.

Osman, R., Weinstein, H. and Green, J. P. (1979). Parameters and methods in quantitative structure-activity relationships. *In* "Computer-Assisted Drug Design" (E. C. Olson and R. E. Christoffersen, eds), pp. 21–77. *Am. Chem. Soc.*, Washington DC.

Overton, K. H. (1979). Concerning stereochemical choice in enzymic reactions. *Chem. Soc. Rev.* **8**, 447–473.

Page, M. I. (1977). Entropy, binding energy, and enzymic catalysis. *Angew. Chem. Inter. Ed.* **16**, 449–459.

Page, M. I. (1983). The energetics of drug-receptor interactions. *In* "Quantitative Approaches to Drug Design" (J. C. Dearden, ed.), pp. 109–119, Elsevier, Amsterdam.

Parascandola, J. (1980). Origins of the receptor theory. *Trends Pharmacol. Sci.* **1**, 189–192.

Park, B. K. and Beckenridge, A. M. (1981). Clinical implications of enzyme induction and enzyme inhibition. *Clin. Pharmacokinet.* **6**, 1–24.

Parke, D. V. (1981). The endoplasmic reticulum: its role in physiological functions and pathological situations. *In* "Concepts in Drug Metabolism" (P. Jenner and B. Testa, eds), part B, pp. 1–52. Dekker, New York.

Paton, W. D. M. and Rang, H. P. (1966). A kinetic approach to the mechanism of drug action. In "Advances in Drug Research" (N. J. Harper and A. B. Simmonds, eds), vol. 3, pp. 57–80. Academic Press, London, Orlando and New York.

Pattee, H. H. (1979). The complementarity principle and the origin of macro-molecular information. *BioSystems* **11**, 217–226.

Paul, S. M., Syapin, P. J., Paugh, B. A., Moncada, V. and Skolnick, P. (1979). Correlation between benzodiazepine receptor occupation and anticonvulsant effects of diazepam. *Nature* **281**, 688–689.

Peinel, G., Frischleder, H. and Birnstock, F. (1980). The electrostatical molecular potential—A tool for the prediction of electrostatic molecular interaction properties. *Theoret. Chim. Acta* **57**, 245–253.

Pelkonen, O. (1980a). Biotransformation of xenobiotics in the fetus. *Pharmacol. Ther.* **10**, 261–281.

Pelkonen, O. (1980b). Developmental drug metabolism. *In* "Concepts in Drug Metabolism" (P. Jenner and B. Testa, eds), part A, pp. 285–309. Dekker, New York.

Pelkonen, O. and Sotaniemi, E. (1982). Drug metabolism in alcoholics. *Pharmacol. Ther.* **16**, 261–268.

Peticolas, W. L. and Kurtz, B. (1980). Transformation of the ϕ-ψ plot for proteins to a new representation with local helicity and peptide torsional angles as variables. *Biopolymers* **19**, 1153–1166.

Philipp, A. H., Humber, L. G. and Voith, K. (1979). Mapping the dopamine receptor. 2. Features derived from modifications in the rings A/B region of the neuroleptic butaclamol. *J. Med. Chem.* **22**, 768–773.

54   B. TESTA

Pincus, M. R. and Scheraga, H. A. (1981). Theoretical calculations of enzyme-substrate complexes: the basis of molecular recognition and catalysis. *Accounts Chem. Res.* **14**, 299–306.

Pitman, I. H. (1981). Pro-drugs of amides, imides, and amines. *Med. Res. Rev.* **1**, 189–214.

Ponnuswamy, P. K., Prabhakaran, M. and Manavalan, P. (1980). Hydrophobic packing and spatial arrangements of amino acid residues in globular proteins. *Biochim. Biophys. Acta* **623**, 301–316.

Pople, J. A. (1976). Structural studies using molecular orbital theory. *Bull. Soc. Chim. Belg.* **85**, 347–361.

Portoghese, P. S. (1971). Translocation of ligand conformational free energy in receptor activation: a possible functional role of conformational isomerism in drug action. *J. Pharm. Sci.* **60**, 806–807.

Portoghese, P. S. (1978). Stereoisomeric ligands as opioid receptor probes. *Accounts Chem. Res.* **11**, 21–29.

Pullman, A. (1977). Bound water in biological systems. A quantum-mechanical investigation. *In* "Search and Discovery—A Tribute to Albert Szent-Györgyi" (B. Kaminer, ed.), pp. 231–249. Academic Press, Orlando, New York and London.

Pullman, B. (1974). The adventures of a quantum-chemist in the kingdom of pharmacophores. *In* "Molecular and Quantum Pharmacology" (E. Bergmann and B. Pullman, eds), pp. 9–36. Reidel, Dordrecht.

Purcell, W. P., Bass, G. E. and Clayton, J. M. (1973). "Strategy of Drug Design: A Guide to Biological Activity." Wiley, New York.

Quistad, G. B., Staiger, L. E. and Schooley, D. A. (1982). Xenobiotic conjugation: a novel role for bile acids. *Nature* **296**, 462–464.

Rahwan, R. G., Piascik, M. F. and Witiak, D. T. (1979). The role of calcium antagonism in the therapeutic action of drugs. *Can. J. Physiol. Pharmacol.* **57**, 443–460.

Reichert, D. (1981). Toxication of foreign substances by conjugation reactions. *Angew. Chem. Inter. Ed.* **20**, 135–142.

Reinberg, A. and Smolensky, M. H. (1982). Circadian changes of drug disposition in man. *Clin. Pharmacokinet.* **7**, 401–420.

Rekker, R. F. (1977). "The Hydrophobic Fragmental Constant. Its Derivation and Applications. A Means of Characterizing Membrane Systems." Elsevier, Amsterdam.

Rekker, R. F. and de Kort, H. M. (1979). The hydrophobic fragmental constant; an extension to a 1000 data point set. *Eur. J. Med. Chem.* **14**, 479–488.

Rekker, R. F., Timmerman, H., Harms, A. F. and Nauta, W. T. (1971). The antihistaminic and anticholinergic activities of optically active diphenhydramine derivatives. *Arzneim.-Forsch.* **21**, 688–691.

Richards, W. G. (1977). Calculation of essential drug conformations and electron distributions. *In* "Drug Action at the Molecular Level" (G. C. K. Roberts, ed.), pp. 41–54. Macmillan Press, London.

Roche, B. (1977). "Design of Biopharmaceutical Properties through Prodrugs and Analogs." American Pharmaceutical Association, Washington DC.

Rossky, P. J. and Karplus, M. (1979). Solvation. A molecular dynamics study of a dipeptide in water. *J. Am. Chem. Soc.* **101**, 1913–1937.

Rothman, R. B. and Westfall, T. C. (1982). Allosteric coupling between morphine and enkephalin receptors in vitro. *Molec. Pharmacol.* **21**, 548–557.

Rowland, M. and Tozer, T. N. (1980). "Clinical Pharmacokinetics: Concepts and Applications." Lea and Febiger, Philadelphia.

Ryan, J. P. (1980). Information-entropy interfaces and different levels of biological organization. *J. Theor. Biol.* **84**, 31–48.

Scheraga, H. A. (1979). Interactions in aqueous solution. *Accounts Chem. Res.* **12**, 7–14.

Schwyzer, R. (1980). Organization and transduction of peptide information. *Trends Pharmacol. Sci.* **1**, 327–331.

Seeman, P. (1972). The membrane actions of anesthetics and tranquilizers. *Pharmacol. Rev.* **24**, 583–655.

Seeman, P. (1982). Nomenclature of central and peripheral dopaminergic sites and receptors. *Biochem. Pharmacol.* **31**, 2563–2568.

Seydel, J. K. (1983). Pharmacokinetics in drug design. *In* "Quantitative Approaches to Drug Design" (J. C. Dearden, ed.), pp. 163–181, Elsevier, Amsterdam.

Seydel, J. K. and Schaper, K. J. (1982). Quantitative structure–pharmacokinetic relationships and drug design. *Pharmacol. Ther.* **15**, 131–182.

Sharma, R. N., Cameron, R. G., Farber, E., Griffin, M. G., Joly, J.-G. and Murray, R. K. (1979). Multiplicity of induction patterns of rat liver microsomal monooxygenases and other polypeptides produced by administration of various xenobiotics. *Biochem. J.* **182**, 317–327.

Sharon, N. and Lis, H. (March 30, 1981). Glycoproteins: research booming on long-ignored, ubiquitous compounds. Knowledge of structure, vital biological roles, applications is growing rapidly. *Chem. Eng. News*, 21–44.

Smith, R. N., Hansch, C. and Ames, M. M. (1975). Selection of a reference partitioning system for drug design work. *J. Pharm. Sci.* **64**, 599–606.

Sokoloff, P., Martres, M. P. and Schwarz, J. C. (1980). Three classes of dopamine receptor (D-2, D-3, D-4) identified by binding studies with ^{3}H-apomorphine and ^{3}H-domperidone. *Naunyn-Schmied. Arch. Pharmacol.* **315**, 89–102.

Soudijn, W. (1982). Angiotensin converting enzyme inhibitors. *Pharm. Weekbl. Sci. Ed.* **4**, 154–158.

Squires, R. F. and Saederup, E. (1982). γ-Aminobutyric acid receptors modulate cation binding sites coupled to independent benzodiazepine, picrotoxin, and anion binding sites. *Molec. Pharmacol.* **22**, 327–334.

Stella, V. J. and Himmelstein, K. J. (1980). Prodrugs and site-specific drug delivery. *J. Med. Chem.* **23**, 1275–1282.

Streich, W. J., Dove, S. and Franke, R. (1980). On the rational selection of test series. *J. Med. Chem.* **23**, 1452–1456.

Symons, M. C. R. (1981). Water structure and reactivity. *Accounts Chem. Res.* **14**, 179–187.

Tapia, O. (1980). Local field representation of surrounding medium effects, from liquid solvent to protein core effects. *In* "Quantum Theory of Chemical Reactions" (R. Daudel, A. Pullman, L. Salem and A. Veillard, eds), vol. II, pp. 25–72. Reidel, Dordrecht.

Testa, B. (1976). Drug metabolism as a mutation—Drug metabolism in mutation. *Drug Metab. Rev.* **5**, i–ii.

Testa, B. (1979). "Principles of Organic Stereochemistry." Dekker, New York.

Testa, B. (1982a). The geometry of molecules: Basic principles and nomenclatures. *In* "Stereochemistry" (Ch. Tamm, ed.), pp. 1–47. Elsevier Biomedical Press, Amsterdam.

Testa, B. (1982b). Nonenzymatic contributions to xenobiotic metabolism. *Drug Metab. Rev.* **13**, 25–50.

Testa, B. and Etter, J. C. (1975). Etude de l'hydrolyse de la procaine dans des hydrogels de Carbopol^R. *Can. J. Pharm. Sci.* **10**, 20–23.

Testa, B. and Jenner, P. (1978). Novel drug metabolites produced by functionalization reactions: chemistry and toxicology. *Drug Metab. Rev.* **7**, 325–369.

Testa, B. and Jenner, P. (1981). Inhibitors of cytochrome P-450s and their mechanisms of action. *Drug Metab. Rev.* **12**, 1–117.

Testa, B. and Mihailova, D. (1978). An *ab initio* study of electronic factors in metabolic hydroxylation of aliphatic carbon atoms. *J. Med. Chem.* **21**, 683–686.

Testa, B. and Purcell, W. P. (1978). A QSAR study of sulfonamide binding to carbonic anhydrase as test of steric models. *Eur. J. Med. Chem.* **13**, 509–514.

Testa, B. and Seiler, P. (1981). Steric and lipophobic components of the hydrophobic fragmental constant. *Arzneim.-Forsch.* **31**, 1053–1058

Testa, B., Di Carlo, F. J. and Jenner, P. (1981). Xenobiotic metabolism: necessity, chance, mishap, or none of the above? *In* "Concepts in Drug Metabolism" (P. Jenner and B. Testa, eds), part B, pp. 515–535. Dekker, New York.

Thornber, C. W. (1979). Isosterism and molecular modification in drug design. *Chem. Soc. Rev.* **8**, 563–580.

Tollenaere, J. P. (1981). Conformational analysis in medicinal chemistry. *Trends Pharmacol. Sci.* **2**, 273–275.

Topliss, J. G. and Edwards, R. P. (1979). Chance factors in studies of quantitative structure–activity relationships. *J. Med. Chem.* **22**, 1238–1244.

Trindle, C. (1980). The quantum mechanical view of molecular structure and the shapes of molecules. *Isr. J. Chem.* **19**, 47–53.

Tute, M. S. (1971). Principles and practice of Hansch analysis: A guide to structure–activity correlation for the medicinal chemist. *In* "Advances in Drug Research" (N. J. Harper and A. B. Simmonds, eds), vol. 6, pp. 1–77. Academic Press, London, Orlando and New York.

Tute, M. S. (1980). Limitations and prospects for the Hansch approach to SAR. *In* "Physical Chemical Properties of Drugs" (S. H. Yalkowsky, A. A. Sinkula and S. C. Valvani, eds), pp. 141–161. Dekker, New York.

Vainio, H. and Hietanen, E. (1980). Role of extrahepatic metabolism in drug disposition and toxicity. *In* "Concepts in Drug Metabolism" (P. Jenner and B. Testa, eds), part A, pp. 251–284. Dekker, New York.

van de Waterbeemd, H. and Testa, B. (1983a). Theoretical conformational studies of some dopamine antagonistic benzamide drugs: 3-pyrrolidyl and 4-piperidyl derivatives. *J. Med. Chem.* **26**, 203–207.

van de Waterbeemd, H. and Testa, B. (1983b). The development of a hydration factor ω and its relation to correction terms in current hydrophobic fragmental systems. *Int. J. Pharmaceut.* **14**, 29–41.

van de Waterbeemd, H., van Bakel, P. and Jansen, A. (1981). Transport in quantitative structure–activity relationships VI: relationship between transport rate constants and partition coefficients. *J. Pharm. Sci.* **70**, 1081–1082.

Van Gompel, P., Geerts, R. and Leysen, J. E. (1982). Differential binding properties of drugs for interactions with sub-unit sites of the rat striatal dopaminergic receptor. *Arch. Int. Pharmacodyn. Ther.* **258**, 327–330.

van Rossum, J. M. (1966). Limitations of molecular pharmacology. Some implications of the basic assumptions underlying calculations on drug-receptor interactions and the significance of biological drug parameters. *In* "Advances in Drug Research" (N. J. Harper and A. B. Simmonds, eds), vol. 3, pp. 189–234. Academic Press, London, Orlando and New York.

Veillard, A. (1976). Small molecules and inorganic compounds. *In* "Quantum Mechanics of Molecular Conformations" (B. Pullman, ed.), pp. 1–115. Wiley, London.

Verloop, A., Hoogenstraaten, W. and Tipker, J. (1976). Development and application of new steric substituent parameters in drug design. *In* "Drug Design" (E. J. Ariëns, ed.), vol. VII, pp. 165–207. Academic Press, Orlando, New York and London.

Wagner, J. G. (1975). "Fundamentals of Clinical Pharmacokinetics." Drug Intelligence. Publ. Co, Hamilton, Illinois, USA.

Walker, C. H. (1980). Species variations in some hepatic microsomal enzymes that metabolize xenobiotics. *In* "Progress in Drug Metabolism" (J. W. Bridges and L. F. Chasseaud, eds), vol. 5, pp. 113–164. Wiley, Chichester.

Warshel, A. (1981). Electrostatic basis of structure–function correlation in proteins. *Accounts Chem. Res.* **14**, 284–290.

Warshel, A. and Weiss, R. M. (1980). As empirical valence bond approach for comparing reactions in solutions and in enzymes. *J. Am. Chem. Soc.* **102**, 6218–6226.

Waud, D. R. (1968). Pharmacological receptors. *Pharmacol. Rev.* **20**, 49–88.

Weiland, G. A., Minneman, K. P. and Molinoff, P. B. (1979). Fundamental difference between the molecular interactions of agonists and antagonists with the β-adrenergic receptor. *Nature* **281**, 114–117.

Weiner, P. K., Langridge, R., Blaney, J. M., Schaefer, R. and Kollman, P. A. (1982). Electrostatic potential molecular surfaces. *Proc. Natl Acad. Sci. USA* **79**, 3754–3758.

Weinstein, H. and Green, J. P. (eds) (1981). "Quantum Chemistry in Biomedical Sciences." *Annals N.Y. Acad. Sci.*, vol. 367. New York Academy of Science, New York.

Weinstein, H., Osman, R., Topiol, S. and Green, J. P. (1981). Quantum chemical studies on molecular determinants for drug action. *In* "Quantum Chemistry in Biomedical Sciences" (H. Weinstein and J. P. Green, eds), *Annals N.Y. Acad. Sci.* vol. 367, pp. 434–451. New York Academy of Science, New York.

Welch, R. M. and Findlay, J. W. A. (1981). Excretion of drugs in human breast milk. *Drug Metab. Rev.* **12**, 261–277.

Wermuth, C. G. (1984). Designing prodrugs and bioprecursors. *In* "Drug Design: Fact or Fantasy?" (G. Jolles and K. R. H. Woolridge, eds), pp. 47–72. Academic Press, London, Orlando, and New York.

Williams, R. J. P. (1980). On first looking into Nature's chemistry. *Chem. Soc. Rev.* **9**, 281–324, 325–364.

Wilson, S. R. and Huffman, J. C. (1980). Cambridge data file in organic chemistry. Applications to transition-state structure. Conformational analysis, and structure/activity studies. *J. Org. Chem.* **45**, 560–566.

Wilson, J. T., Brown, R. D., Cherek, D. R., Dailey, J. W., Hilman, B., Jobe, P. C., Manno, B. R., Manno, J. E., Redetzki, H. M. and Stewart, J. J. (1980). Drug excretion in human breast milk: principles, pharmacokinetics and projected consequences. *Clin. Pharmacokinet.* **5**, 1–66.

Wodak, S. J. and Janin, J. (1981). Location of structural domains in proteins. *Biochemistry* **20**, 6544–6552.

Wolfenden, R., Andersson, L., Cullis, P. M. and Southgate, C. C. B. (1981). Affinities of amino acid side chains for solvent water. *Biochemistry* **20**, 849–855

Wolley, R. G. (1978). Must a molecule have a shape? *J. Am. Chem. Soc.* **100**, 1073–1078.

Wooldridge, K. R. H. (1980). A rational substituent set for structure–activity studies. *Eur. J. Med. Chem.* **15**, 63–66.

Yates, F. E. (1982). Outline of a physical theory of physiological systems. *Can. J. Physiol. Pharmacol.* **60**, 217–248.

Zadeh, L. A. (1965). Fuzzy sets and systems. "Proceedings of the Symposium on System Theory," pp. 29–39. Polytechnic Press, New York.

The Binding of Drugs to Blood Plasma Macromolecules: Recent Advances and Therapeutic Significance[1,2]

JEAN-PAUL TILLEMENT, GEORGES HOUIN, ROLAND ZINI,
SAÏK URIEN, EDITH ALBENGRES, JÉRÔME BARRÉ,
MICHEL LECOMTE, PHILIPPE D'ATHIS, and BERNARD SEBILLE

*Département de Pharmacologie, Faculté de Médecine de Paris XII,
Créteil, France*

[1]This review is dedicated to Professor Uwe Wollert, head of the Department of Pharmacology at Mainz University, who died February 26, 1981.

[2]The work was subsidized by grants from the University of Paris XII and from "La Direction de la Recherche au Ministere de l'Education Nationale" (France).

ADVANCES IN DRUG RESEARCH VOL. 13
0-12-013313-X

1 Introduction

Drug–protein interactions have only recently been acknowledged as one of the main topics of general pharmacology. However, many reasons would have supported the interest of the pharmacologist for these studies. Indeed, the most significant events occurring after a drug has penetrated into the body imply that it first binds to adequate protein structures. Thus, according to Schanker's theory (1961), each pharmacological effect requires the preliminary drug's binding to receptors, while storage represents binding to acceptors and metabolic transformation supposes binding to one or several successive enzymes. In almost every case, these binding processes fulfil the criteria of a reversible equilibrium to which the law of mass action is applicable. So drug protein interactions have to be considered as a general phenomenon which can often be measured and which has many possible implications according to the role and nature of the binding protein.

In many cases, it is possible to determine the binding parameters of the interaction, i.e. n, the number of drug binding sites per mole of a given protein and K, the relevant association constant. For plasma proteins, these parameters are estimated according to the following relationship derived from the law of mass action:

$$\frac{B}{R} = \sum \frac{n_i K_i F}{1 + K_i F} \tag{1}$$

where B, F and R are the concentration of bound drug, of free drug, and of total protein, respectively. Many authors use the linearization procedure of Scatchard (1949) in order to determine the binding parameters graphically.

A variety of methods have been developed in order to measure the protein binding of drugs. Some of them are based on a physical separation of the unbound drug from the bound form, e.g. equilibrium dialysis, ultracentrifugation, ultrafiltration and gel filtration (Chignell, 1971). These methods have been reviewed and criticized by Rowland (1980). Other methods deal with specific spectroscopic properties of the ligand–macromolecule complexes; they include fluorescence spectroscopy, optical rotatory dispersion, circular dichroism, nuclear magnetic resonance and electron spin resonance spectroscopy (Chignell, 1971). These methods are useful for examining the qualitative nature of the interaction or for determining the macromolecule and/or ligand binding site. Finally, the interaction between drugs and macromolecules has also been studied by microcalorimetry, which gives information on the nature of the binding forces involved (Coassolo *et al.*, 1978; Tanford, 1980; Briand *et al.*, 1981).

When applied to the study of different experimental diseases, these methods have shown among other results that the number of binding sites of a given tissue for a given drug is not constant, but can be modified either by physiological, pharmacological or pathological factors. It has also been possible to show that, in some cases, the ligand modifies the structure of the binding protein, giving it new biological properties (see section 2.1).

The binding of a drug to plasma proteins requires a particular attention. For instance, some effects of drugs on coagulation can be explained by their binding to circulating clotting proteins such as prothrombin, thromboplastins, or fibrinogen. But it has also a more general role due to the fact that blood is the main carrier of drugs to tissues. Hence a drug bound to blood components is to be considered as a transport form to the cells. Assuming that membrane transport of a drug is a passive diffusion, the bound drug is too large a complex to easily cross cell membranes. As a consequence, drug penetration can be impaired by plasma protein binding, and the tissue diffusion of a drug is limited by the stability of its blood or plasma bound form.

Moreover, in some pathological states, drug antibodies can be characterized in blood, be it in plasma or on circulating cells, leucocytes, platelets or red blood cells.

At present, most available results refer to plasma protein binding of drugs and to their pharmacological consequences, a topic making up most of the present chapter.

2 Classification of drugs according to their interaction with plasma proteins

The binding of drugs to plasma proteins is not a general phenomenon. If most drugs are bound, others are not, at least not detectably. Amikacin, atenolol, ethambutol, isoniazid, lithium salts and ouabain are examples of the latter case, which appears to be related to the polarity and hydrophilicity of these molecules. In contrast, highly ionized but lipophilic substances are often bound, the binding forces involving electrostatic and/or hydrophobic interactions.

The binding proteins may be different ones according to the nature of the drug. Human serum albumin (HSA), α_1-acid glycoprotein (α_1-AGP), lipoproteins (high density lipoproteins, HDL; low density lipoproteins, LDL; very low density lipoproteins, VLDL) and immunoglobulins (IgG) may bind drugs. *Albumin*, the major plasma protein, is a single peptide chain of about 580 amino acid residues with a molecular weight of 66 000. Plasma albumin has been assigned numerous physiological roles. It is the main component responsible for the osmotic pressure of the blood and for the transport of both endogenous and exogenous compounds (Müller and Wollert, 1979). HSA is mainly involved in the transport of free fatty acids, bilirubin, tryptophan, cystine, pyridoxal phosphate, calcium, and various hormones such as thyroxine and steroids when specific transport proteins are saturated. Most drugs are bound to HSA, be they acidic, basic and neutral compounds (Chignell, 1971; Gillette, 1973; Lindup 1975; Jusko and Gretch, 1976). α_1-*AGP* is a globulin with molecular weight of 44 000 which can be distinguished from the other plasma proteins by a number of physicochemical properties: a very high carbohydrate content, a large number of sialyl residues, a very acidic isoelectric point, a peripheral microheterogeneity probably due to the different sialyl–galactosyl linkages, a large number of amino acid substitutions and a significant degree of homology with the immunoglobulins (Schmid, 1975). α_1-AGP shows large fluctuations due both to physiological and pathological conditions, but little is known about the physiological role of this glycoprotein, which plays a major role in the binding of several basic drugs (Piafsky *et al.*, 1978).

Lipoproteins are macromolecular complexes displaying characteristic sizes, densities and compositions. All lipoproteins contain protein components, called apoproteins, and polar lipids (phospholipids) in a surface film surrounding a neutral core (free and esterified cholesterol, triglycerides). The serum lipoproteins vary in composition with respect to the lipid component because their principal physiological function is to transport lipids in a water-soluble form, but also with respect to polypeptide chain composition. Lipoprotein plasma levels may show 5- to 10-fold variations. A large number of xenobiotic compounds can be transported by lipoproteins, for example carcinogens (Shu and Nichols, 1981) and cationic drugs (Tillement *et al.*, 1974; Vallner and Chen, 1977; Pike *et al.*, 1982). Relatively little work has been reported on the binding of drugs to γ-*globulins* and other plasma globulins. They generally only marginally account for the plasma binding of drugs (Piafsky, 1980), but can be involved in some immunopathological reactions due to antibody formation.

When examining plasma protein binding, it is of utmost importance to consider the drug concentrations used. It is clear that for very high drug concentrations, many interactions with various plasma proteins can be observed. For example, the distribution of bound thiamine varies during perfusion in the rabbit (Tillement, 1968). At low concentrations, nearly all the bound thiamine is HSA-linked. When the concentration increases, some binding to the different globulins occurs beginning with α-, β-, and γ-globulins. Similarly, azapropazone is bound to α_1-AGP and HSA in serum; as shown in Fig. 1, the relative saturation of each binding protein varies according to the total concentration of the drug (Urien, unpublished results). This phenomenon may also occur in physiological situations for some hormones such as thyroxine or cortisol which bind to HSA when their respective and specific transport proteins are saturated. The description to follow will include only clinically relevant concentrations. In these conditions, the different plasma drug–protein interactions can be classified according to the physicochemical properties of the drugs.

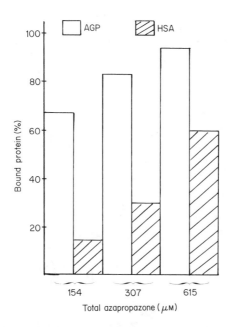

FIG. 1. Degrees of occupancy of α_1-acid glycoprotein (α_1-AGP) and albumin (HSA) binding sites by azapropazone. α_1-AGP and HSA concentrations are 20 and 600 μM, respectively.

2.1 BINDING OF ACIDIC DRUGS (TYPES I, II, AND III)

Acidic drugs are classified as type I, II, or III, according to their ionization, the kinetics, saturable or not saturable, of their overall plasma binding, and the relevant association constants (Table 1).

Most of the binding of highly ionized acidic drugs can be accounted for by association with HSA. Their pK_a values vary from 3·6 to 6, and the binding forces involve both electrostatic and hydrophobic bonds. In this case, the binding is saturable and HSA binding sites are located at the few electropositive poles of the macromolecule. These drugs are classified here as Type I.

TABLE 1

Classification of acidic drug protein interactions in human plasma

Types of drugs	I	II	III
Reference drugs	Warfarin and Diazepam	Indomethacin	Phenytoin
pK_a	5·05 and 3·4	4·5	8·33
Binding proteins	HSA $\alpha_1 GPA^a$	HSA	HSA
Binding processes	saturable	saturable and non-saturable	non-saturable
Association constants[b] in M^{-1}	$10^4–10^6$	$10^3–10^5$	$10^2–10^3$
Binding sites per mole of protein	1 to 3	6	many
Drug–HSA saturation[c]	possible	no	no
FFA-induced drug displacement[c]	possible	possible	possible

[a]Only for some acidic drugs.
[b]It concerns the lone class of binding sites or those of the highest affinity.
[c]At therapeutic levels of drugs and physiological concentrations of HSA.

2.1.1 Type I drugs

Type I drugs can bind to two separate and specific binding sites on HSA (Sudlow *et al.*, 1976; Sjöholm *et al.*, 1979; Fehske *et al.*, 1981). The first is the warfarin binding site, which involves Try and Lys 199 as amino acid residues. As regards the indol and benzodiazepine binding site, it is made up of the following amino acids: Tyr 411, His 146, Lys 194, and Arg 149 (see Fig. 2). Drugs that specifically bind to each site are listed in Table 2. Although these two sites are distinct, their respective bindings can influence each other. Typical binding plots of these drugs are presented in Fig. 3. For acidic drugs, HSA binding is often the only one occurring in human plasma. Nevertheless some of them, warfarin and acenocoumarol for example, are also bound to α_1-AGP; such drugs have no free carboxylic group, and the only binding forces involved seem to be hydrophobic ones (Urien *et al.*, 1982a). Recently, Wanwimolruk *et al.* (1982) have shown that some basic compounds chemically related to phenylbutazone are also bound to the warfarin site.

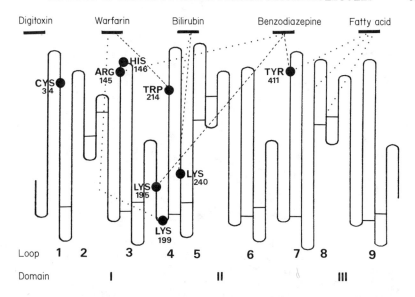

FIG. 2. The structure of human serum albumin and the possible location of drug binding sites. Amino acid residues (●) involved in the five most important binding sites of the protein are indicated by the dashed line (– – –). Other ones possibly involved are indicated by the pointed line (· · ·). Modified after Feshke *et al.* (1981). For further details, see this reference.

TABLE 2

Specific binding of drugs to HSA (compiled from Sudlow *et al.*, 1976, Sjöholm *et al.*, 1979 and Feshke *et al.*, 1981)

Warfarin site	Benzodiazepine site
Warfarin	Diazepam
Acenocoumarol	Benzodiazepines
Azapropazone	Clofibric acid
Dansylamide	Dansylsarcosine
Dicoumarol	Dicoumarol
Furosemide	Ethacrynic acid
Glibenclamide	Flufenamic acid
Iodopamide	Flurbiprofen
Iophenoxic acid	Glibenclamide
Oxyphenylbutazone	Ibuprofen
Phenprocoumon	Iopanoic acid
Phenylbutazone	Ketoprofen
Sulfinpyrazone	Naproxen
Tolbutamide	
Valproic acid	

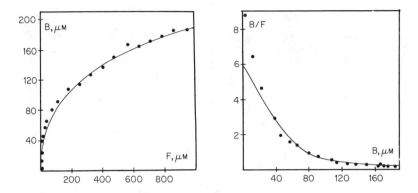

FIG. 3. Binding curves for the interaction of warfarin with human serum albumin: two successive saturable processes. In the left panel is represented the direct plot of bound (B) versus free (F) warfarin concentrations. In the right panel, the transformation of Scatchard is used. The curves are drawn according to the parameters estimated by nonlinear regression of the nontransformed values (bound and free concentrations). They clearly show that an estimation based on the Scatchard plot may lead to different results. This representation is nevertheless useful to qualitatively assess the binding process, in this case two saturable classes of binding sites.

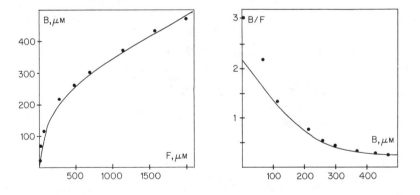

FIG. 4. Binding curves for the interaction of indomethacin with human serum albumin: successive saturable and nonsaturable processes. Left panel: direct plot of bound versus free indomethacin concentrations. Right panel: Scatchard transformation. The binding process is first saturable, then nonsaturable. See legend of Fig. 3 for commentary on the different binding representations.

2.1.2 Type II drugs

The real importance of this group is still questionable since in our opinion it currently contains only three drugs, namely indomethacin, its positional isomer clometacin (Zini et al., 1979), and diclofenac (Barré et al., unpublished results). As shown in Fig. 4, HSA binding of these drugs follows a characteristic pattern with two successive processes, the first one being saturable, the second not.

The saturable process seems to involve a large number (6) of equivalent binding sites: this is in close agreement with a lack of displacement of these drugs in therapeutic conditions. However, recent findings indicate that some of these sites have a very high affinity and may therefore be common with the binding sites of Type I drugs. These results were obtained by circular dichroism for indomethacin (Ekman et al., 1980) and diclofenac.

2.1.3 Type III drugs

Phenytoin is the reference drug of this type. It appears that in the range of clinical concentrations, its binding is not saturable (Lecomte et al., 1979). So the drug binding percentages remain constant whatever the dose. From a theoretical viewpoint, it becomes impossible to calculate the respective n and K values of the binding process, but only their product, nK. The latter is always low, suggesting that the relevant K is low. This can be due to the small degree of ionization of phenytoin at physiological pH. Phenobarbital thiopental, pentobarbital (Zini et al., unpublished results), chlortetracycline, demethylchlortetracycline, doxycycline, minocycline, and tetracycline (Fabre et al., 1971) follow these binding characteristics.

2.1.4 Free fatty acids and bilirubin binding sites

Although free fatty acids (FFA) and bilirubin are not drugs, they must be reviewed together with acidic drugs since they can modify the HSA binding of the latter due to interacting binding sites (Sjöholm et al., 1976). The location of the FFA binding site is probably in the third domain of the HSA structure (see Fig. 2) around amino acid residue 422 (Geisow and Beaven, 1977; Heaney-Kieras and King, 1977; Berde et al., 1979). The effects of FFA on the binding of most drugs bound to the diazepam site indicate that the FFA and diazepam sites are located close together (Sjödin, 1977). This explains the occurrence of allosteric interactions between both sites which result in noncompetitive inhibition of drug binding, that is a decrease in the apparent n, the number of sites (Urien et al., 1980). Regarding the warfarin site, FFA are able both to enhance or to inhibit the binding of anionic ligands (Soltys and Hsia, 1977). Wilding *et al.* (1977) have shown that the warfarin affinity constant increases from $0.85 \times 10^5 \, \text{M}^{-1}$ to $3.66 \times 10^5 \, \text{M}^{-1}$ as the oleic acid concentration increases from zero to three moles per mole of HSA, and that larger amounts of FFA progressively decrease the amount of warfarin bound in a noncompetitive fashion. All these results suggest that the binding of FFA affects the conformational state of HSA.

The bilirubin binding site is fairly independent of the benzodiazepine site (Roosdorp *et al.*, 1977; Brodersen *et al.*, 1977), and bilirubin is capable of competitively displacing some drugs bound to the warfarin site, e.g. warfarin (Sjöholm *et al.*, 1979), phenylbutazone (Brodersen, 1974) azapropazone (Fehske *et al.*, 1980), and valproic acid (Urien *et al.*, 1981). It is thus concluded that one bilirubin binding site overlaps with the warfarin binding area.

Table 1 shows (lower part) the pharmacological consequences of these bindings. Type I drugs bind to a limited number of sites; hence protein saturation may occur when effective doses are high enough (Bridgam *et al.*, 1972; Urien *et al.*, 1981). In the same way, drug–drug interactions can take place if HSA binding sites are common to both drugs. However, exceptions to this rule do exist. Indeed, drugs specific to diazepam site will bind to the warfarin site in the presence of greater than 2/1 ratios of FFA to HSA, this effect being due to FFA-induced conformational adaptations in the HSA molecule (Birkett *et al.*, 1977). As an example, clofibrate has been shown to displace warfarin from plasma proteins *in vivo*, despite it being primarily bound to the benzodiazepine site (Bjornsson *et al.*, 1979).

TABLE 3

Classification of non-ionized and basic drug protein interactions in human plasma

Types of interaction	IV	V	VI
Reference drugs	Digitoxin	Erythromycin	Imipramine
pK_a	—	8·8	9·5
Binding proteins	HSA (NS)[a]	HSA (NS) α_1-AGP (S)[b]	HSA (NS) α_1-AGP (S) HDL (NS) VLDL (NS) LDL (NS)
Drug plasma saturation	no	possible	no
Drug-induced free plasma level increase	no	possible	no
FFA-induced free plasma level increase	possible	no	no

[a]NS: non-saturable binding.
[b]S: saturable binding.

2.2 BINDING OF NON-IONIZABLE DRUGS (TYPE IV)

Digitalis glycosides are the main drugs of this group (Tillement *et al.*, 1980a). In human plasma, they are bound only to HSA, in a nonsaturable way. Their binding percentages thus remain constant whatever the dose used, provided the HSA concentrations remain within normal range. Their binding cannot be modified by other known drugs. FFA are the only molecules to decrease their binding (Table 3). Nevertheless, some authors (Lukas *et al.*, 1969; Kober *et al.*, 1979) have determined that digitoxin binds to a specific site with high affinity. But their studies agree with the fact that displacement of digitoxin by other drugs is uncommon (Sjöholm *et al.*, 1979). Typical binding curves of digitoxin are depicted in Fig. 5.

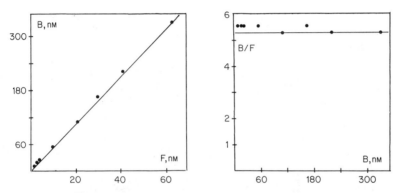

FIG. 5. Binding curves for the interaction of digitoxin with human serum albumin: one nonsaturable process. *Left panel:* Direct plot of bound versus free digitoxin concentrations. *Right panel:* Scatchard transformation. See legend of Fig. 3 for commentary on the different binding representations.

2.3 BINDING OF BASIC DRUGS (TYPES V AND VI)

Saturable binding to α_1-AGP and nonsaturable binding (see Fig. 6) to HSA are a common feature of many basic drugs (Piafsky, 1980; Prandota *et al.*, 1980; Schley *et al.*, 1980), though certain basic drugs such as bepridil (Albengres *et al.*, 1984) exhibit a saturable binding to HSA (Table 4). Saturable binding involves a higher association constant than the nonsaturable one. When drugs are also liposoluble, binding to circulating lipoproteins is observed. The binding occurs on each class of lipoproteins, VLDL, HDL, and LDL. Nonsaturable processes are observed with binding capacities (nK) which decrease from VLDL to LDL to HDL, suggesting that these drugs

TABLE 4

Classification of basic drugs

Type V drugs	Reference	Type VI drugs	Reference
Bupivacaine	Piafsky and Knoppert (1978)	Alprenolol	Piafsky (1980)
Dipyridamole	Hinderling and Garrett (1976)	Bepridil	Albengres et al. (1984)
	Piafsky (1980)	Chlorpromazine	Tillement et al. (1974); Bickel (1975)
Erythromycin	Prandota et al. (1980)	Disopyramide	Piafsky (1980)
Etidocaine	Piafsky and Knoppert (1978)	Imipramine	Tillement et al. (1974)
Lidocaine	Routledge et al. (1981a); Routledge	Nortriptyline	Tillement et al. (1974); Bickel (1975)
	et al. (1981b)	Pindolol	Lemaire and Tillement (1982a)
Methadone	Abramson (1982)	Propranolol	Scott et al. (1979); Glasson et al. (1980);
Minaprine	Barré et al. (1983)[a]		Sager et al. (1981)
Perazine	Schley et al. (1980)	Quinidine	Fremstad et al. (1979)
		Ticlopidine	Glasson et al. (1982)
		Tinoridine	Zini et al. (1983)[a]

[a] Unpublished results from our laboratory.

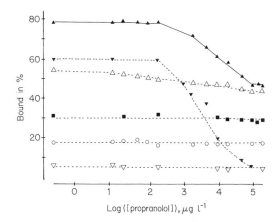

FIG. 6. Propranolol binding to different serum proteins. Serum (▲—▲); α_1-AGP at 22·5 μM (▼ ... ▼); HSA at 580 μM (△ ... △); HDL at 13 μM (■ ... ■); LDL at 1 μM (○ ... ○); VLDL at 0·2 μM (▽ ... ▽). After Glasson *et al.* (1980).

distribute into the lipid moiety of lipoproteins. This has been demonstrated for propranolol (Glasson *et al.*, 1980), ticlopidine (Glasson *et al.*, 1982), pindolol (Lemaire and Tillement, 1982a) and some carcinogens (Shu and Nichols, 1981). Multiple binding of erythromycin and propranolol are depicted in Fig. 6 and Fig. 7.

With basic drugs, additional binding can be observed to immunoglobulins, red blood cells, leucocytes and platelets. Specific receptors for some basic drugs have been identified on human blood cells: α-adrenergic receptors on platelets, β-adrenergic receptors on granulocytes, lymphocytes (Motulsky and Insel, 1982), and erythrocytes (Sager, 1982). Although propranolol can interact with specific receptors on erythrocytes, at therapeutic blood levels the nonspecific binding predominates (Sager, 1982). Chlorpromazine, thioridazine, diazepam, desmethyldiazepam, ticlopidine and bepridil also distribute in erythrocytes (Jadot *et al.*, 1981; Albengres *et al.*, 1984). Chlorpromazine and ticlopidine have been shown to interact with blood cells membranes by means of solubilization of the drug in lipidic regions (Schwendener and Weder, 1978; Daveloose *et al.*, 1982).

It is clear that when a drug such as the one above has multiple plasma- and blood-bound forms involving some nonsaturable processes, an increase of the free form by a drug displacement is unlikely to occur. This increase, however, has been shown to arise for erythromycin (Prandota *et al.*, 1980) and CM 7857 (Zini *et al.*, unpublished results) which have mainly one saturable binding site (on α_1-AGP) of high affinity.

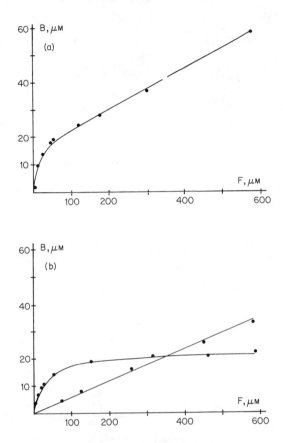

FIG. 7. Erythromycin binding to different serum proteins. (a) Bound versus free concentrations in serum. (b) Bound versus free concentrations for erythromycin interaction with α_1-AGP (hyperbola) and HSA (straight line), at macromolecular concentrations prevailing in serum. Note that the sum of the two curves of (b) will give the curve of (a). (After Prandota *et al.*, 1980.)

2.4 BINDING OF OTHER TYPES OF DRUGS

Probucol, a highly apolar and hydrophobic drug, binds practically to the sole lipoproteins in blood (Urien *et al.*, 1982b). Cyclosporin, a cyclic poly-peptidic drug of high hydrophobic character, binds mainly to plasma lipoproteins and erythrocytes (Lemaire and Tillement, 1982b). Steroids, including corticosteroids, oestrogens, progestagens, androgens, and their synthetic derivatives are HSA-bound according to a saturable process with n varying from 1 to 10 and K ranging between 10^4 and 10^5 M^{-1}. Most of the physiological steroids are transported primarily by the specific corticosteroid-binding globulin which binds them with a very high affinity constant (10^7 to 10^9 M^{-1}), but they also interact with α_1-AGP with an affinity constant of about 10^5 M^{-1}. Steroid binding to plasma proteins has been extensively reviewed by Westphal (1971). Finally, some polyene macrolide antibiotics have been found to associate to a large extent with human plasma lipoproteins (Brajtburg et al., 1984). The binding characteristics and influencing structural features of these compounds remain to be better assessed before a categorization can be proposed.

3 Pharmacological consequences of plasma protein binding

As a drug bound to plasma proteins is practically nondiffusible, the stability of the plasma drug–protein complex is the main impairing factor of drug tissue distribution. Hence plasma binding affects the apparent volume of distribution (V_D) and in some cases also the clearance (Cl) of a drug.

3.1 PLASMA PROTEIN BINDING AND DRUG DISTRIBUTION

The first consequence of drug–protein binding is to create a new molecular species, the drug–protein complex, which is believed to follow the distribution of the protein. Conversely, only the free drug is thought to be capable of diffusion across the membranes. But binding is a reversible phenomenon and the rates of association and dissociation are usually very rapid. So, as soon as the free drug crosses the membrane, a new equilibrium is reached both in plasma and in tissue, providing the latter also contains drug binding proteins. From theoretical considerations it can be demonstrated (Tillement et al., 1979) that at equilibrium the ratio of bound drug concentrations between a tissue and plasma at a determined time is related to the ratio of their corresponding drug binding capacities. This parameter is expressed as NK, N being the tissue (or plasma) concentration of binding sites and K the relevant association constant (Fig. 8).

As a consequence of the above, different situations can be observed. The plasma drug binding capacity can be higher or lower than that of tissues, or it can have an intermediate value, higher than that of some tissues but lower than that of others (Table 5).

Plasma retention of a drug is seen when blood binding capacity is far higher than that of other tissues. This is observed mainly for type I and II drugs of acidic character which are almost totally ionized at plasma pH and highly

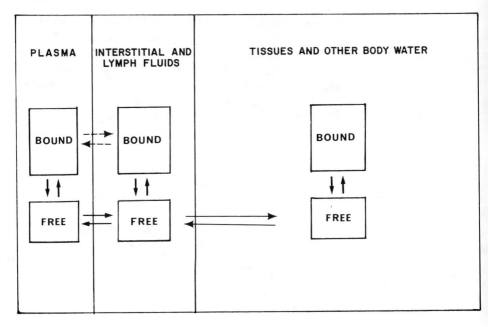

Fig. 8. Liquid compartments in humans and drug distribution. Plasma, 4% of body weight; interstitial and lymph fluids, 12% of body weight; tissues and other body water, 42% of body weight. (Modified after Jusko and Gretch, 1976.)

TABLE 5

Drug distribution as a result of its relative binding capacities in plasma and tissues

The binding capacity is expressed as NK, the product of binding site concentration times the affinity constant. The apparent volume of distribution is an index of the extent of drug diffusion in tissues

	Binding capacity		
Drugs	Plasma > tissues Types I, II	Intermediate Propranolol	Tissues > plasma Phenothiazines
Plasma binding (%)	>90	>90	>80
NK (plasma)	>50	3·8	>10
Apparent distribution volume (l kg^{-1})	0·1–0·5	3·62	>20

bound to HSA. Some examples of these drugs are given in Table 6. Their V_D values are low, they do not differ statistically and they are superimposable to the V_D of injected HSA, 0.1 l kg^{-1}. This clearly shows that, in this case, the drug V_D is governed by that of its main binding protein (Houin and

TABLE 6

Incidence of high plasma protein affinity on drug distribution (data from Tillement, 1978)

	Clofibric acid	Fluoro-phenindione	Phenyl-butazone	Warfarin
Plasma protein binding percentage	97	95	99	97
Apparent volume of distribution (l kg^{-1})	0·09	0·09	0·09	0·13
Half-life (h)	13	31	75	44

Tillement, 1981). Numerous drugs exhibit the same particularity to a smaller or larger extent (Table 7). Their V_D values are dependent upon the fraction of unbound drug in plasma (fu): an increase in the unbound plasma fraction results in an elevation of the relevant V_D.

TABLE 7

Examples of drugs for which body diffusion is limited by plasma binding. All these drugs are bound to HSA (see Goodman-Gilman et al., 1980, and Avery, 1980)

Drugs	Plasma free drug (%)	Apparent volume of distribution l kg^{-1}	Clearance ml min^{-1}
Carbenoxolone	1	0·10	5·8
Ibuprofen	1	0·14	57·0
Phenylbutazone	1	0·10	8·0
Naproxen	2	0·09	5·2
Clofibric acid	3	0·09	6·1
Fusidic acid	3	0·15	12·0
Warfarin	3	0·10	3·8
Bumetamide	4	0·18	48·5
Dicloxacillin	4	0·29	114·0
Furosemide	4	0·20	190·0
Tolbutamide	4	0·14	16·2
Cloxacillin	5	0·34	160·0
Fluorophenindione	5	0·09	2·3
Nalidixic acid	5	0·35	162·0
Sulfaphenazole	5	0·29	23·0
Chlorpropamide	8	0·20	6·8
Oxacillin	8	0·44	210·0
Nafcillin	10	0·63	160·0

Tissue retention of a drug is observed, conversely, when the plasma binding capacity is low as compared to those of the tissues. In this case, the drug is mostly located in tissues. The corresponding V_D values are large and do not correspond to physiological compartments (Table 8), but they are positively correlated with tissue affinity.

TABLE 8

Examples of drugs for which tissue distribution is apparently independent from plasma protein binding (data from Tillement et al., 1980b)

	Plasma protein binding percentage	Apparent volume of distribution $(l\ kg^{-1})$	Half-life (h)
Desipramine	92	40	33
Imipramine	95	30	12
Nortriptyline	94	39	52
Vinblastine	70	35	28
Vincristine	70	11	144

The preferential tissue distribution of a drug is relevant to a particular case where plasma binding capacity is higher than that of most tissues except one or two. This is observed mainly for propranolol, whose protein binding in plasma is lower than in liver and lungs but higher than in other tissues (Evans et al., 1973). Liver and perhaps lungs are also the tissues where its biotransformation takes place. Pharmacokinetic parameters of this drug vary in different species (see Table 9). Despite clearance differences, the V_D increases as the bound drug concentration decreases, showing that plasma binding is a limiting factor for the tissue diffusion of this drug. The low value of the liver blood flow observed in man explains the lower clearance and the longer half-life as compared to the other species. Thus, when the appropriate correction for clearance differences is made, an increase in drug binding still results in a relative shortening of drug half-life, i.e. an augmentation of drug elimination rate. These considerations demonstrate that plasma binding of propranolol increases the rate of elimination by delivering more drug to tissues with higher binding capacity (mainly the liver) and limits its diffusion to other tissues.

Although it is currently difficult to measure the drug binding capacity of a tissue, this parameter is easily checked in plasma. It is with type I bound drugs that V_D are the lowest, i.e. with drugs exhibiting the highest affinity for HSA. Up to now, the kinetic dependency of a drug to its plasma binding

TABLE 9

Variations of plasma protein binding, apparent distribution volume and half-life of propranolol in different species (data from Evans et al., 1973)

	Monkey	Dog	Man	Rat
Plasma protein binding (%)	99·2	96·6	93·2	92·2
Apparent volume of distribution (l kg^{-1})	0·60	1·71	3·62	5·30
Clearance (ml min^{-1} kg^{-1})	14	34	16	93
Half-life (min)	30	35	167	40
Hepatic extraction ratio	0·46	0·90	0·90	0·97
Liver blood flow (ml min^{-1} kg^{-1})	50	43	22	48

Note: The apparent volume of distribution (V_D), the liver blood flow (Q_H), the extraction ratio (E) and the drug half-life ($t_{\frac{1}{2}}$) are related by the equation

$$t_{\frac{1}{2}} = \frac{V_D \times 0·693}{Q_H E} .$$

proteins is only demonstrated with HSA. It is easy to imagine that in the future similar dependencies will be checked for drugs bound to other circulating proteins with a high association constant, namely α_1-AGP and lipoproteins.

3.2 PLASMA PROTEIN BINDING AND DRUG CLEARANCE

Total drug clearance can be expressed as follows:

$$Cl = Q \cdot E \tag{2}$$

where Q is the blood flow through the clearing tissue and E the extraction ratio of the drug. The latter is defined as:

$$E = \frac{C_A - C_V}{C_A} \tag{3}$$

where C_A and C_V are the drug concentrations in the artery and the vein of the clearing tissue, respectively (see Wilkinson and Shand, 1975).

When E is high (more than 0·7) clearance tends to depend only on Q: the drug, whatever its form (free or bound), is cleared from blood by the tissue. In this case, plasma binding has little incidence on clearance values. As seen in Fig. 9, it is evident that the blood clearance of propranolol ($E = 0·9$) is not dependent on the fraction of free drug in plasma. In contrast, only the free blood fraction of slowly cleared drugs ($E < 0·3$) is trapped by the clearing tissue. In this case, total clearance is obviously dependent upon free plasma

TABLE 10

Various effects of blood protein binding upon total clearance of drugs

Different examples have been chosen according to their extraction ratio and to their plasma binding

Drug	Binding protein	Plasma binding	Hepatic-extraction ratio	Clearance	Reference
Clofibric acid	HSA	variable	low	variable[a]	Houin (1981)
Phenylbutazone	HSA	variable	low	variable[a]	Sjöqvist et al. (1980)
Salicylic acid	HSA	variable	low	variable[a]	Furst et al. (1979)
Valproic acid	HSA	variable	low	variable[a]	Bowdle et al. (1980)
Glibenclamide	HSA	constant	low	constant	Goodman-Gilman et al. (1980)
Indomethacin	HSA	constant	low	constant	Goodman-Gilman et al. (1980)
Erythromycin	α_1-AGP	variable	low	variable[b]	Austin et al. (1980)
Disopyramide	α_1-AGP	variable	low	variable[b]	Giacomini et al. (1982)
Propranolol	α_1-AGP	variable	high	constant	Evans et al. (1973)
Imipramine	α_1-AGP	variable	high	constant	Goodman-Gilman et al. (1980)

[a]Total clearance positively correlated with *fu.*
[b]Renal clearance positively correlated with *fu.*

fraction (fu) of the drug and may vary according to it. In Fig. 10(a) and (b), the warfarin and phenytoin clearances are plotted against their free fraction in plasma, showing that changes in the plasma binding produce proportional changes in the clearance of these drugs with low extraction ratio. Table 10 gives some examples of such drugs: they are highly HSA-bound, i.e. of type I.

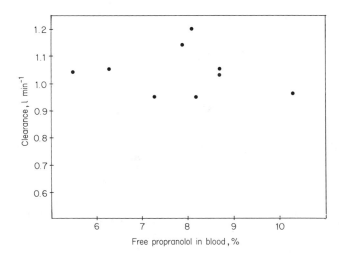

FIG. 9. Clearance and free fraction of a drug with high hepatic extraction ratio. Note the absence of correlation. (After the data of Evans, 1973.)

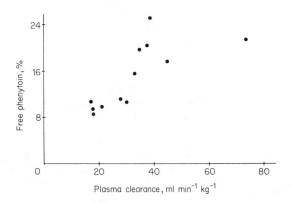

FIG. 10a. Clearance and free fraction of phenytoin with low hepatic extraction ratio, according to Rowland (1980). $p < 0.01$. (Reproduced by permission of Raven Press, New York.)

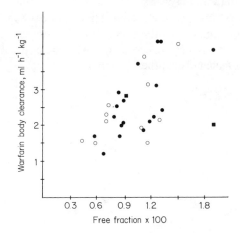

FIG. 10b. Clearance and free fraction of warfarin with low hepatic extraction ratio, according to Yacobi *et al.* (1976). $p < 0.001$. (Reproduced by permission of the C. V. Mosby Company, St. Louis.)

3.3 PLASMA PROTEIN BINDING AND DOSE-DEPENDENT KINETICS

Dose-dependent pharmacokinetics arises from the fact that high association constant and limited number of binding sites in plasma are often linked. Especially for type I acidic drugs, plasma binding can be quickly saturated at concentrations which include the therapeutic range. As a consequence, the kinetic parameters of a given drug differ according to the dose used, be it below or beyond plasma protein saturation levels (see Table 11).

TABLE 11

Dose-dependent pharmacokinetics of valproic acid as related to plasma protein binding

The kinetic parameters are different for different doses. Note the correlation between dose, plasma free drug percentage, and kinetic parameters. Data from Bowdle et al. (1980)

Dose (mg day⁻¹)	Plasma free drug (%)	Apparent volume of distribution (l kg⁻¹)	Clearance (ml h⁻¹ kg⁻¹)	Elimination rate (h⁻¹)
500	7·0	0·132	6·67	0·0510
1000	8·2	0·147	6·74	0·0498
1500	9·3	0·177	8·20	0·0479

4 Factors influencing plasma protein binding

4.1 PHYSIOLOGICAL STATES

Modified plasma protein binding of drugs may result from differences in age, genetics, sex, and from pregnancy. The observed variations in binding are caused mainly by differences in the plasma concentrations of proteins (HSA and α_1-AGP), FFA and bilirubin. Table 12 summarizes some data available on this subject. In addition, a qualitative difference in HSA structure has been reported to cause a smaller binding of acidic drugs in the newborn as compared to adults (Wallace, 1977).

4.2 PHARMACOLOGICAL INTERACTIONS

The inhibition of binding or the displacement of a bound drug may occur under different circumstances. Binding antagonism can result either from a competitive or a noncompetitive interaction. The first case is observed between drugs which share the same binding site (see classification above). For instance, competition between warfarin and clofibric acid (Bjornsson, 1979), or between two or several sulfonamides (Christensen et al., 1963) may be observed in therapy. The probability of interaction will depend mainly on the relative concentrations of the binding protein and of the drugs. A further condition is that both drugs bind to a limited number of sites, implying saturable binding at therapeutic levels. The interaction is likely to occur when at least one of the competing drugs occupies most or all of the available binding sites, leaving only few or no free sites. Hence the degree of binding site occupancy is an important parameter to predict such an interaction. It is with drugs of low activity that such interactions are most common because the efficiency of these compounds requires high doses which usually correspond to high levels in plasma. Table 13 gives some examples showing major differences in the occupancy of HSA and α_1-AGP sites.

In most cases, the phenomenon is further complicated by the fact that ligand binding involves also a modification of protein structure, especially with the relatively flexible HSA. The resulting allosteric effect may affect the binding of other drugs.

In summary, different situations exist where the levels of free drug may increase, and the pharmacokinetic parameters of the displaced drug may be modified. If the drug has a high liver extraction ratio, increased fu will result in increased V_D without change of its hepatic clearance, its half-life being prolonged. On the other hand, for a drug with a low E, both hepatic clearance and V_D will increase, the corresponding half-life being either unchanged or only slightly increased (Rowland and Tozer, 1980).

TABLE 12

Physiological states influencing the plasma protein binding of drugs

Factors of variation	Drugs studied	Plasma binding	Causal factor	Reference
Age				
Newborn	HSA bound drugs	Decreased	↓ HSA level Qualitative difference in HSA	Wallace (1976) Wallace (1977)
	Lidocaine Metocurine ⎱ Propranolol ⎰ d-Tubocurarine	Decreased	↓ α_1-AGP level	Wood and Wood (1981)
Aging	Phenytoin	Decreased	↑ FFA, bilirubin levels	Fredholm et al. (1975)
	Tolbutamide	Decreased	↓ HSA level	Adir et al. (1982)
Genetics	Warfarin	Increased	↑ FFA level	Abel et al. (1982)
	Diazepam	Decreased		
Pregnancy	Acidic drugs ⎱ Basic drugs ⎰ Dexamethasone	Decreased	↓ HSA level ↓ α_1-AGP level ?	Perucca and Crema (1982)
Sex (female compared to male)	Lidocaine	Decreased	↓ α_1-AGP level ↓ HSA, ↓ α_1-AGP ↑ FFA level	Routledge et al. (1981b)
	Diazepam	Decreased		Abel et al. (1979)

TABLE 13

Maximal plasma levels and binding site concentrations for some drugs highly bound to plasma

HSA and α_1-AGP concentrations are assumed to be 600 and 20 μM

Drug	Maximal drug plasma level (μM)	Binding protein	N^a (μM)	Degree of occupancy
Acenocoumarol	28	HSA	1200	0·02
Clofibric acid	600	HSA	400	1·33
Diazepam	11	HSA	400	0·02
Dicloxacillin	42	HSA	600	0·07
Dicoumarol	60	HSA	1200	0·05
Digitoxin	0·05	HSA	600	0·0001
Disopyramide	12	α_1-AGP	20	0·60
Erythromycin	5	α_1-AGP	20	0·25
Fenofibric acid	83	HSA	2400	0·03
Imipramine	0·5	α_1-AGP	20	0·03
Indomethacin	0·5	HSA	20	0·03
Methadone	10	α_1-AGP	20	0·50
Oxacillin	10	HSA	600	0·02
Phenylbutazone	300	HSA	600	0·50
Propranolol	1	α_1-AGP	20	0·05
Salicylic acid	724	HSA	900	0·80
Valproic acid	903	HSA	1200	0·75
Warfarin	16	HSA	1200	0·04

[a]N is the binding site concentration in plasma. The degree of occupancy is the ratio of the maximal drug plasma level to the binding site concentration in plasma (N).

Table 14 exemplifies the modifications of the pharmacokinetic parameters of warfarin when partly displaced by clofibrate in man (Bjornsson *et al.*, 1979). The pharmacological consequences of these variations are clear. These authors concluded that since the free levels of warfarin in liver are increased, this interaction can explain the observed potentiation of anti-coagulant effect. But another mechanism, probably an inhibition of warfarin inactivation in liver, may also help explain the increase in activity.

From a general point of view, it is admitted that displacement of plasma protein binding generally leads to a minor potentiation in the therapeutic effects of the displaced drug. This can be explained by the larger V_D of the free drug as compared to that of the bound drug: the total plasma concentration is quickly decreasing as the free drug disappears from blood and distributes to tissues. However, new adverse reactions may result from increased levels in tissues otherwise poorly reached.

TABLE 14

Effect of clofibrate on the disposition of warfarin (data from Bjornsson et al., 1979)

Warfarin kinetic parameters

Subject	Plasma free drug (in %)		Apparent volume of distribution ($l\,kg^{-1}$)		Clearance ($l\,h^{-1}$)		Half-life (h)	
	CP	IP	CP	IP	CP	IP	CP	IP
1	1·20	1·45	0·108	0·129	0·226	0·286	24·2	24·0
2	1·76	1·89	0·157	0·168	0·195	0·195	38·5	41·4
3	1·67	1·90	0·138	0·168	0·344	0·466	21·5	20·0
4	1·67	1·86	0·116	0·148	0·182	0·225	33·1	34·9

CP, control period; IP, interaction period (effect of clofibrate). Note that increase in percentage of free drug correlates with an increase in apparent volume of distribution and clearance, the half-life being unaffected.

An increase of fu may produce an increase in renal clearance, leading to a quicker drug elimination and thus limiting the effects of potentiation. The overall modifications of the respective plasma concentrations of both free and bound drug, when displacement occurs, are depicted in Fig. 11 according to Sellers *et al.* (1978). This type of drug interaction thus leads to an instantaneous higher free fraction in tissues but also to an increase in drug elimination by kidneys. The pharmacological consequences may vary according to the kinetics of the effects, immediate or delayed, of the displaced drug. In the first case, potentiation may be observed, while in the second the response is not clear. These problems need to be better studied if we are to acquire a deeper knowledge of their pharmacological consequences.

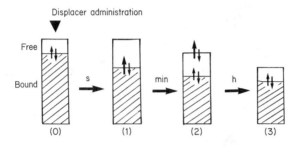

FIG. 11. Effect of drug displacement on the bound, unbound and total plasma concentrations of the displaced drug. (0) prior to displacement, (1) intravascular displacement, (2) redistribution of displaced drug, (3) increased elimination. (Modified after Sellers, 1978.)

Whatever the displacement mechanism, modifications of plasma free drug concentrations can be predicted by *in vitro* experiments using pure solutions of binding proteins or human plasma and therapeutic concentrations of associated drugs. Plasma obtained under different pathological conditions including for instance icterus, cirrhosis, or renal chronic insufficiency, may also be used to investigate drug binding in these diseases. The interest of such studies is to measure the possible increase in free drug plasma levels in an attempt to assess the relevant pharmacokinetic consequences.

Drug interactions at the plasma binding level may also occur by nondirect displacement mechanism. Naranjo *et al.* (1982) have shown that heparin, by raising FFA levels, produces an increase in free diazepam and a decrease in free warfarin (see section 2 for mechanism); in contrast, the increase in propranolol fu was unrelated to FFA levels. Similarly, Sager *et al.* (1981) have demonstrated that heparin activation of lipoprotein–lipase induces a decrease in the triglycerid-rich lipoprotein which corresponds closely to a decrease in propranolol binding.

TABLE 15

Modifications of drug effects induced by altered plasma protein binding

Drug	Cause	Plasma free drug	Pharmacological consequences	References
Clofibrate	Nephrotic syndrome Uremia (hypoalbuminemia)	↑	Induced myopathy in nearly all patients	Pierides et al. (1975)
Warfarin	Displacement by clofibrate	↑	Increased anticoagulant effect	Bjornsson et al. (1979)
Diazepam Chlordiazepoxide	Hypoalbuminemia	↑	Increased frequency of unwanted CNS depression	Greenblatt and Koch-Weser (1974)
Phenytoin	Hypoalbuminemia	↑	Increased frequency of adverse effects	Boston Collaborative Drug Surveillance Program (1973)
Prednisone	Hypoalbuminemia	↑	Increased frequency of adverse effects	Lewis et al. (1971)
Methadone	Cancer ($\nearrow \alpha_1$-AGP)	↓	Decreased analgesic effect	Abramson (1982)

4.3 PATHOLOGICAL STATES

Plasma binding of drugs is altered in various pathological states, the variations observed being due to three main mechanisms: (a) the structure of the binding protein can be modified, thus altering its drug binding capacities, (b) its plasma concentration may vary leading to a modification of plasma binding capacity (NK), and (c) plasma binding inhibitors may appear or increase, antagonizing drug binding. These inhibitors are either physiological compounds at high, abnormal concentrations like bilirubin, or endogenous substances resulting from an abnormal pathological metabolism.

Hypoalbuminemia may be the reflection either of a decrease of HSA total amount or of an altered distribution in the body (see Fig. 8). Concomitantly or not, concentrations of various acidic endogenous substances may increase, e.g. FFA, bilirubin, and uric acid. In all these cases, the plasma binding of acidic drugs (mainly type I) is decreased. This matter has been extensively developed elsewhere (Tillement et al., 1974), and some examples are summarized in Table 15. Moreover, other endogenous binding inhibitors have been recently identified, such as cyanate (Bachmann et al., 1980) and abnormal peptides in plasma of uremic patients (Kinniburgh and Boyd, 1981). Finally, evidence has been presented that elevated urea and creatinine levels may explain the binding defect of valproic acid seen in uremic patients (Brewster and Muir, 1980).

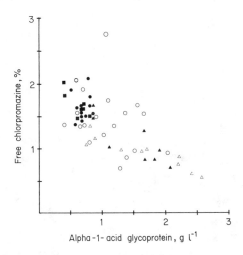

FIG. 12. Relationship between α_1-AGP level and free drug percentage in plasma. The free drug percentage is negatively correlated with the α_1-AGP level ($p < 0.001$). (According to Piafsky et al., 1978; reproduced by permission of The New England Journal of Medicine.)

In contrast to albumin, the plasma concentrations of other main binding proteins (α_1-AGP and lipoproteins) may show large fluctuations due both to physiological (see above) or pathological conditions. Interestingly, the variations encountered are often an increase in the protein concentrations. The results will be an increased binding of those basic drugs which have affinity for α_1-AGP and/or for lipoproteins. As an example, the relationship between the free fraction of propranolol or chlorpromazine and the corresponding α_1-AGP levels is depicted in Fig. 12 (Piafsky *et al.*, 1978). For a detailed review of disease-induced changes in plasma binding of basic drugs, see Piafsky (1980). Additional studies have recently focused on this subject. Routledge *et al.* (1981) have studied the disposition of lidocaine in myocardial infarction in relation with α_1-AGP levels, and Abramson *et al.* (1982) have demonstrated altered plasma binding of propranolol and lidocaine in cancer as a result of increased α_1-AGP levels. Finally, the role of lipoproteins has been recently evaluated in the serum binding variations of amitriptyline, nortriptyline and quinidine (Pike *et al.*, 1982).

5 Therapeutic applications of drug binding to plasma proteins

Drug response may be affected by plasma protein binding, both in physiological conditions, i.e. at normal plasma protein concentrations, and in pathological states leading to an altered binding. Measurement of plasma binding capacity may thus be a useful means for selecting and monitoring dosage regimens, and for avoiding untoward effects.

5.1 RATIONAL DOSAGE REGIMEN

When the tissue distribution of a drug is impaired by its plasma binding the percentage of this binding may be considered as an index of instantaneous inactivation if drug effects are supposed to take place in tissues. These drugs belong to types I and II and some others like digitoxin to type IV: all of them are characterized by a high HSA binding capacity. This implies that the major part of the first dose will be HSA-bound, hence almost immediately inactivated. When initiating a treatment with these drugs, the first doses will be ineffective in so far as the corresponding plasma-free drug concentrations will not be high enough.

As a consequence, the first dose will usually be a high, loading dose whose goal is first to provide the plasma bound drug, and second to lead to an effective free drug concentration. On the other hand, the maintenance doses will be lower. They compensate the fraction of drug eliminated by metabolism and thus maintain the initial intensity of the effects. So all above drugs should be administered according to this scheme. This necessity was early recognized for oral anticoagulants at a time when the phenomenon was not really understood. It is now commonly accepted that steroidal and nonsteroidal antiinflammatory drugs as well as some acidic antibiotics must be administered starting with a loading dose.

5.2 DOSAGE ADJUSTMENT ACCORDING TO PLASMA BINDING CAPACITY

A loading dose refers to the total number of HSA binding sites available in plasma, i.e. the protein concentration. As previously shown, it is only when the total amount of HSA is decreased in the body that the loading dose must be decreased to the same extent. It is also in such cases that, for pathological reasons, the degree of occupancy may increase, thus enhancing the possibility of drug interactions. This phenomenon has been described in different pathological situations (see Table 15).

In contrast to the above, the pharmacological effects of normal doses of basic drugs should decrease when α_1-AGP and/or lipoprotein concentrations are increased. So an increase of dosage of these drugs is warranted in such pathological states. Currently, however, this hypothesis is not verified with enough clinical data.

5.3 DRUG MONITORING USING PLASMA FREE DRUG CONCENTRATIONS

For all drugs associating a high plasma binding percentage and a relatively low apparent volume of distribution, the free drug plasma concentration is a good reflection of the diffusible drug, i.e. the active concentration. In such cases, drug responses may be better correlated with the plasma-free drug concentration (see Table 15). For these drugs, therapeutic monitoring should thus rely on plasma-free drug concentration instead of total ones. This is especially useful when pathological states involve large modifications of drug plasma binding capacity. Conversely, when drugs are highly bound to tissue proteins, the concentration of free drug in plasma has no value *per se*, because drug diffusion in tissues is not impaired to a great extent by plasma binding capacity.

6 Conclusion

Although indirect, much evidence leads to the conclusion that plasma protein binding may influence the pharmacokinetic behaviour of a drug. It thus seems reasonable to admit that plasma binding capacity, when high enough, controls the drug distribution either by limiting tissue diffusion or by directing it.

This conclusion can be a source of inspiration for those whose aim is to modify the generally unspecific distribution of most drugs in the body. The concept of new drugs with a plasma binding capacity high enough to prevent their dissemination to the entire body, but lower than that of target cells, has to be investigated in the future.

At present, the effect of plasma protein binding in directing drug distribution has been characterized mainly for HSA-bound drugs. All of them are acidic compounds which in plasma bind only to HSA. As other drugs are known to be bound to other circulating proteins with a high binding capacity, it would be interesting to examine whether their distribution pattern is superimposable on, or similar to, that of their binding proteins.

The evaluation of plasma protein binding effectiveness supposes an adequate measurement of the binding capacity of body tissues. If this measurement is now possible in some specific cases, no general method is available. Problems are numerous, including the selection of basic materials (unaltered tissue, homogenates or highly purified extracts), the necessity for radioligands of high specific radioactivity, and the determination of an experimental scheme to overcome the so-called "nonspecific" binding. In the future, a decisive step will be made when such a method becomes available.

In therapy, the extent of drug plasma binding may be a valuable parameter in various circumstances. But it is now well established that plasma protein binding capacity has no significance *per se*, and that it cannot be used independently of other pharmacokinetic parameters, especially V_D and Cl. Only so can it help in the choice of an appropriate drug, in the selection of the best dosage regimen, and in its monitoring. Moreover, in pathological states, taking into account altered plasma protein binding can lead to dosage adjustments and can thus help to avoid unwanted interactions and untoward effects.

References

Aarons, L., Schary, W. L. and Rowland, M. (1979). *J. Pharm. Pharmac.* **31**, 322–330.
Abel, J. G., Sellers, E. M., Naranjo, C. A., Shaw, J., Kadar, D. and Romach, M. K. (1979). *Clin. Pharmac. Ther.* **26**, 247–255.
Abel, J. G., Roth, E. A., Sellers, E. M. and Ray, A. K. (1982). *Clin. Pharmac. Ther.* **31**, 436–441.
Abramson, F. P. (1982). *Clin. Pharmac. Ther.* **32**, 652–658.
Albengres, E., Urien, S., Pognat, J. F. and Tillement, J. P. (1984). *Pharmacology* **28**, 139–149.
Austin, K. L., Mather, L. E., Philpot, C. R. and McDonald, P. J. (1980). *Br. J. Clin. Pharmac.* **10**, 273–289.
Avery, G. S. (1980). "Drug treatment—Principles and Practice of Clinical Pharmacology and Therapeutics." 2nd edition. Churchill Livingstone, Edinburgh and London.

Bachmann, K., Valentovic, M. and Shapiro, R. (1980). *Biochem. Pharmac.* **29**, 1598–1601.

Berde, C. B., Hudson, B. S., Simoni, R. D. and Sklar, L. A. (1979). *J. Biol. Chem.* **254**, 391–399.

Bickel, M. H. (1975). *J. Pharm. Pharmac.* **27**, 733–738.

Birkett, D. J., Myers, P. and Sudlow, G. (1977). *Molec. Pharmac.* **13**, 987–992.

Bjornsson, T. D., Meffin, P. J., Swezey, S. and Blaschke, T. F. (1979). *J. Pharmac. Exp. Ther.* **210**, 316–321.

Boston Collaborative Drug Surveillance Program. (1973). Diphenylhydantoin side effects and serum albumin levels. *Clin. Pharmac. Ther.* **14**, 529–532.

Bowdle, T. A., Patel, I. H., Levy, R. H. and Wilensky, A. J. (1980). *Clin. Pharmac. Ther.* **28**, 486–492.

Brajtburg, J., Bolard, J., Levy, R. A., Ostlund, R. E., Jr, Elberg, S. and Medoff, G. (1984). *J. Infect. Dis.* In press.

Brewster, D. and Muir, N. C. (1980). *Clin. Pharmac. Ther.* **27**, 76–82.

Briand, C., Sarrazin, M., Peyrot, V., Gilli, R., Bourdeaux M. and Sari, J. C. (1981). *Molec. Pharmac.* **21**, 92–99.

Bridgman, J. F., Rosen, S. M. and Thorp, J. M. (1972). *Lancet* **ii**, 506–509.

Brodersen, R. (1974). *J. Clin. Invest.* **54**, 1353–1363.

Brodersen, R., Sjödin, T. and Sjöholm, I. (1977). *J. Biol. Chem.* **252**, 5067–5072.

Chignell, C. F. (1971). Physical methods for studying drug–protein binding. *In* "Concepts in Biochemical Pharmacology" (B. B. Brodie and J. R. Gillette, eds), Part 1. Springer-Verlag, Berlin, Heidelberg, New York.

Christensen, L. K., Hansen, J. M. and Kristensen, M. (1963). *Lancet* **ii**, 1298–1301.

Coassolo, P., Sarrazin, M., Sari, J. C. and Briand, C. (1978). *Biochem. Pharmac.* **27**, 2787–2792.

Daveloose, D., Sablayrolles, M., Molle, D. and Leterrier, F. (1982). *Biochem. Pharmac.* **31**, 3949–3954.

Ekman, B., Sjödin, T. and Sjöholm, I. (1982). *Biochem. Pharmac.* **29**, 1759–1765.

Evans, G. H., Nies, A. S. and Shand, D. G. (1973). *J. Pharmac. Exp. Ther.* **186**, 114–122.

Fabre, J., Milek, E., Kalfopoulos, P., and Merier, G. (1971). *Schweiz. Med. Wschr.* **101**, 625–633.

Fehske, K. J., Jähnchen, E., Müller, W. E. and Stillbauer, A. (1980). *Naunyn-Schmiedeberg's Arch. Pharmacol.* **313**, 159–163.

Fehske, K. J., Müller, W. E. and Wollert, U. (1981). *Biochem. Pharmac.* **30**, 687–692.

Fredholm, B. B., Rane, A. and Persson, B. (1975). *Pediatric Res.* **9**, 26–30.

Fremstad, D., Nilsen, O. G., Storstein, L., Amlie, J. and Jacobsen, S. (1979). *Eur. J. Clin. Pharmac.* **15**, 187–192.

Furst, D. E., Tozer, T. N. and Melmon, K. L. (1979). *Clin. Pharmac. Ther.* **26**, 380–389.

Geisow, M. J. and Beaven, G. H. (1977). *Biochem. J.* **163**, 477–484.

Giacomini, K. M., Swezey, S. E., Turner-Tamiyasu, K. and Blaschke, T. F. (1982). *J. Pharmacokin. Biopharm.* **10**, 1–14.

Gillette, J. R. (1973). *Ann. N.Y. Acad. Sci.* **226**, 6–17.

Glasson, S., Zini, R., D'Athis, P., Tillement, J. P. and Boissier, J. R. (1980). *Molec. Pharmacol.* **17**, 187–191.

Glasson, S., Zini, R. and Tillement, J. P. (1982). *Biochem. Pharmac.* **31**, 831–835.

Goodman-Gilman, A., Goodman, L. S. and Gilman, A. (1980). "The Pharmacological Basis of Therapeutics." 6th edition. Baillière Tindall, London.

Greenblatt, D. J. and Koch-Weser, J. (1974). *Eur. J. Clin. Pharmac.* 7, 259–262.

Heaney-Kieras, J. and King, J. (1977). *J. Biol. Chem.* 252, 4326–4329.

Hinderling, P. H. and Garrett, E. R. (1976). *J. Pharmacokin. Biopharm*, 4, 199–230.

Houin, G. (1981). Les caractéristiques pharmacocinétiques du clofibrate chez l'homme après administration unique et répétée: un exemple de dose-dépendance. Thèse de Sciences Pharmaceutiques, Université Paris-Sud, Paris.

Houin, G. and Tillement, J. P. (1981). *Méd. et Hyg.* 39, 913–921.

Jackson, P. R., Tucker, G. T. and Woods, H. F. (1982). *Clin. Pharmac. Ther.* 32, 295–302.

Jadot, G., Valli, M., Bruguerolle, P. and Bouyard, P. (1981). *Nouv. Press. Méd.* 10, 3369–3370.

Jusko, J. and Gretch, M. (1976). *Drug Metab. Rev.* 5, 43–140.

Kinniburgh, D. W. and Boyd, N. D. (1981). *Clin. Pharmac. Ther.* 30, 276–280.

Kober, A., Sjöholm, I., Borgå, O. and Odar-Cederlöf. (1979). *Biochem. Pharmac.* 28, 1037–1042.

Lecomte, M., Zini, R., D'Athis, P. and Tillement, J. P. (1979). *Eur. J. Drug Metab. Pharmacokin.* 4, 23–28.

Lemaire, M. and Tillement, J. P. (1982a). *Biochem. Pharmac.* 31, 359–362.

Lemaire, M. and Tillement, J. P. (1982b). *J. Pharm. Pharmac.* 34, 715–718.

Lewis, G. P., Jusko, W. J., Burke, C. W. and Graves, L. (1971). *Lancet* ii, 778–781.

Lindup, W. E. (1975). *Biochem. Soc. Trans.* 3, 635–640.

Lukas, D. S. and DeMartino, A. G. (1969). *J. Clin. Invest.* 48, 1041–1053.

Motulsky, H. J. and Insel, P. A. (1982). *N. Engl. J. Med.* 307, 18–29.

Müller, W. E. and Wollert, U. (1979). *Pharmacology* 19, 59–67.

Naranjo, C. A., Khouw, V. and Sellers, E. M. (1982). *Clin. Pharmac. Ther.* 31, 746–752.

Perucca, E. and Crema, A. (1982). *Clin. Pharmacokin.* 7, 336–352.

Piafsky, K. M. (1980). *Clin. Pharmacokin.* 5, 246–262.

Piafsky, K. M. and Knoppert, D. (1978). *Clin. Res.* 26, 836A.

Piafsky, K. M., Borgå, O., Odar-Cederlöf, I., Johansson, C. and Sjöqvist, F. (1978). *N. Engl. J. Med.* 299, 1435–1439.

Pierides, A. M., Alvarez-Ude, F., Kerr, D. N. S. and Skillen, A. W. (1975). *Lancet* ii, 1279–1282.

Pike, E., Skuterud, B., Kierulf, P. and Lunde, P. K. M. (1982). *Clin. Pharmac. Ther.* 32, 599–606.

Prandota, J., Tillement, J. P., D'Athis, P., Campos, H. and Barré, J. (1980). *J. Int. Med. Res.*, 8, Supplement (2) 1–8.

Roodsdorp, N., Wänn, B. and Sjöholm, I. (1977). *J. Biol. Chem.* 252, 3876–3880.

Routledge, P. A., Shand, D. G., Barchowsky, A., Wagner, G. and Stargel, W. W. (1981a). *Clin. Pharmac. Ther.* 30, 154–157.

Routledge, P. A., Stargel, W. W., Kitchell, B. B., Barchowsky, A. and Shand, D. G. (1981b). *Br. J. Clin. Pharmac.* 11, 245–250.

Rowland, M. (1980). *Ther. Drug Monitoring*, 2, 29–37.

Rowland, M. and Tozer, T. N. (1980). "Clinical Pharmacokinetics—Concepts and Application." Lea and Febiger, Philadelphia.

Sager, G. and Jacobsen, S. (1979). *Biochem. Pharmac.* 28, 2167–2173.

Sager, G., Hansteen, V., Aakesson, I. and Jacobsen, S. (1981). *Br. J. Clin. Pharmac.* 12, 613–620.

Scatchard, G. (1949). *Ann. N.Y. Acad. Sci.* **51**, 660–672.

Schanker, L. S. (1961) *Ann. Rev. Pharmac.* **1**, 29–44.

Schley, J., Siegert, M. and Müller-Oerlinghausen, B. (1980). *Eur. J. Clin. Pharmac.* **18**, 501–504.

Schmid, K. (1975). α_1-acid glycoprotein. *In* "The Plasma Proteins" (F. W. Putnam, ed.), pp. 183–228. Academic Press, New York.

Schwendener, R. A. and Weder, H. G. (1978). *Biochem. Pharmac.* **27**, 2721–2727.

Scott, B. J., Bradwell, A. R., Schneider, R. E. and Bishop, H. (1979). *Lancet* **i**, 930.

Sellers, E. M. (1978). The clinical importance of interaction based on displacement of protein bound drugs. *In* "Advances in Pharmacology and Therapeutics. Biochemical Pharmacology" (J. P. Tillement, ed.), vol. 7, pp. 153–162. Pergamon Press, Oxford and New York.

Shu, H. P. and Nichols, A. V. (1981). *Biochim. Biophys, Acta,* **665**, 376–384.

Sjödin, T. (1977). *Biochem. Pharmac.* **26**, 2157–2161.

Sjöholm, I., Kober, A., Odar-Cederlöf, I. and Borgå, O. (1976). *Biochem. Pharmac.* **25**, 1205–1213.

Sjöholm, I., Ekman, B., Kober, A., Lungstedt-Påhlman, I., Seiving, B. and Sjödin, T. (1979). *Molec. Pharmac.* **16**, 767–777.

Sjöqvist, F., Borgå, O. and L'E Orme, M. (1980). Fundamentals of clinical pharmacology. *In* "Drug Treatment" (G. S. Avery, ed.). Churchill Livingstone, Edinburgh and London.

Soltys, B. J. and Hsia, J. C. (1977). *J. Biol. Chem.* **252**, 4043–4048.

Sudlow, G., Birkett, D. J. and Wade, D. N. (1976). *Molec. Pharmac.* **12**, 1052–1061.

Tanford, C. (1980). "The Hydrophobic Effect: Formation of Micelles and Biological Membranes." John Wiley, Chichester, Brisbane, Toronto, New York.

Tillement, J. P. (1968). "Contribution à l'étude des effets métaboliques, pharmacologiques et toxicologiques de la thiamine". R. Foulon et Cie, Paris.

Tillement, J. P. (1978). The relationship between plasma protein binding, distribution and pharmacokinetics of drugs. *In* "Advances in Pharmacology and Therapeutics", vol. 7, pp. 103–111. Pergamon Press, Oxford and New York.

Tillement, J. P., Zini, R., D'Athis, P. and Boissier, J. R. (1974). *J. Pharmac. Clin.* **1**, 227–233.

Tillement, J. P., Lhoste, F. and Giudicelli, J. F. (1978). *Clin. Pharmacokin.* **3**, 144–154.

Tillement, J. P., Albengres, E. and Urien, S. (1979). *Eur. J. Drug. Metab. Pharmacokin.* **3**, 123–127.

Tillement, J. P., Zini, R., Lecomte, M. and D'Athis, P. (1980a). *Eur. J. Drug. Metab. Pharmacokin.* **5**, 129–134.

Tillement, J. P., Albengres, E. and Urien, S. (1980b). *Pharmacy International* **1**, 64–65.

Urien, S., Albengres, E., Zini, R., D'Athis, P. and Tillement, J. P. (1980). Serum binding and interactions of chlorophenoxyisobutyric acid, itanoxone and fenofibric acid according to their different HSA binding sites. *In* "Drugs Affecting Lipid Metabolism", pp. 201–209. Elsevier North Holland Biomedical Press, Amsterdam.

Urien, S., Albengres, E. and Tillement, J. P. (1981). *Int. J. Clin. Pharmac. Ther. Toxicol.* **19**, 319–325.

Urien, S., Albengres, E. and Tillement, J. P. (1982a). *Biochem. Pharmac.* **31**, 3687–3689.

Urien, S., Albengres, E. and Tillement, J. P. (1982b). Determination of the probucol-plasma lipoproteins interaction parameters. 6th International Symposium on atherosclerosis, International Atherosclerosis Society, Abstract no 252P, June 13th–17th, Berlin (West).

Vallner, J. J. and Chen, L. (1977). *J. Pharm. Sci.* **66**, 420–421.

Wallace, S. (1976). *Br. J. Clin. Pharmac.* **3**, 510–512.

Wallace, S. (1977). *Br. J. Clin. Pharmac.* **4**, 82–84.

Wanwimolruk, S., Birkett, D. J. and Brooks, P. M. (1982). *Biochem. Pharmac.* **31**, 3737–3743.

Westphal, U. (1971). Steroid-protein Interactions. Springer Verlag, Berlin, Heidelberg, New York.

Wilding, G., Feldhoff, R. C. and Vesell, E. S. (1977). *Biochem. Pharmac.* **26**, 1143–1146.

Wilkinson, G. R. and Shand, D. G. (1975). *Clin. Pharmac. Ther.* **18**, 377–390.

Wood, M. and Wood, A. J. J. (1981). *Clin. Pharmac. Ther.* **29**, 522–526.

Yacobi, A., Udall, J. A. and Levy, G. (1976). *Clin. Pharmac. Ther.* **19**, 552–558.

Zini, R., D'Athis, P., Barré, J. and Tillement, J. P. (1979). *Biochem. Pharmac.* **28**, 2661–2665.

Xenobiotic Metabolism by Brain Monooxygenases and Other Cerebral Enzymes

MARCEL MESNIL, BERNARD TESTA

School of Pharmacy, University of Lausanne, Switzerland

PETER JENNER

University Department of Neurology, Institute of Psychiatry and King's College Hospital Medical School, Denmark Hill, London, UK

ADVANCES IN DRUG RESEARCH VOL. 13
0-12-013313-X

1 Introduction

In the current stage of development of the biological and therapeutic sciences, it is no longer appropriate to administer a drug without a sufficient understanding of its disposition and effects in the organism. Recent interest has centered on the ability of extrahepatic organs to metabolize drugs and the consequences of this action. Evidence has accumulated that the most intricate and delicate of the major organs, namely the brain, might also possess this capability. The results of cerebral metabolism of xenobiotics may be far reaching in both causing disruption of neuronal function and in contributing to drug action.

Compounds acting on the central nervous system can produce effects which may not be fully reversible, e.g. dependence to opiates or benzodiazepines, tardive dyskinesia following prolonged treatment with neuroleptics, depression and psychosis due to amphetamine withdrawal, drug-induced Parkinsonism (Grimes, 1982), or the direct neurotoxicity of some antibiotics and environmental carcinogens also require a full understanding of their effects on the brain, with particular emphasis on accumulation, enzyme induction and inhibition, or even synergism with other toxic agents.

Damage to the brain is all the more serious as this organ has limited regenerative ability, and as its aging appears to a large extent to dictate the life span of the organism.

In addition to its potential toxicological consequences, cerebral metabolism of xenobiotics may also contribute to the pharmacological and therapeutic effects of centrally acting drugs. The generation of active metabolites within the brain, or the inactivation of active drugs, can clearly be expected to influence drug action quantitatively, kinetically and even qualitatively. For example, Horn et al. (1982) have elegantly demonstrated the cerebral activation of prodrugs of the dopamine agonist 2-amino-6,7-dihydroxytetrahydronaphthalene (ADTN) (section 4.4.2). The complexity of the brain is such that our current knowledge of its functioning is inevitably simplistic with an unavoidable inconsistency of the available data. The brain functions to synchronize all vital functions of the body culminating in the existence of life and the human mind. There is a need to integrate knowledge on cerebral mechanisms in order to demonstrate their infinitely complex interdependence but such a task is beyond our present comprehension. Even at the biochemical level with which we are presently concerned, the fragmental observations made *in vitro* are only partially relevant to the *in vivo* situation where a higher order of organization predominates. The reductionistic approach to brain biology is currently the only one available, and imposes itself in the present review. Hence many of the findings discussed here, although perfectly correct in their experimental context, may well have to be interpreted differently when placed in a broader and more complex context.

Only recently has the brain appeared as an organ able to metabolize xenobiotics. Major analytical advances increasing the limits of sensitivity and specificity partly explain this new awareness. However, the intense interest in all aspects of xenobiotic metabolism has focused attention on many extrahepatic tissues. The ability of cerebral tissue to metabolize drugs, although generally weaker than that of the liver, the lungs and some other organs, appears quite diversified and versatile and is of clear pharmacological and toxicological interest. At this time it thus appears appropriate to review the currently available data on cerebral biotransformation pathways with particular emphasis on monooxygenase-mediated reactions.

A rigid and arbitrary delineation between exogenous and endogenous substrates (Testa *et al.*, 1981) is misleading in all tissues and impossible in brain. Thus, many endogenous compounds are administered as such (hormones, peptides) or as bioprecursors (e.g. L-DOPA) and hence also have an exogenous origin. Some xenobiotics so much resemble endogenous compounds (e.g. synthetic peptides) that the discrimination is not desirable, while other compounds (e.g. ethanol) cannot be categorized. The aims of the present review are sufficiently broad to avoid falling into this dichotomic trap.

2 Cerebral enzymatic systems (potentially) able to metabolize xenobiotics

Few, if any, enzyme systems have a rigorous substrate specificity. Should an exogenous compound offer—from the point of view of the enzyme—sufficient similarities with the natural substrate, then a reaction will occur. Besides cerebral metabolic pathways known to transform xenobiotics, this section will also consider those other enzyme systems likely to utilize xenobiotics as substrates.

2.1 OXYGENASES

2.1.1 Flavin-dependent enzymes

2.1.1.1 Monoamine oxidase (MAO, EC 1.4.3.4)

Monoamine oxidases have been extensively investigated in brain due to their involvement in the catabolism of catecholamines. MAOs are localized in the external membrane of mitochondria and convert neuroactive monoamines into inactive aldehydes according to Fig. 1 (Walsh, 1977, p. 402). Of particular interest is the formation of H_2O_2 as a reaction product; the implications of this reactive metabolite will be considered in subsequent sections.

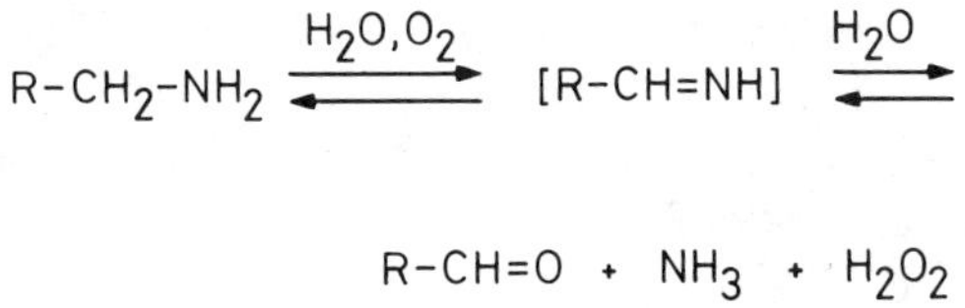

$$R-CH_2-NH_2 \underset{}{\overset{H_2O,O_2}{\rightleftharpoons}} [R-CH=NH] \underset{}{\overset{H_2O}{\rightleftharpoons}}$$

$$R-CH=O + NH_3 + H_2O_2$$

FIG. 1. General reaction scheme of monoamine oxidase (Walsh, 1977, p. 402).

Various forms of MAO exist in human brain (Johnston, 1968; Kamyshanskaya and Moskovitina, 1981). MAO A and B are differentiated by substrate affinity (Schoepp and Azzaro, 1981; Cawthon et al., 1981; Leung et al., 1982) and appear to be sexually differentiated in the rat (Vaccari et al., 1981). MAO type A from human brain and liver mitochondria metabolizes serotonin, while type B has a high affinity for β-phenylethylamine (White and Glassman, 1977). The different MAO types may be distinct binding sites on the same large molecular complex which may be embedded in the outer mitochondrial membrane. The idea that human brain MAO may be one molecular entity with multiple binding sites also has been proposed by Schurr et al. (1981).

Liver MAO displays broad substrate selectivity which allows it to metabolize a number of xenobiotics. Substrates are primary amines, or secondary and tertiary N-methylated amines. The amino function must be attached to an unsubstituted methylene group. While some lipophilic aliphatic amines are oxidized, the best substrates are arylalkylamines, especially benzylamine and phenylethylamine derivatives (Tipton, 1980). In contrast, little, if anything, is known of the ability of brain MAO to metabolize xenobiotics. However, in view of the analogies existing between liver and brain MAO types (see in particular the comparisons made by White and Glassman, 1977) it is reasonable to speculate that the substrate selectivities of liver MAO towards xenobiotics are essentially maintained for the brain enzyme. This entire field of research remains to be explored.

In this context, it is interesting to compare MAO activity towards *para*-tyramine and its *meta*- and *ortho*-isomers. As shown in Table 1, the activity decreases in the series *para* ≥ *meta* > *ortho*, with little difference between the various brain regions investigated (Yu and Boulton, 1980).

TABLE 1

Monoamine oxidase activity towards tyramine isomers by rat brain mitochondrial preparations (Yu and Boulton, 1980)

Rat brain regions	Specific MAO activity (nmol mg^{-1} protein min^{-1})		
	para-tyramine	*meta*-tyramine	*ortho*-tyramine
Hypothalamus	2·91 ± 0·21(6)	2·70 ± 0·26(5)	0·64 ± 0·09(5)
Striatum	2·48 ± 0·09(8)	2·08 ± 0·13(8)	0·29 ± 0·03(8)
Cortex	2·21 ± 0·18(6)	1·19 ± 0·21(6)	0·26 ± 0·01(6)
Cerebellum	1·97 ± 0·16(6)	1·69 ± 0·13(6)	0·31 ± 0·03(6)
Brain stem	2·15 ± 0·60(6)	1·68 ± 0·08(6)	0·28 ± 0·03(6)

The results are expressed as the mean values ± S.E.M., with the numbers of experiments in parentheses.

Monoamine oxidase, as pointed out earlier, produces H_2O_2. This metabolite has the potential of acting on xenobiotics in addition to endogenous molecules; this may help explain the presence of glutathione peroxidase in mitochondria (see section 2.1.6) (Maker *et al.*, 1981).

2.1.1.2 Flavin-dependent monooxygenases (EC 1.14.13.8)
Flavin-dependent monooxygenases have been well characterized in the liver and some other tissues (Ziegler, 1980) but nothing appears known of their presence in brain. However, a cerebral location may be indicated by the metabolism of *N,N*-dimethyltryptamine (I) in whole rat brain homogenates (Barker *et al.*, 1980). This hallucinogen is metabolized by MAO to indole-acetic acid (II), and by uncharacterized enzyme(s) to *N*-methyltryptamine (III) and to dimethyltryptamine *N*-oxide (IV). As expected, the MAO inhibitor iproniazid inhibits II formation by 83%, but unexpectedly the formation of III and IV is inhibited by 90%. This inhibition may be indicative of the involvement of flavin-adenine dinucleotide containing monooxygenases.

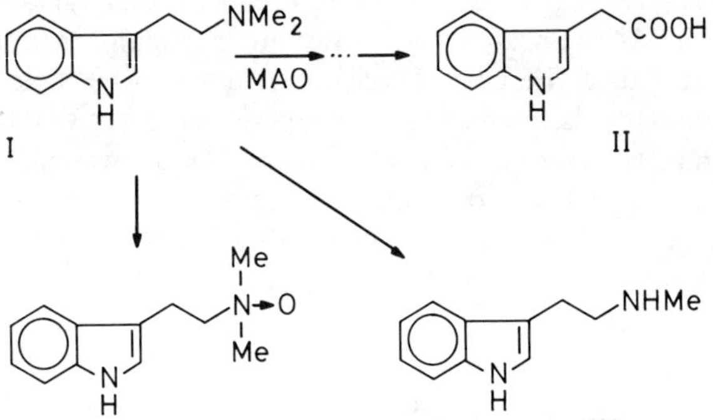

2.1.2 Pterin-dependent monooxygenases

2.1.2.1 Phenylalanine hydroxylase (EC 1.14.16.1)

This well characterized enzyme system (Goodwin, 1979; Walsh, 1980) catalyses the para-hydroxylation of phenylalanine in a NADPH-dependent manner with characteristic hydrogen migration (NIH shift) consistent with an arene oxide intermediate. It is generally accepted that brain does not contain phenylalanine hydroxylase (Goodwin, 1979), but recently a 2000-g rat brain supernatant preparation fortified with the 6,7-dimethyl-5,6,7,8-tetrahydropteridine cofactor was shown to yield comparable amounts of ortho-, meta- and para-tyrosine from phenylalanine (Ishimitsu et al., 1980).

A deficiency of phenylalanine hydroxylase is responsible for phenylketonuria, but increased proportions of the ortho and meta isomers of tyrosine might account for CNS dysfunction. The regulation of the biopterin cofactor and of the pterin-requiring monooxygenases may be intimately linked to the biosynthesis of monoamines (Nagatsu, 1981). The relationship to brain disease states is clear as seen, for example, in the greatly decreased biopterin levels found in the brain of Parkinsonian patients.

2.1.2.2 Tyrosine hydroxylase (tyrosine 3-monooxygenase, EC 1.14.16.2)

Another critical enzyme in the regulation of catecholamines is tyrosine hydroxylase, which is located in the adrenal medulla and in catecholaminergic neurones, and which catalyses the formation of 3,4-dihydroxyphenylalanine (DOPA) from tyrosine (McGeer, 1967; Weiner, 1979). Tyrosine hydroxylase shows circadian rhythm (Cahill and Ehret, 1981), and is inhibited by catechols (feedback mechanisms) and by biopterin (Mann and Gordon, 1979). Interestingly, para-chlorophenylalanine alters the activity of this enzyme (Crespi et al., 1980); the mechanism of this interaction remains unexplained but may be a direct one.

2.1.2.3 Tryptophan 5-monooxygenase (EC 1.14.16.4)

This essentially cerebral enzyme catalyses the 5-hydroxylation of tryptophan by a reaction mechanism comparable to that of the two above enzymes (Hamon *et al.*, 1979). Similarly, no exogenous substrate appears to be known. Catecholamines and *para*-chlorophenylalanine are effective inhibitors.

2.1.3 Copper-dependent monooxygenases

2.1.3.1 Dopamine β-hydroxylase (EC 1.14.17.1)

Dopamine β-hydroxylase mediates the synthesis of norepinephrine by hydroxylation of the benzylic position of dopamine. The reaction cycle is understood as shown in Fig. 2 (Walsh, 1977; pp. 458–460; Diliberto and Allen, 1980). However, the form in which oxygen is activated is not yet known. The enzyme is located in a variety of mammalian tissues, including brain where its distribution was established some years ago (Reis and Molinoff, 1972).

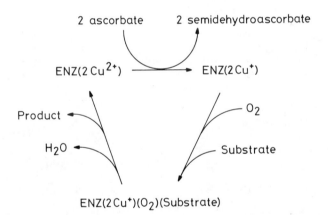

FIG. 2. General reaction scheme of dopamine β-hydroxylase (Walsh, 1977, pp. 459–460; Diliberto and Allen, 1980).

Dopamine β-hydroxylase appears as an enzyme with comparatively low substrate selectivity, as opposed to high product stereoselectivity. Table 2 illustrates the relatively broad structural range of phenylethylamine substrates, many of which are xenobiotics, e.g. 4-hydroxyamphetamine (no. 8) and mescaline (no. 20) (van der Schoot and Creveling, 1965).

Rat brain shows a marked ability to metabolize amphetamine (V) both *in vivo* and *in vitro*. After intracisternal administration of amphetamine,

TABLE 2

Relative activity of phenylethylamine substrates of dopamine β-hydroxylase
(van der Schoot and Creveling, 1965)

Substrate	Relative activity
1. Phenylethylamine (PEA)	63
2. 4-Hydroxy-PEA	100
3. 3-Hydroxy-PEA	77 ± 3
4. 2-Hydroxy-PEA	0
5. 4-Methoxy-PEA	3 ± 1
6. 4-Hydroxy-N-methyl-PEA	25
7. 4-Hydroxy-N,N-dimethyl-PEA	0
8. 4-Hydroxy-α-methyl-PEA	65
9. 4-Hydroxy-α-ethyl-PEA	37
10. 4-Hydroxy-β-methyl-PEA	8 ± 3
11. 3-Hydroxy-α-methyl-PEA	50
12. 3,4-Dihydroxy-PEA	93
13. 4-Hydroxy-3-methoxy-PEA	70
14. 3-Hydroxy-4-methoxy-PEA	2 ± 3
15. 3,4-Dimethoxy-PEA	2 ± 3
16. 3,4-Dihydroxy-N-methyl-PEA	25
17. 3,4-Dihydroxy-α-methyl-PEA	58 ± 2
18. 4-Hydroxy-3-methoxy-α-methyl-PEA	8 ± 3
19. 4-Hydroxy-3,5-dimethoxy-PEA	28 ± 2
20. 3,4,5-Trimethoxy-PEA	3 ± 2
21. 2,4,5-Trimethoxy-PEA	0

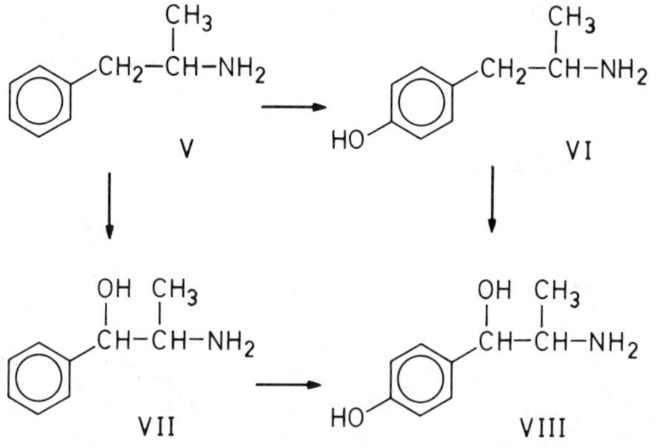

para-hydroxyamphetamine (V), norephedrine (VII) and *para*-hydroxynor-ephedrine (VIII) were isolated from brain tissue. These metabolites could not be detected in brain after intraperitoneal administration, indicating their formation within brain tissue after intracisternal administration. This was confirmed by the generation of the three metabolites in brain slices incubated for 30 min with amphetamine. Relevant to the present context is the fact that U-14614, an inhibitor of dopamine β-hydroxylase, or 6-hydroxyamphetamine, which destroys catecholamine nerve terminals, caused a marked reduction in VII and VIII formation, indicating the involvement of dopamine β-hydroxylase (Kuhn *et al.*, 1978) (see also section 4.4.1).

The strict product stereoselectivity of dopamine β-hydroxylase is seen in the exclusive (R)-hydroxylation of 2-phenylethylamines (Taylor, 1974; Battersby *et al.*, 1976). This stereoselectivity is consistent with the recently demonstrated (May *et al.*, 1981) hydroxylation of the unnatural (S)-octo-pamine (IX) enantiomer. Attack by dopamine β-hydroxylase at the pro-R position in phenylethylamines yields a gem-diol (X) which readily dehydrates to *para*-hydroxy-α-aminoacetophenone (XI). This interesting pathway may help explain the weak adrenergic activity of (S)-octopamine and (S)-nor-epinephrine.

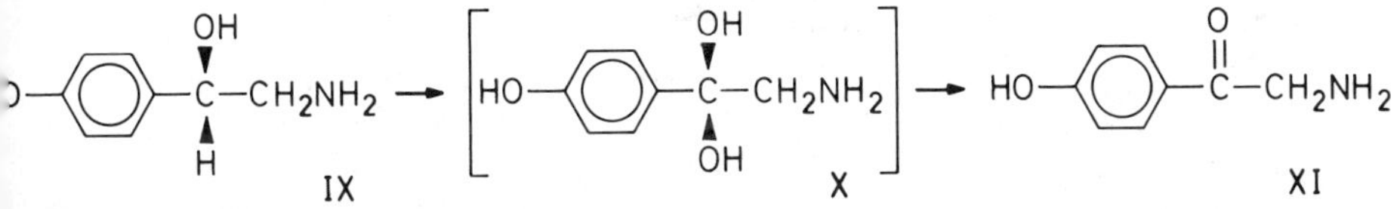

The range of potential substrates of dopamine β-hydroxylase underwent a dramatic increase when May and Phillips (1980) demonstrated the capacity of the enzyme to catalyse sulfoxidation. In the presence of dopamine β-hydroxylase isolated and purified from bovine adrenals, phenyl 2-aminoethyl sulfide (XII) yields the laevorotatory sulfoxide XIII with high stereoselec-tivity. Although the enzyme used was not of cerebral origin, this example is intriguing with regard to xenobiotic metabolism in brain.

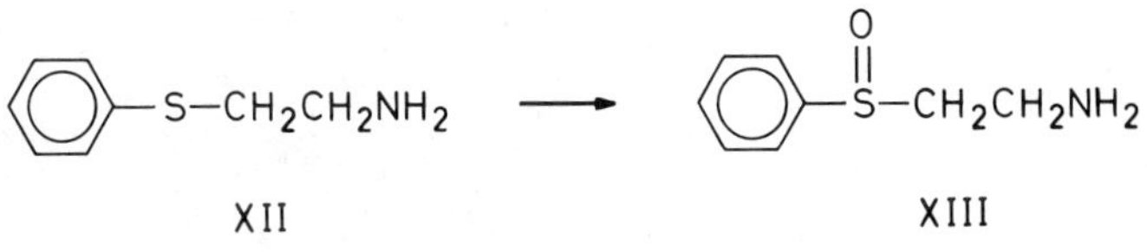

2.1.3.2 Tyrosinase (monophenol monooxygenase, EC 1.14.18.1)

A number of copper-containing oxygenases are collectively known as phenolases or tyrosinases. They catalyse the conversion of phenols and catechols to *ortho*-quinones (monophenolase and diphenolase activity). It appears that the monophenolase activity may be a hydroxylation of a monophenol (XIV) to a catechol (XVI) coupled to the oxidation of a catechol (XV) to an *ortho*-quinone (XVII) (Gunsalus *et al.*, 1975). Recently, the post-enzymatic reactivity of *ortho*-dopaquinone formed by tyrosinase has been investigated (Canovas *et al.*, 1982). While the final products are always dopachrome and then melanins, it appears that the nature of intermediate products is pH-dependent (see also sections 2.1.9.1., 2.1.9.2. and 2.1.10).

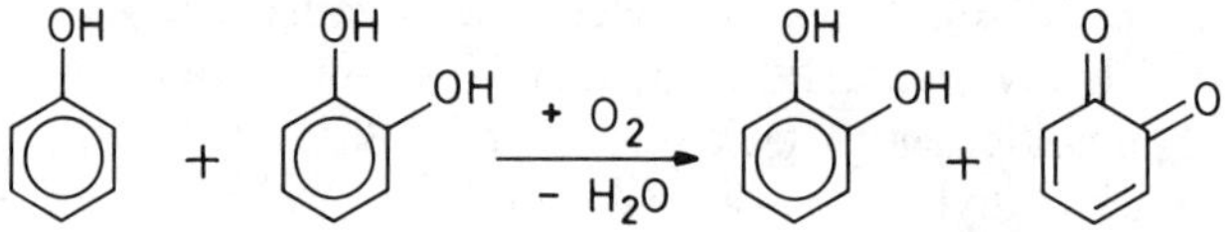

XIV   XV   XVI   XVII

The potential of tyrosinase to metabolize xenobiotics appears unexplored. It is our belief that the entire field of quinone metabolites deserves a much greater interest than it is currently receiving. Several years ago, the metabolism of morphine to form a 2,3-catechol type of metabolite was detected in the rat (Misra *et al.*, 1971, 1973). This product appears to be in equilibrium with its zwitterionic tautomer 2-hydroxymorphine-3-one and with its product of oxidation, morphine 2,3-quinone (XVIII). Incubation of morphine with either rat brain or live homogenates yielded 6–7% of XVIII. This metabolite may be of pharmacological importance, since it has central stimulant properties which can override the depressant effects of morphine when the two compounds are administered intracisternally in equivalent amounts (Misra *et al.*, 1974). The production of the catechol metabolite could also account for the persistence of radioactivity in brain tissues following administration of labelled morphine since it exhibits more marked covalent binding to proteins than morphine (Misra *et al.*, 1974) (see also section 4.5.1).

XVIII

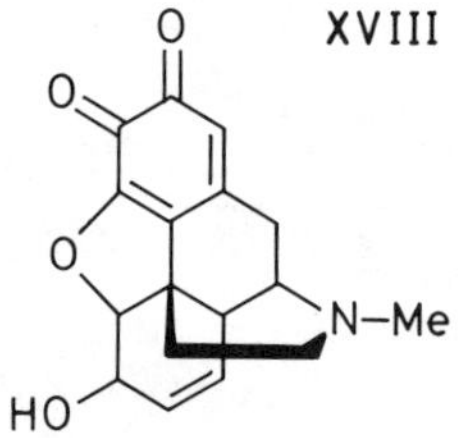

Although the formation of morphine 2,3-quinone might be due to enzymes other than phenolases, or might even be non-enzymatic, this example illustrates the potential pharmacological and toxicological significance of quinones and the metabolic routes leading to their formation.

2.1.4 Haemoprotein monooxygenases

Cytochrome P-450 (EC 1.14.14.1)

The last three decades have seen a progressive understanding of cytochrome P-450. A critical observation was the characterization of a complex with carbon monoxide with a maximum absorbance at 450 nm (Klingenberg, 1958). Omura and Sato (1962) revealed the haemoprotein nature of the pigment and named it cytochrome P-450. The interest shown in cytochrome P-450 is due in part to the wide variety of xenobiotics with which it interacts, to the numerous classes of endogenous molecules which are substrates for the enzyme, to the variety of chemical reactions carried out, and to its ubiquity and multiplicity (Testa *et al.*, 1981; Jenner *et al.*, 1981; Alvares, 1981; Nebert and Negishi, 1982). Excellent reviews on cytochrome P-450 have been published, in particular those of Coon and Persson (1980) and of Mannering (1981).

The mechanism of cytochrome P-450 catalysed reactions is now well understood (Schenkman and Gibson, 1981; Alexander and Goff, 1982). A scheme summarizing the main chemical steps of the monooxygenation catalytic cycle is shown in Fig. 3. Two electrons enter the catalytic cycle. The first is transferred to the substrate-ferricytochrome P-450 complex by NADPH-cytochrome c (P-450) reductase (EC 1.6.2.4). This transfer is modulated by the spin state of the iron atom; in the microsomal membrane the monooxygenase is present mainly in the low spin form (midpoint potential -350 mV) for which electron transfer from NADPH (redox potential -365 mV) is not favoured. Substrate binding increases the proportion of the high spin form (-175 mV) and thus considerably favours reduction. Substrates, temperature, and the micro-environment of cytochrome P-450, in particular phospholipids, control the spin-state and hence the reaction rate (Sligar *et al.*, 1979; Gander and Mannering, 1980; Schenkman and Gibson, 1981; Mannering, 1981).

The second electron reduces the substrate-oxyferrocytochrome P-450 complex, and according to substrates and/or isozymes originates either from NADPH-cytochrome P-450 reductase or from NADH-cytochrome b_5 reductase (EC 1.6.2.2) via cytochrome b_5. A wealth of information on these electron transport systems is available in recent reviews and research papers (e.g. Masters and Okita, 1980; Bonfils *et al.*, 1981; Mannering, 1981; Strittmatter and Dailey, 1982; Black and Coon, 1982).

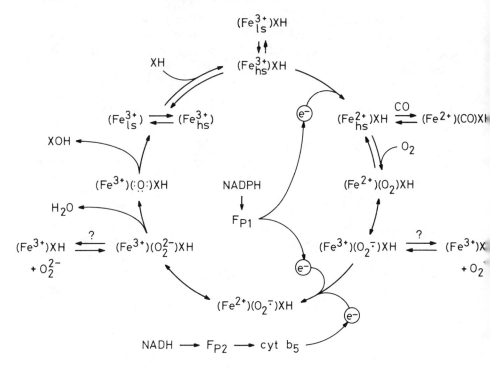

FIG. 3. Catalytic cycle of cytochrome P-450 associated with monooxygenation reactions. (Fe^{3+}) = ferricytochrome P-450; hs = high spin, ls = low spin; (Fe^{2+}) = ferrocytochrome P-450; F_{P1} = NADPH-cytochrome P-450 reductase; F_{P2} = NADH-cytochrome b_5 reductase; cyt b_5 = cytochrome b_5; XH = substrate. (Modified from Gander and Mannering, 1980; Schenkman and Gibson, 1981.)

Three forms of activated oxygen are to be seen in Fig. 3, namely the superoxide anion-radical, the peroxy anion, and the monoatomic oxene species which is postulated to be the actual activated form involved in the reaction of monooxygenation (Trager, 1980; Mannering, 1981). The activated forms of oxygen, and their post-enzymatic chemistry, have been authoritatively reviewed by O'Brien (1978) and Trager (1982). This problem will be considered again in sections 2.1.9 and 2.1.10.

For many years, no attention was paid to cytochrome P-450 in extrahepatic tissues. The sixties saw a growing awareness of the existence and role of extrahepatic monooxygenases, and the seventies witnessed an exponential growth of data (Testa and Jenner, 1976, pp. 419–453; Vainio and Hietanen, 1980). In the brain, it has been difficult to detect cytochrome P-450 with the analytic instruments available before 1970. Ichikawa and Yamano (1967) failed to detect this enzyme in the cerebellum, but recorded low levels (0.07

nmol mg^{-1} protein) in the bovine pituitary gland. Norman and Neal (1976) demonstrated that the oxidative desulfuration of parathion to paraoxon in rat brain microsomes is mediated by cytochrome P-450 but were not able to spectrally detect this enzyme in any rat brain region.

It was in 1977 that Cohn and colleagues (Cohn *et al.*, 1977), and Sasame and colleagues (Sasame *et al.*, 1977) provided spectroscopic evidence for the existence of cytochrome P-450 in brain. Sections 3 and 4 are dedicated to cerebral cytochrome P-450, the enzymes of the electron transport chains (Fig. 3), and cytochrome P-450 linked enzymatic activities.

2.1.5 Peroxidasic haemoproteins

Catalase (EC 1.11.1.6)

Catalase mediates the dismutation of hydrogen peroxide into molecular oxygen and water (Walsh, 1977; pp. 488–494). Thus it has a clear protective role in preventing H_2O_2 generated by MAO or a number of other enzymatic and post-enzymatic routes (see section 2.1.10) from inducing damage to tissue constituents by oxidizing thiol groups or initiating lipid peroxidation. Compared to other mammalian tissues, the brain contains only small amounts of catalase (e.g. Table 3) (Sinet *et al.*, 1980 and references therein). Activity is associated with subcellular particles termed microperoxisomes (Gaunt and de Duve, 1976). The reaction mechanism of catalase occurs according to equations (1) and (2):

$$\text{catalase} + H_2O_2 \rightleftarrows \text{compound I} \qquad (1)$$

$$\text{compound I} + H_2O_2 \rightarrow \text{catalase} + O_2 + 2H_2O \qquad (2)$$

Compound I is a catalase-H_2O_2 complex where the enzyme has the formal Fe(IV) oxidation state (Walsh, 1977, p. 493). The reaction of compound I with H_2O_2 (equation 2) represents the physiological catalytic activity of this enzyme.

Compound I is also of interest since it can oxidize some alcohols by a peroxidatic reaction (equation 3):

$$\text{Compound I} + R\text{-}CH_2OH \rightarrow \text{catalase} + R\text{-}CHO + 2H_2O \qquad (3)$$

The oxidation of ethanol to acetaldehyde is well documented (see Sinet *et al.*, 1980 and references therein). Recently, Tampier (1978) investigated the oxidation of methanol to formaldehyde in rat brain preparations. Activity appears essentially located in the cortex (0.41 $\pm$ 0.05 μmol g^{-1}h^{-1}) and the corpus striatum (0.20 $\pm$ 0.04 μmol g^{-1}h^{-1}). Subcellular fractionation showed activity to be essentially localized in the mitochondrial suspension and cytosol. The oxidative activity was essentially catalase-mediated, but the

TABLE 3

Specific activities of catalase, glutathione peroxidase and Cu,Zn-superoxide dismutase in rat liver and brain (Mavelli et al., 1982)

	$10^4 \times$ Catalase specific activity (units mg^{-1} protein)	$10^4 \times$ Glutathione peroxidase activity (units mg^{-1} protein)	Cu,Zn-superoxide dismutase (μg mg^{-1} protein)
Rat hepatocytes (total homogenates)			
Newborn	$1\cdot30 \pm 0\cdot10$	$0\cdot29 \pm 0\cdot05$	$0\cdot40 \pm 0\cdot07$
Adult	$3\cdot00 \pm 0\cdot60$	$2\cdot81 \pm 0\cdot63$	$1\cdot74 \pm 0\cdot42$
Rat brain (total homogenates)			
Newborn	$0\cdot07 \pm 0\cdot01$	$0\cdot08 \pm 0\cdot01$	$0\cdot27 \pm 0\cdot09$
Adult	$0\cdot40 \pm 0\cdot005$	$0\cdot10 \pm 0\cdot01$	$0\cdot50 \pm 0\cdot05$

level of enzyme activity was about 15 times lower than that found in the liver. Interestingly, ethanol and to a lesser extent butanol inhibited the reaction, suggesting a competitive interaction.

2.1.6 Glutathione peroxidase (EC 1.11.1.9)

As with catalase, the cerebral levels of this selenium-containing enzyme are low compared with other tissues (e.g. Table 3) (Prohaska and Ganther, 1976; Savolainen, 1978). However, its distribution appears coincidental with the need to remove H_2O_2 that can arise from the deamination of dopamine by MAO, mainly in the substantia nigra and caudate nucleus (Brannan et al., 1980). The enzyme reduces hydrogen peroxide according to equation (4):

$$H_2O_2 + 2GSH \rightarrow 2H_2O + GSSG \qquad (4)$$

where GSH is glutathione. The discovery of the reduction by GSH-peroxidase of organic hydroperoxides formed from unsaturated fatty acids (Christophersen, 1968; Little and O'Brien, 1968; Wendel, 1980) enhanced interest in the enzyme in relation to xenobiotic metabolism. The general catalytic reaction is thus:

$$R\text{-}OOH + 2GSH \rightarrow ROH + H_2O + GSSG \qquad (5)$$

The existence of a non-selenium-dependent GSH-peroxidase, the marked differences in organ distribution among species, the rather limited number of known substrates, combine to make it difficult to predict a possible role of these enzymes in cerebral xenobiotic metabolism.

2.1.7 Metalloflavoproteins

2.1.7.1 Xanthine oxidase (EC 1.2.3.2) and aldehyde oxidase (EC 1.2.3.1)

These two very similar enzymes contain molybdenum, FAD and iron as prosthetic groups. They catalyse a unique reaction of hydroxylation in which the oxygen atom is derived from water. The electrons derived from the substrate are transferred to any of a number of possible acceptors (Rajagopalan, 1980). The general reaction is

$$R - \underset{\underset{H}{|}}{C} = X + H_2O \rightarrow R + \underset{\underset{OH}{|}}{C} = X + 2e^- + 2H^+ \qquad (6)$$

where X is NR' or O. Mammalian enzymes always use O_2 as the electron acceptor; hence a product of the reaction (6) is H_2O_2.

In vitro xanthine oxidase and aldehyde oxidase oxidize aldehydes with a low affinity and it is not known whether such reactions occur in vivo (Weiner, 1980). Their actions in vivo are probably concerned with the oxidation of purines, pteridines and pyrimidines, i.e. nitrogen-containing heterocycles. Several xenobiotic azaheterocycles are also oxidized, although most data available have been obtained with hepatic enzymes (Stubley et al., 1979; Stubley and Stell, 1980; Rajagopalan, 1980).

Another reaction mediated by xanthine oxidase is the reduction of aromatic nitro groups, a reaction in which the nitro derivative accepts electrons from the reduced form of the enzyme. This reaction has considerable toxicological consequences in view of the strong mutagenicity of some polycyclic aromatic nitro derivatives. For example, the covalent binding of 1-nitropyrene is catalysed by xanthine oxidase (Howard and Beland, 1982). Up to now, there is contradictory evidence as to the presence of xanthine oxidase in brain (Guroff, 1980, p. 227), although this would seem indicated by the degradation of purines (Villela, 1968).

2.1.7.2 Superoxide dismutase (EC 1.15.1.1)

Superoxide dismutase plays a vital protective role by destroying the superoxide anion-radical according to equation (7):

$$2O_2^- + 2H^+ \rightarrow H_2O_2 + O_2 \qquad (7)$$

To the best of our knowledge, no substrate other than superoxide has been described. Nevertheless, the enzyme has some relevance to xenobiotic metabolism in relation with superoxide generation. Indeed, this activated oxygen species is generated during autoxidation of numerous compounds including hydroquinones, catecholamines, thiols, and haemoproteins. Superoxide is also produced during the action of oxidative enzymes such as xanthine oxidase and aldehyde oxidase (Hassan and Fridovich, 1980, and references therein). It has been further established that superoxide is the oxygenating species in some cytochrome P-450 mediated reactions, while the uncoupling phenomenon, which releases superoxide prior to substrate oxidation, is another distinct possibility (see also section 2.1.9.2) (O'Brien, 1978; White and Coon, 1980; Mannering, 1981; Trager, 1982). Superoxide formation is also believed to occur through the reduction of quinones mediated by NADH-reductases such as mitochondrial ubiquinone oxidoreductase and microsomal cytochrome b_5 reductase. In this reaction, one electron is transferred to the quinone, forming a semiquinone radical which reduces O_2 (Powis *et al.*, 1981).

Eucaryote cells contain two major groups of superoxide dismutases, namely those containing both copper and zinc, which are cytosolic enzymes, and those containing manganese, which are essentially mitochondrial enzymes (Hassan and Fridovich, 1980). Many tissues contain these enzymes, among them the brain (e.g. Table 3). As degenerative changes occur with age, variation in superoxide dismutase levels occur. An interesting study by Vanella and colleagues (1982) showed the variations with age of Cu-Zn and Mn containing enzymes in rat cerebral cortex (Fig. 4). While the activity of Cu-Zn containing enzymes markedly decreased, those of the Mn containing enzyme increase. But because the Mn-activity represents only a fraction of total dismutase activity, the compensation is only partial and this may be a major factor involved in cerebral senescence (Vanella *et al.*, 1982).

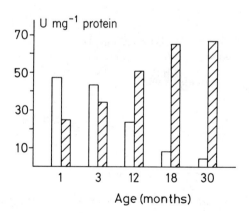

FIG. 4. Variation with age of specific superoxide dismutase activities in the rat cerebral cortex. Empty boxes: Cu,Zn-superoxide dismutase specific activity in the 100 000 g supernatant. Striped boxes: Mn-superoxide dismutase specific activity in purified mitochondria. (Replotted from Vanella *et al.*, 1982. Reproduced with the permission of S. Karger AG, Basel, Switzerland.)

Superoxide dismutase levels also have been compared in various brain regions in the developing rat (Ledig *et al.*, 1982). The Cu-Zn and Mn activity were comparable in the neocortex, striatum and hypothalamus, but activity in the medulla-pons was higher.

2.1.8 Dioxygenases

2.1.8.1 Tryptophan 2,3-dioxygenase (EC 1.13.11.11)

Among dioxygenases, tryptophan 2,3-dioxygenase has been characterized in the liver. This enzyme functions in the catabolism of tryptophan, converting the indole derivative into a substituted anthranilate derivative, N-formyl-kynurenine (Walsh, 1977, p. 513). The presence of this enzyme in the brain has not been established directly, but may be postulated from the discovery in rat brain of kynurenine 3-hydroxylase (EC 1.14.13.9), a downstream enzyme in the catabolism of tryptophan (Battie and Verity, 1981). As stated by Guroff (1980, p. 126), the problem of tryptophan degradation in brain might be profitably re-explored. This may be of consequence to the understanding of cerebral xenobiotic metabolism.

2.1.8.2 Fatty acid cyclooxygenase (EC 1.14.99.1)

Prostaglandin synthetase consists of two enzymatic components: fatty acid cyclooxygenase (prostaglandin endoperoxide synthetase) and a hydroperoxidase. Fatty acid cyclooxygenase converts arachidonic acid to PGG_2 by introducing a cyclic endoperoxide and a hydroperoxide moiety. The hydroperoxidase reduces PGG_2 to PGH_2 (Walsh, 1977, p. 514). For further details, the reader is referred to the excellent short review by Nelson and colleagues (1982).

Prostaglandin synthetase exists in a number of tissues (e.g. platelets, blood vessels, kidneys and lungs). Recently, two distinct forms have been characterized in rabbit brain by monitoring the levels of two direct metabolites of PGH_2, namely PGE_2 generated by isomerization, and $PGF_{2\alpha}$ produced by reduction (Lysz and Needleman, 1982). Table 4 shows as an example the concentrations of these two prostaglandins after 5-min incubation of arachidonic acid with rabbit brain microsomes. After 30-min incubation the levels of PGE_2 were not further increased, whereas those of $PGF_{2\alpha}$ had increased two- to five-fold.

There are indications that cyclooxygenase could be involved in brain damage following hypoxia and ischaemia. Indeed, ischaemia is known to increase the tissue concentration of arachidonic acid, and elevated levels persist for relatively long periods after restoration of blood flow. The restoration of circulation is accompanied by a burst of prostaglandin and prostacyclin synthesis. Following this activation the oxygenase acts as a suicidal enzyme by self-destructing (Siesjö *et al.*, 1980).

TABLE 4

Regional comparison of arachidonate metabolism after 5-min incubations with rabbit brain microsomes (Lysz and Needleman, 1982)

Brain area	pmol PG produced per mg protein	
	PGE_2	$PGF_{2\alpha}$
Medulla	820 ± 46	263 ± 14
Cortex	703 ± 119	118 ± 74
Hippocampal formation	464 ± 56	197 ± 57
Pons	427 ± 88	132 ± 21
Cerebellum	184 ± 18	215 ± 61

In the present context, prostaglandin synthetase is of interest because of its ability to oxidize xenobiotics. More precisely, co-oxidation of xenobiotics is observed during prostaglandin biosynthesis at the hydroperoxidasic step (Lasker et al., 1981; Boyd and Eling, 1981) although the exact mechanism has yet to be established (Marnett, 1981). Known xenobiotic substrates include polycyclic aromatic hydrocarbons, N-methylamines, antiinflammatory agents such as aminopyrine and phenylbutazone, nitrofurans, and aromatic amines (Marnett, 1981; Lasker et al., 1981; Boyd and Eling, 1981; Sivarajah et al., 1982). While none of these co-oxidation reactions has been shown to occur in brain, they could be of considerable potential in terms of cerebral metabolism.

2.1.9 Oxidation reactions with uncertain classification

2.1.9.1 Melanin-forming mitochondrial catecholamine oxidase
Vander Wende and Spoerlein (1963) reported the presence of a mitochondrial enzyme in rat brain which catalyses the oxidation of dopamine, and to a lesser extent norepinephrine, to melanin. Their experimental methodology, however, left open the possibility of a post-enzymatic oxidation mediated by H_2O_2 released by MAO. Barrass and colleagues (1973, 1974) have suggested that catecholamine oxidase activity may control the relative levels of catecholamines. Løvstad (1979) has observed that various centrally active drugs (phenothiazine, butyrophenone and iminodibenzyl derivatives) inhibited catecholamine oxidase in a non-specific manner. Obviously more studies are required to establish the existence and characteristics of this enzyme in connection with tyrosinases (section 2.1.3.2) and to assess its potential in xenobiotic metabolism.

2.1.9.2 Unclassified microsomal oxidations
Microsomes from brain or liver oxidized adrenaline to *adrenochrome* in the

presence of NADPH or organic hydroperoxides (Savov *et al.*, 1980). All reactions were prevented by superoxide dismutase, indicating a role for the superoxide radical. However, there is some evidence to suggest that the organic hydroperoxides may generate singlet oxygen since quenchers of this species exerted a weak inhibitory action. It was suggested that cytochrome P-450 might generate the superoxide radical, but no proof exists that this is so.

Hepatic and cerebral microsomes in the presence of NADPH and O_2 also formed *melanin-like pigments* from indole derivatives such as 5-hydroxy-tryptamine and 5-hydroxyindolacetic acid (Uemura *et al.*, 1980). This microsomal melanogenesis was inhibited by superoxide dismutase, but the involvement of cytochrome P-450 remains a possibility.

2.1.9.3 Lipid peroxidation

Lipid peroxidation is a process of membrane denaturation arising essentially from an imbalance in the mechanisms protecting against activated species of oxygen. It is certainly not a "normal" process in physiological terms, its consequences being disastrous. For this reason and the connection of lipid peroxidation with oxidative metabolism, we include this short section.

Lipid peroxidation occurs in the liver and in other organs, among which the brain must be singled out for its high lipid content. Brain lipoperoxidation has been extensively studied. In rat cortical slices in a normal atmosphere (0.2 atm O_2), the indicator of lipoperoxidation, malonaldehyde, reached total levels of *c.* 140 nmol g^{-1} wet tissue (Kovachich and Mishra, 1980). Increasing O_2 pressure up to 10 atm markedly increased lipoperoxidation, as shown in Fig. 5.

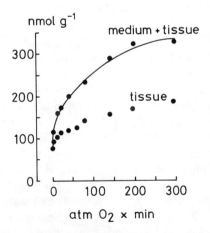

FIG. 5. Liberation of malonaldehyde (nmol g^{-1} wet tissue) by rat brain cortical slices as a combined function of time and O_2 pressure (Kovachich and Mishra, 1980. Reproduced with the permission of Raven Press, New York).

Malonaldehyde production by rat brain microsomes is also a function of NADPH concentration, levels of c. 7 nmol mg^{-1} protein min^{-1} being reached at a NADPH concentration of 0.4 mM (Player and Horton, 1981). However, the overall rate of reaction in brain microsomal systems was only approximately 10% of that found for hepatic NADPH-dependent lipoperoxidation. The involvement of cytochrome P-450 and/or NADPH-cytochrome c reductase appears probable. However, cerebral lipoperoxidation, in contrast to the liver, also occurs in the absence of NADPH and this accounts for about 40% of the maximum activity observed in the presence of NADPH (Player and Horton, 1981). Clearly an important non-enzymatic lipoperoxidation takes place in brain microsomes (see below).

The superoxide anion-radical is considered a major initiator of lipoperoxidation (Kellogg and Fridovich, 1975; Trager, 1982), be it generated enzymatically by monooxygenases (acting here as oxidases, see Testa et al., 1981) or by autoxidation of various compounds (see section 2.1.10). However, other mechanisms of lipoperoxidation initiation exist, such as the generation of radicals from xenobiotics, e.g. CCl$_4$, or non-enzymatic processes such as lipoperoxidation induced by iron or ascorbic acid.

Carbon tetrachloride is activated by cytochrome P-450 to a reactive metabolite, the trichloromethyl radical, which is able to initiate lipoperoxidation (Recknagel et al., 1977). However, recent investigations have failed to detect CCl$_4$-induced lipoperoxidation in rat brain (Kornbrust and Mavis, 1980a) presumably due to only slight conversion to the trichloromethyl radical.

Iron-initiated lipoperoxidation has been shown to be due to free Fe^{2+} (Kornbrust and Mavis, 1980b). In brain microsomes in the presence of NADPH, iron markedly influences lipoperoxidation increasing the reaction rate by four-fold (Player and Horton, 1981). Interestingly the reaction rates in the absence of NADPH but in the presence of FeCl$_3$ (which should be inactive as such, see above) are practically the same as those observed in the presence of NADPH and absence of FeCl$_3$ (Player and Horton, 1981). This indeed might suggest alternative mechanisms; but clearly the role of iron is complex (Gutteridge et al., 1982), since it is involved in both the initiation and the propagation phases (Svingen et al., 1979).

A further type of lipoperoxidation is the non-enzymatic reaction induced by ascorbic acid. This process was characterized in rat brain mitochondria and shown to be markedly influenced by the ascorbic acid concentration (Thyagarajan, 1981a). The total amount of malonaldehyde formed was approximately 11 nmol mg^{-1} protein at the optimum ascorbic acid concentration of 1 mM. Higher levels of ascorbic acid resulted in a much slower reaction rate, while polyamines (spermine and spermidine) increased the reaction rate several-fold.

2.1.9.4 *Retinoic acid 5,6-epoxidation*

DeLuca *et al.* (1981) have recently described a biochemical reaction in which retinoic acid (XIX) is oxidized to the 5,6-epoxide (XX). This activity is quite marked in the brain, with *in vitro* activity of a few pmol mg^{-1} tissue min^{-1}. The highest activity was found in the kidney, followed by intestine, liver, brain, spleen and testes; no activity was detectable in muscle and lung.

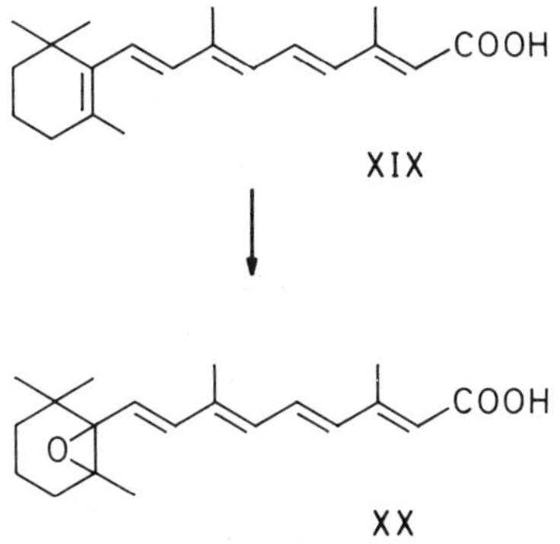

XIX

XX

The properties of the renal epoxidase activity were rigorously investigated (DeLuca *et al.*, 1981; Sietsema and DeLuca, 1982), and they will be briefly described here on the reasonable assumption that the renal and cerebral activities resemble each other. The microsomal and the mitochondrial fractions in the kidney have identical activities on a mg of protein basis; the nuclear fraction possesses some activity, possibly due to mitochondrial contamination, while cytosol is completely inactive.

The particulate nature of this enzyme, the chemical nature of the reaction and the requirement for O_2 and NADPH are all suggestive of a cytochrome P-450 mediated process. However, the lack of inhibition to carbon monoxide, metyrapone and α-naphthoflavone, which are classical cytochrome P-450 inhibitors, rule out this possibility. Epoxidation of retinoic acid does not appear to occur by the same mechanism as it does for vitamin K, since the latter system has no strict requirement for NADPH. Similarly, fatty acid cyclooxygenase has no requirement for ATP or NADPH and therefore is not a candidate.

In contrast, there are some similarities between retinoic acid epoxidation and some lipid peroxidation reactions. EDTA, a divalent metal ion chelator, completely inhibited the epoxidation reaction. A difference with lipoperoxidation systems was the strict requirement for ATP, which could not be replaced by ADP, PO_4^{3-} or $P_2O_7^{4-}$.

Retinoic acid epoxidase certainly involves a free radical intermediate in the reaction, since it is blocked by *N,N'*-diphenyl-*para*-phenylenediamine, a free radical scavenger. It thus has properties close to those of some lipid peroxidases. The discovery of this activity raises a number of questions regarding its nature, its physiological role (it is not required for retinoic acid function), and its substrate selectivity. While the 13-*cis* isomer of retinoic acid is also a substrate, nothing appears known about the ability of this epoxidase to metabolize xenobiotics.

2.1.10 Non-enzymatic and post-enzymatic oxidation reactions

These reactions can be due to oxidizing agents such as organic hydroperoxides, to reduced forms of oxygen such as $O_2^{\bar{}}$ and H_2O_2 released by various enzymes, or to other activated forms produced from the oxygen metabolites by various reactions, e.g. singlet oxygen ($^1O_2$) and the hydroxyl radical (HO˙) (Trager, 1982; see also Gorman and Rodgers, 1981; Sawyer and Valentine, 1981; Malmström, 1982). The post-tyrosinase oxidation of dopaquinone has already been mentioned (section 2.1.3.2).

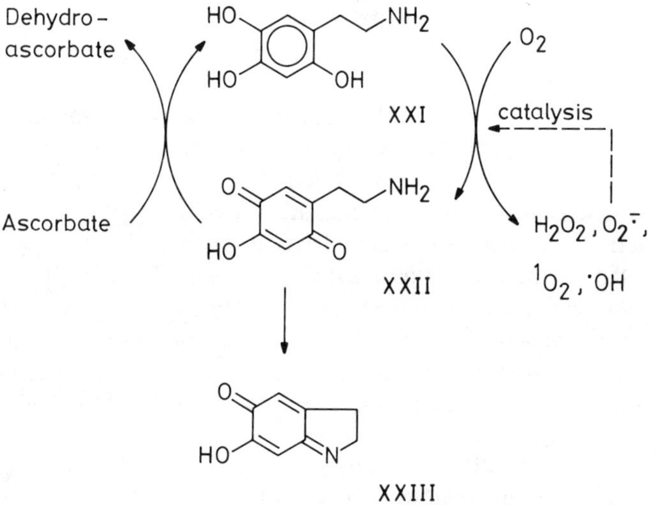

FIG. 6. Autoxidation of 6-hydroxydopamine (from Jonsson, 1980. Reproduced with the permission of Annual Reviews Inc., Palo Alto, California.)

Another mechanism exists, namely the autoxidation of a number of compounds, e.g. catecholamines (Hassan and Fridovich, 1980). One of the best known and most reactive compounds is 6-hydroxydopamine (XXI), which autoxidizes as shown (Fig. 6) to a para-quinone (XXII) with the formation of various reduced oxygen species (see also Perez-Reyes and Mason, 1981). The *para*-quinone itself can be reduced back to 6-hydroxydopamine by ascorbic acid or cyclize to aminochrome (XXIII), ultimately leading to melanins (Jonsson, 1980, and references therein). The participation of active oxygen species in 6-hydroxydopamine toxicity has recently been further evaluated (Tiffany-Castiglioni et al, 1982). Other catecholamines acting in a very similar manner are 5,6- and 5,7-dihydroxytryptamine (XXIV) (Jonsson, 1980).

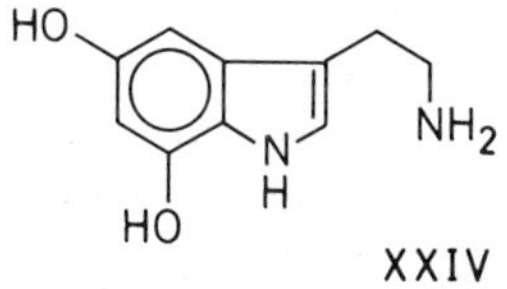

XXIV

The autoxidation of catecholamines is markedly increased by cations such as Mn^{2+}, Cu^{2+}, Fe^{2+} which act as catalysts, causing covalent binding as shown with norepinephrine (Maguire et al., 1974). Similarly, Donaldson and colleagues (1980) have postulated that the neurotoxicity of manganese is due to enhanced dopamine autoxidation associated with increased generation of activated oxygen species. Indeed, manganism (manganese-induced dyskinesia) and Parkinsonism display remarkable neurochemical, neuro-pathological and symptomatological similarities (see also section 4.3.3). The ability of metallic cations to promote dopamine autoxidation to amino-chrome is closely related to their redox potential: Mn > Cu > Ni > Zn ≫ Mg > Ca (Donaldson et al., 1980, and references therein).

2.2 REDUCTASES AND DEHYDROGENASES

2.2.1 Alcohol dehydrogenase (EC 1.1.1.1), aldehyde reductases and ketone reductases

Alcohol dehydrogenase, which catalyses the oxidation of alcohols to aldehydes, is a NADH-dependent cytosolic enzyme found mainly in the liver (Bosron and Li, 1980). Its presence in the brain has been controversial (e.g. Guroff, 1980, p. 444; Bosron and Li, 1980), but it now appears that a moderate alcohol dehydrogenase activity resides in this organ (Raskin and Sokoloff, 1970) and may be inducible (Raskin and Sokoloff, 1974). This finding has clear consequences, be it for the metabolism of ethanol, or for that of other alcohols which are substrates of the enzyme (Bosron and Li, 1980). Other cerebral dehydrogenases exist and may in later studies be assigned a role in drug metabolism, e.g. sorbitol dehydrogenase (O'Brien et al., 1983).

Steroidal secondary alcohols are substrates of a number of oxidoreductases yielding the corresponding ketones. For example, testosterone was found to be dehydrogenated to androstenedione in rabbit brain, the cortex being equiactive with the hypothalamus and limbic system (Naftolin *et al.*, 1975a).

Aldehyde reductases are a family of NADPH-linked cytosolic enzymes comprising aldehyde reductase (EC 1.1.1.2) and many others such as aldose reductase (EC 1.1.1.21) and lactaldehyde reductase (EC 1.1.1.55). The substrate selectivity of these enzymes is relatively low and overlaps considerably with that of ketone reductases to be discussed below (von Wartburg and Wermuth, 1980). Aldehyde reductases are widely distributed, and many publications report their presence in the brain (von Warburg and Wermuth, 1980, and references therein). Recent studies include the purification of a high affinity aldehyde reductase from rat and ox brain (Rivett *et al.*, 1981) and the purification from human brain of two aldehyde reductases which reduce succinic semialdehyde to 4-hydroxybutyrate (Cash *et al.*, 1979). These human enzymes, designated DE1 and DE2, behave quite differently towards exogenous aldehyde. While the DE1 reduces most, DE2 is fairly selective for the physiological substrate (Table 5).

TABLE 5

Substrate selectivity of two aldehyde reductases (DE1 and DE2) purified from human brain (Cash *et al.*, 1979)

Substrate	Relative activities	
	DE1	DE2
Succinic semialdehyde	63	100
Acetaldehyde	2·6	ND[a]
D-Lactaldehyde	12	ND
D,L-Lactaldehyde	5·9	ND
D,L-Glyceraldehyde	4·7	1·4
Benzaldehyde (B)	2·8	ND
4-Hydroxy-B	ND	ND
4-Carboxy-B	62	5
4-Nitro-B	100	11
3-Nitro-B	11	11
p-Anisaldehyde	1·6	ND
3-Pyridine carboxaldehyde	27	ND
Benzyl methyl ketone	0·5	ND

[a]Not detected.

Another aldehyde reductase is the mitochondrial NADH-dependent form. Recently, an enzyme of this type found in rat brain was shown to be inducible by barbiturates, as opposed to the cytosolic NADPH-dependent form(s), the activity of which remained unaffected (Satoh *et al.*, 1979).

Ketone reductases are a family of generally poorly characterized enzymes, most of which are NADPH-dependent and which are found in the cytosol (Felsted and Bachur, 1980). These enzymes, like the aldehyde reductases which they so closely resemble, have been detected in virtually every mammalian tissue examined, including brain. Substrates include ketonic steroids and a number of xenobiotics, e.g. *para*-nitroacetophenone, daunorubicin and oxisuran (Ahmed *et al.*, 1979; Felsted and Bachur, 1980).

The close similarities and overlapping substrate selectivities of aldehyde and ketone reductases have led to the suggestion that overall they can be considered as non-specific carbonyl reductases (Wermuth, 1981). Some forms have been purified from human brain and found to reduce quinones such as menadione and tocopherolquinone, ketones such as some prostaglandins, ketosteroids and daunorubicin, and activated aldehydes such as *para*-nitrobenzaldehyde (Wermuth, 1981).

Carbonyl reductases are not the only enzymes capable of reducing quinones. Indeed, the flavoprotein *DT-diaphorase* (EC 1.6.99.2) also has this capacity and has been shown to serve as a cellular device against quinone toxicity by controlling semiquinone and superoxide formation (Lind *et al.*, 1982). Quinone formation and metabolic fate (see also sections 2.1.3.2, 2.1.9, 2.1.10, 2.2.3 and 2.2.6) is thus a highly complex and important biochemical area which deserves much attention.

2.2.2 Aldehyde dehydrogenase (EC 1.2.1.3)

Dehydrogenases act by removing a hydride anion from the substrate, while reductases transfer it to the substrate. Aldehyde dehydrogenase is no exception to this rule, and removes the carbonyl hydrogen as a hydride ion. The acceptor of the hydride ion is either NAD or flavin (Weiner, 1980).

Aldehyde dehydrogenase occurs in most organs, but mainly in the liver and brain. It is found in cytosol, mitochondria, and microsomes, and its subcellular distribution in human brain has been investigated (Inoue and Lindros, 1982). This enzyme has a broad substrate selectivity. Acetaldehyde entering the brain or formed within it is rapidly oxidized. Thus, acetaldehyde could not be detected in the whole brain of rats dosed with ethanol unless the animals were pre-treated with disulfiram (a well-known inhibitor of the enzyme), and despite the fact that relatively high levels were detectable in blood (Westcott *et al.*, 1980).

Aldehydes of varied chemical structure are substrates for the enzyme. In derivatives of the general structure $X-CH_2-CHO$, a substituent X increases the velocity of oxidation in relation to its electron-withdrawing character. A number of aromatic aldehydes are also dehydrogenated (Weiner, 1980, and references therein).

2.2.3 Dihydrodiol dehydrogenase

A poorly studied enzyme is dihydrodiol dehydrogenase which converts dihydrodiols (XXV, generated from arene oxides by epoxide hydrolase) to catechols (XXVI) (see Bolcsak and Nerland, 1983, and references therein). Using NADP as a cofactor and benzene dihydrodiol as substrate, the activity of this cytosolic enzyme was quantified in various tissues of the male rat (Vogel et al., 1982). The brain displayed distinct activity but this was only 2.4% of that found in the liver.

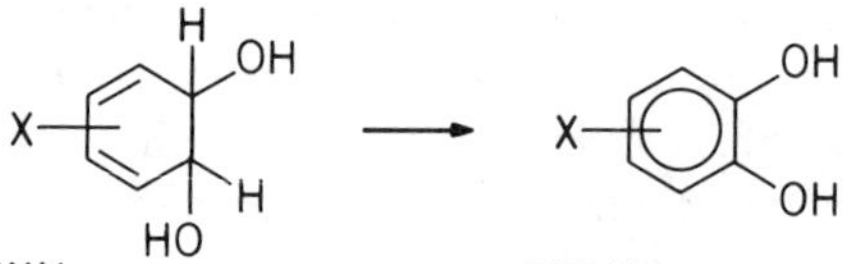

$$XXV \longrightarrow XXVI$$

The physiological role of the enzyme may relate to steroid metabolism, since the 3α-hydroxy group of certain steroids is oxidized, and the 3-keto group of 4,5-saturated steroids is reduced (Vogel et al., 1982). With regard to xenobiotics, a very broad substrate selectivity is apparent in the dehydrogenation or hydrogenation not only of dihydrodiols, but also of aldehydes and ketones, of ortho-quinones and of para-quinones. Even more intriguing is the loss of mutagenicity of benz[a]anthracene 8,9-diol 10,11-oxide in the presence of highly purified dihydrodiol dehydrogenase (Glatt et al., 1982). Its activity, in fact, was greater than that of epoxide hydrolase, pointing to an important role for this enzyme in the control of diol epoxides. The presence of dihydrodiol dehydrogenase in the brain, even if a modest one, may be of toxicological importance.

2.2.4 Reduction of carbon-carbon double bonds

Few examples of C-C double bond reduction are known in xenobiotic metabolism (see Testa and Jenner, 1976, p. 121). This reaction is a significant pathway in the metabolism of suitable steroids, especially Δ^4-steroids (both endogenous and exogenous).

In the brain, the only known substrates of C-C double bond reduction are endogenous steroids, and a number of publications describe Δ^4-steroid 5α-reductase activity. Thus, the hypothalamus of the female Rhesus monkey is able to reduce progesterone to 5α-dihydroprogesterone, the highest activity being found in the membrane fraction (supernatant of nuclei), followed by the nuclear fraction (Billiar et al., 1981). Similarly, testosterone is reduced to 5α-dihydrotestosterone, the activity being found, e.g. in hypothalamus and pituitary from infantile and adolescent rats of both sexes

(Degtiar *et al.*, 1981). In a further study, testosterone 5α-reductase was quantified in various cerebral regions of the adult male rat. The activity decreased in the order midbrain tegmentum, hypothalamus, cerebellum, dorsal hippocampus, amygdala and cerebral cortex (Snipes and Shore, 1982). The significance of these findings to the cerebral metabolism of exogenous steroids remains to be assessed.

2.2.5 Nitro- and N-oxide reductases

A number of enzymes catalyse nitro reduction, namely NADPH-dependent enzymes in the endoplasmic reticulum (cytochrome P-450 and cytochrome P-450 reductase), and cytosolic enzymes such as xanthine oxidase and aldehyde oxidase (Mitchard, 1971; Testa and Jenner, 1976, pp. 123–131, 304–307, and references therein).

Little is known of nitro reduction in brain, a remarkable exception being the study of Köchli *et al.* (1980), who found a mitochondrial NADH-dependent nitro reductase system in the liver and brain of the rat. The enzyme was active towards a number of aromatic nitro derivatives (Table 6), the best substrates carrying a neutral, electron-withdrawing substituent. As opposed to the microsomal enzyme, the mitochondrial enzyme did not catalyse the reduction to the amine. This implies that reactive nitroso and hydroxylamino metabolites may accumulate with obvious toxicological consequences. These important findings warrant further study.

TABLE 6

Substrate selectivity of nitro reductase from rat brain mitochondria
(Köchli *et al.*, 1980)

Substrate	Relative activity
1,3-Dinitrobenzene	100
1,4-Dinitrobenzene	226
Niridazole	198
4-Nitrobenzaldehyde	110
2-Nitrobenzaldehyde	70
3-Nitrobenzaldehyde	10
4-Nitrobenzyl alcohol	37
2,4-Dichloronitrobenzene	27
4-Nitrobenzyl chloride	21
4-Nitroacetophenone	16
Nitrobenzene	8
4-Nitrobenzoate	0
3-Nitrophenol	0
N,N-Dimethyl-3-nitroaniline	0
1-Nitropropane	0

In connection with dopamine antagonistic effects of some, but not all, amine oxides of phenothiazine antipsychotics, the ability of the brain to reduce N-oxides was investigated (Lewis *et al.*, 1983). Chlorpromazine N-oxide was used as substrate, with negative results. Indeed, neither *in vivo* nor *in vitro* did the rat brain demonstrate any N-oxide reductase activity. However, this result awaits confirmation from more systematic investigations.

2.2.6 Non-enzymatic reductions

Nitrosobenzene in a neutral buffer solution can be converted quantitatively by NADH or NADPH to phenylhydroxylamine (Becker and Sternson, 1980). Such a reaction may perhaps have relevance for cerebral xenobiotic metabolism, and is interesting in relation to the previous section.

Of greater interest for brain metabolism is the ascorbate-mediated non-enzymatic reduction of quinones generated from catecholamines (Tse *et al.*, 1976). The importance of catecholamine-quinones has already been mentioned in sections 2.1.9 and 2.1.10. These quinones can undergo a number of reactions as shown in Fig. 7. Intramolecular nucleophilic cyclization produces aminochromes (e.g. adrenochrome, "dopamine-chrome") via leucochromes. Much more rapid (Tse *et al.*, 1976) is the addition of strong nucleophilic sulfhydryl compounds such as glutathione and cysteine. However, the reduction of the *ortho*-quinone back to the catecholamine as catalysed by ascorbic acid has been found to efficiently compete with nucleophilic attacks. This finding is particularly important in view of the relatively high levels of ascorbate in brain (Tse *et al.*, 1976; Milby *et al.*, 1982). Curiously enough, the concentration of ascorbate in the developing rat brain is much higher than that in the adult (Thyagarajan, 1981b), raising speculation as to the effect this might have on catecholamine catabolism.

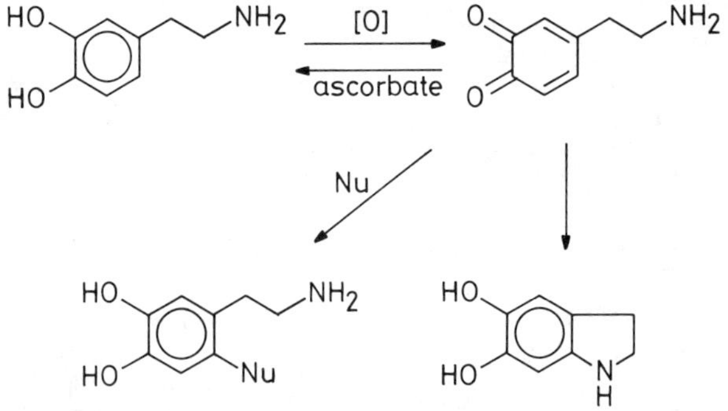

FIG. 7. The chemical reactivity of *ortho*-quinones generated from catecholamines (here, dopamine-*o*-quinone). From right to left: intramolecular nucleophilic cyclization to a leucochrome, addition of an external nucleophile, and reduction to the parent catecholamine. (From Tse *et al.*, 1976.)

2.3 DECARBOXYLASES (EC 4.1.1.–)

A variety of amino acid decarboxylases exist in brain, in particular those involved in the synthesis of neurotransmitters from amino acid precursors (Guroff, 1980, pp. 161–213):

> —aromatic L-amino acid decarboxylase
> (EC 4.1.1.28), which includes the L-DOPA and
> L-5-hydroxytryptophan decarboxylase activities
> —L-histidine decarboxylase (EC 4.1.1.22)
> —L-glutamate 1-decarboxylase
> (EC 4.1.1.15)
> —L-cysteine-sulfinate decarboxylase
> (EC 4.1.1.29)

The substrate selectivity of these pyridoxine-dependent enzymes is rather narrow, since their mechanism of action is specific for α-amino acids. Hence they can be expected to act on a very limited number of xenobiotics only, although this has not been systematically explored. L-DOPA is a typical endogenous substrate, but it is also a drug when administered in large doses; its cerebral decarboxylation is the key reaction permitting treatment of Parkinsonian patients since dopamine itself cannot penetrate the brain (Hefti and Melamed, 1980). To give but one example, administering L-DOPA to rats (150 mg kg^{-1} ip) increases the brain dopamine levels by 130% one hour after injection (Doshi and Edwards, 1981). Interesting findings are also reported in a recent study on the cerebral decarboxylation of *meta*- and *para*-tyrosine (Boulton and Juorio, 1983).

One well-known xenobiotic substrate of DOPA decarboxylase is the drug α-methyl-DOPA (XXVII), which is transformed to α-methyldopamine (XXVIII) (Marshall and Castagnoli, 1973; Walsh 1977, p. 804).

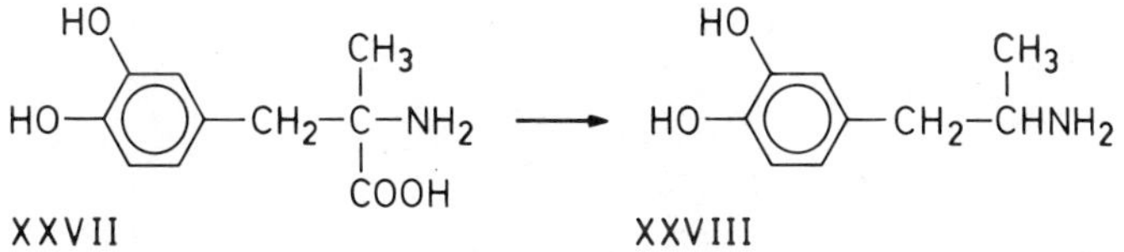

XXVII   XXVIII

2.4 HYDROLASES

Hydrolases catalyse the transfer of a molecule of water to hydrolyse ester linkages (esterases), amide bonds (amidases, peptidases), or epoxides (epoxide hydrolases), among others.

2.4.1 Epoxide hydrolase (EC 3.3.2.3)

Epoxide hydrolase (also still designated epoxide hydrase or epoxide hydratase) transforms electrophilic oxiranes (XXIX) to vicinal *trans*-diols (XXX) that are no longer electrophilically reactive. Two major chemical classes of substrate epoxides exist, namely arene oxides (XXIXa) generated by epoxidation of aromatic rings, and those oxiranes (XXIXb) derived from olefinic compounds.

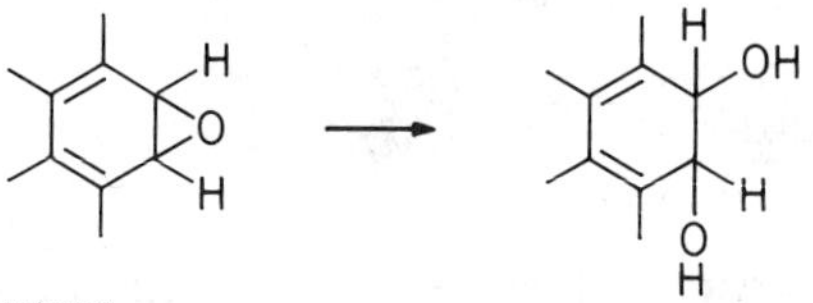

XXIXa

XXXa

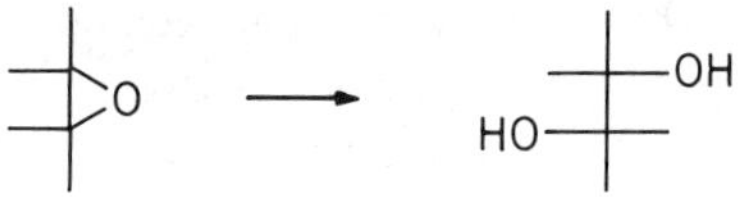

XXIXb

XXXb

Considerable attention has been paid to the molecular mechanism of action of epoxide hydrolase. Converging evidence indicates that the enzyme activates a molecule of water by a general base catalysis (Hanzlik *et al.*, 1976; Westkaemper and Hanzlik, 1981); acid catalysis by oxygen protonation has been excluded (Bellucci *et al.*, 1981). The mechanism of action is thus understood as shown in Fig. 8.

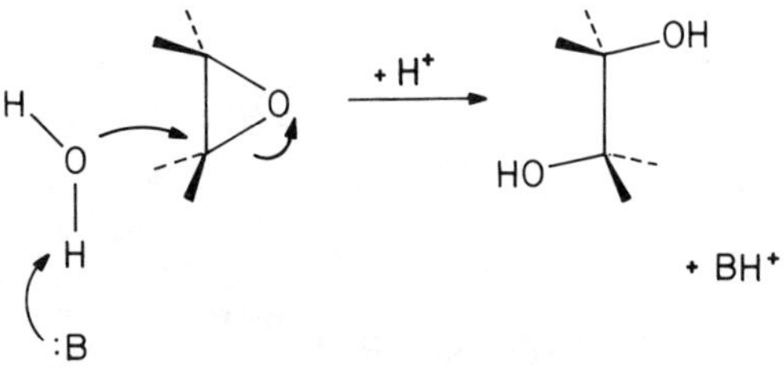

FIG. 8. General mechanism of the reaction catalysed by epoxide hydrolase.

The most characterized form of epoxide hydrolase is located in the endoplasmic reticulum, where it can act on substrates generated by cytochrome P-450 (Oesch, 1979, 1980). However, more than one form of microsomal epoxide hydrolase appears to exist (Guenthner et al., 1982). In addition, a cytosolic and a nuclear form of the enzyme also occur in liver (Guenthner et al., 1981; Garattini et al., 1981).

Epoxide hydrolase activity is found mainly in the liver, but also in many organs and tissues including brain. In male rats for example, the level of activity in the brain was found to be 1/60th that of the liver on a mg of protein basis (Oesch, 1979). In pregnant mice and rats and in their fetuses (Table 7), the differences are 30-to-100 fold, i.e. comparable to that noted for male rats (Rouet et al., 1981). Pretreatment with 5,6-benzoflavone is without effect on the activity of brain epoxide hydrolase activity.

TABLE 7

Effect of 5,6-benzoflavone (BF) on epoxide hydrolase and GSH S-transferase activities in cerebral and hepatic microsomes from pregnant dams and fetuses (19 days old) of mouse and rat (Rouet et al., 1981)

	Epoxide hydrolase[a]		GSH S-Transferase[b]	
	Brain	Liver	Brain	Liver
Mice				
Pregnant dams				
control	0·04 ± 0·001	2·2 ± 0.1	0·67 ± 0·31	3·95 ± 0·23
BF	0·05 ± 0·01	5·3 ± 1·0	0·98 ± 0·01	8·6 ± 0·37
Fetuses				
control	0·010 ± 0·005	0·66 ± 0·02	0·11 ± 0·03	1·5 ± 0·02
BF	0·010 ± 0·004	1·35 ± 0·25	0·20 ± 0·04	1·4 ± 0·17
Rats				
Pregnant dams				
control	0·12 ± 0·005	8·55 ± 0·75	0·69 ± 0·03	9·11 ± 0·36
BF	0·14 ± 0·04	11·0 ± 6·3	0·57 ± 0·06	14·0 ± 0·5
Fetuses				
control	0·010 ± 0·003	0·31 ± 0·09	0·11 ± 0·01	0·41 ± 0·17
BF	0·010 ± 0·005	0·23 ± 0·05	0·24 ± 0·02	0·51 ± 0·21

TABLE 8

[a]Substrate: benzo[a]pyrene 4,5-epoxide; activity expressed as nmol product mg^{-1} protein min^{-1}.
[b]Substrate: 1-chloro-2,4-dinitrobenzene; activity expressed as μmol product mg^{-1} protein min^{-1}.

Using epoxide hydrolase of hepatic origin, structure–activity relationships of substrates and inducers have been investigated in a number of studies (Oesch, 1979, 1980). Much more remains to be done with the cerebral enzyme to assess its role in the detoxication or activation of xenobiotics penetrating into brain.

2.4.2 Esterases

As authoritatively reviewed by Heymann (1980), enzymes catalysing the hydrolysis of esters (XXXI) or amides (XXXII) have substrate selectivities which are dependent more on the nature of the groups R,R' and R'' than on the atom (O,N, or even S) adjacent to the C=O group. Consequently, the traditional classification of esterases and amidases often neglects the marked overlaps which exist in the substrate selectivity of many of these enzymes. We will therefore focus attention on enzyme activity (the nature of substrates) as much as on the enzymes themselves.

$$R-\overset{\overset{\displaystyle O}{\|}}{C}-O-R' \: + \: H_2O \: \longrightarrow \: R-COOH \: + \: HOR'$$

XXXI

$$R-\overset{\overset{\displaystyle O}{\|}}{C}-NR'R'' \: + \: H_2O \: \longrightarrow \: R-COOH \: + \: HNR'R''$$

XXXII

The *non-specific carboxylesterase* (EC 3.1.1.1), with broad substrate selectivity, is located mainly in liver microsomes (although some activity exists also in the cytosol) and in many other organs and tissues. In rat brain for example, the enzyme hydrolyses approximately 23 nmol *para*-nitrophenyl acetate per mg protein per min, an activity identical to that of the liver cytosol enzyme, but 18 times lower than that found in liver microsomes. However, as opposed to the hepatic enzyme, the cerebral enzyme was not inducible by phenobarbital (Nousiainen and Hänninen, 1981). In contrast, meperidine esterase activity, which comprises a group of carboxylesterase isozymes, has been detected in rat liver microsomes but not in brain preparations (Yeh, 1982).

One of the physiologically most important esterases of the nervous system is acetylcholinesterase (EC 3.1.1.7), the substrate selectivity of which is rather narrow (Heymann, 1980). Organophosphorous esters such as phosphate (XXXIII) and phosphonate (XXXIV) esters are irreversible inhibitors of this enzyme because they bind covalently to it (Walsh, 1977, pp. 125–126). The heterogeneity of this enzyme in rat brain has been investigated (Rakonczay et al., 1981).

XXXIII 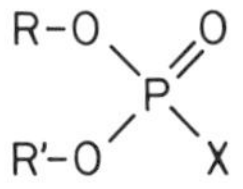 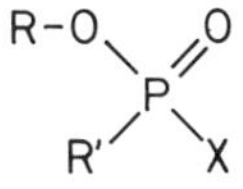
$$\begin{array}{c} R\text{-}O \\ \diagdown \\ R'\text{-}O \diagup \end{array} P \begin{array}{c} O \\ \diagup\diagup \\ \diagdown X \end{array}$$
$$\begin{array}{c} R\text{-}O \\ \diagdown \\ R' \diagup \end{array} P \begin{array}{c} O \\ \diagup\diagup \\ \diagdown X \end{array}$$ XXXIV

Organophosphorus esters react with another enzyme designated "neurotoxic esterase". The inhibited enzyme (enzyme-ester adduct) degrades to become toxic, causing delayed neurotoxicity (Johnson, 1975; Lotti and Johnson, 1980). An excellent review, including extensive structure–activity relationships of the neurotoxic esters, has been published by Johnson (1975). Two phenyl valerate hydrolysing carboxylesterases of hen brain have recently been identified as neurotoxic esterase isozymes. Designated A and B, these two forms account for 2 and 10%, respectively, of total hen brain phenyl valerate hydrolysing activity (Chemnitius et al., 1983).

Cholesterol ester hydrolase (EC 3.1.1.13) has been studied in rat and human brain (Ogino and Suzuki, 1981; Johnson and Shah, 1981). Two forms have been characterized in human cerebrospinal fluid, one probably a microsomal enzyme and the other a myelin enzyme; the myelin enzyme, but not the microsomal enzyme, was significantly lower in patients suffering from multiple sclerosis (Johnson and Shah, 1981).

The brain contains many other esterases, e.g. phosphatases (phosphoric monoester hydrolases, EC 3.1.3.–, and phosphoric diester hydrolases, EC 3.1.4.–), β-glucuronidase (EC 3.2.1.31) (Alvares and Balasubramanian, 1982), β-galactosidase (EC 3.2.1.23), β-N-acetyl-D-hexosaminidase (EC 3.2.1.52), and aryl sulfatases (EC 3.1.6.1) (Guroff, 1980, p. 44). At least some of these enzymes have the potential to hydrolyse xenobiotic esters.

Cerebral esterases are of particular interest in relation to the activation of prodrug esters within brain. For example, a number of oxazepam esters (XXXV, R = CH_3, CH_2CH_3, CH_2CH_2COOH, $CH_2CH_2C_6H_5$, $CH(CH_2CH_3)_2$, $C(CH_3)_2CH_2C_6H_5$) appear to be hydrolysed by rat brain preparations (Maksay et al., 1981). A detailed study (Horn et al., 1982) examined the levels of 2-amino-6,7-dihydroxytetrahydronaphthalene (6,7-ADTN) in the rat corpus striatum and cerebellum following ip administration of diester prodrugs (XXXVI). This example is discussed further in section 4.4.2.

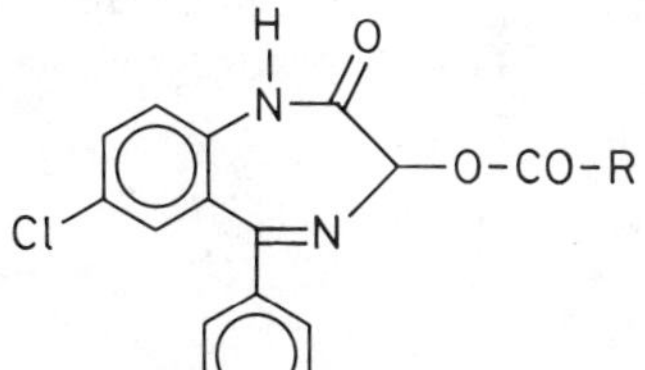

XXXV

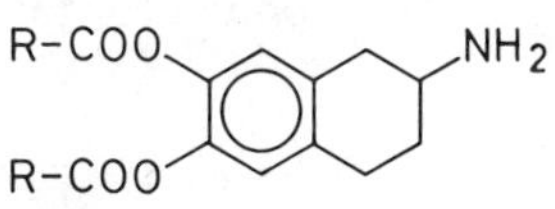

XXXVI

There is obviously a field of considerable potential in the design of brain-targeted prodrugs. The existence of cerebral *lipases* (EC 3.1.1.3) (e.g. Rousseau and Gatt, 1979) may be of interest to the design of fatty acid or glycerol prodrug esters.

The *blood* is rich in esterases (Heymann, 1980). Additionally, hemoglobin (Elbaum and Nagel, 1981) and serum albumin (Kurono *et al.*, 1979) have esterase activity. As a consequence, blood circulating in the brain should contribute to the overall esterasic activity of this organ. *In vivo*, the brain and blood-in-brain enzymatic activities can be expected to have different consequences since they are separated by the blood–brain barrier. *In vitro* on the other hand, blood contamination must be avoided if meaningful cerebral activities are sought.

2.4.3 Amidases

There is some evidence to suggest the cerebral hydrolysis of various amides, although little is known of the enzymes implicated. Thus, *N*-deacetylation of phenacetin (XXXVII) occurs in monkey brain, the activity being high in cerebellum, and in the nuclear fraction of whole brain (Oommen *et al.*, 1980). The enzyme responsible for this degradation was not arylacylamidase (EC 3.5.1.13), an enzyme of broad substrate selectivity (Heymann, 1980) several forms of which have been characterized in rat brain (Hsu *et al.*, 1982).

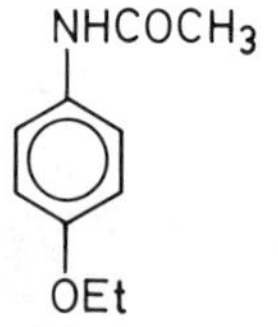

$$NHCOCH_3$$

XXXVII

A lactam, 2-pyrrolidinone (XXXVIII), which penetrates into mouse brain, undergoes *in vivo* conversion to gamma-aminobutyric acid (XXXIX, GABA) (Callery *et al.*, 1979). GABA itself does not cross the blood–brain barrier, and deuterium labelling of XXXVIII provided definitive proof that the hydrolytic reaction was occurring within the brain. Although the rate of hydrolysis was slow and limited in extent, 2-pyrrolidinone appears as an interesting lead compound for the design of GABA prodrugs (Callery *et al.*, 1982).

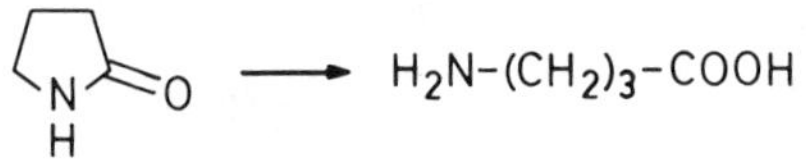

$$\longrightarrow \quad H_2N-(CH_2)_3-COOH$$

XXXVIII   XXXIX

The hydrolysis of aminoacyl derivatives of benzocaine (XL) was investigated in homogenates of various rat tissues (Slojkowska *et al.*, 1982). The analytical method used being specific for aromatic primary amines, the authors may have monitored the appearance of benzocaine (XLII) from XL (as they claim they did) as well as the appearance of *para*-aminobenzoic acid (XLIII) from XLI (a likely alternative). With this reservation in mind, the results (Table 8) are nevertheless interesting. The highest activity was found in the kidney, while a number of other organs including the brain showed comparable activity. With the exception of the dimethylglycine derivative, a poor substrate, all other compounds were hydrolysed at astonishingly similar rates, and no structure–metabolism relationships were apparent.

TABLE 8

Rate of amide bond hydrolysis of aminoacyl benzocaine derivatives in rat organ homogenates (Slojkowska *et al.*, 1982)

Aminoacyl derivative (XL)	Rate of hydrolysis (nmol mg^{-1} protein min^{-1})	
	Brain	Kidney
Glycine		
(R = R' = H)	2·01 ± 0·04	22·99 ± 0·80
N,N-Dimethylglycine		
(R = Me, R' = H)	0·20 ± 0·01	1·72 ± 0·02
Alanine		
(R = H, R' = Me)	3·20 ± 0·01	26·38 ± 0·92
N,N-Dimethylalanine		
(R = R' = Me)	4·08 ± 0·14	13·47 ± 0·70
Valine		
(R = H, R' = CHMe$_2$)	4·02 ± 0·08	28·84 ± 1·00
Leucine		
(R = H, R' = CH$_2$CHMe$_2$)	3·85 ± 0·14	38·17 ± 0·98
γ-Methylglutamic acid		
(R = H, R' = CH$_2$CHMeCOOH)	2·25 ± 0·01	12·95 ± 0·50

The enzymes hypothesized to be operative are α-aminoacylpeptide hydrolases (EC 3.4.11.–) in the case of the aminoacyl amides, and acylamide hydrolases (EC 3.5.1.–) in the case of the N,N-dimethyl derivatives (Slojkowska *et al.*, 1982).

TRH (thyrotropin-releasing hormone) contains a primary carboxamide group, as does its synthetic analog MK-771. When the latter compound was incubated in rat brain homogenates, fast and extensive hydrolysis of the carboxamide group occurred, whereas the reaction was much slower in rat gut homogenates (Vickers *et al.*, 1983). MK-771 may have been metabolized by an amidase specific for TRH, or by a less specific enzyme. In any case, this recent example stresses the significance of cerebral amidases.

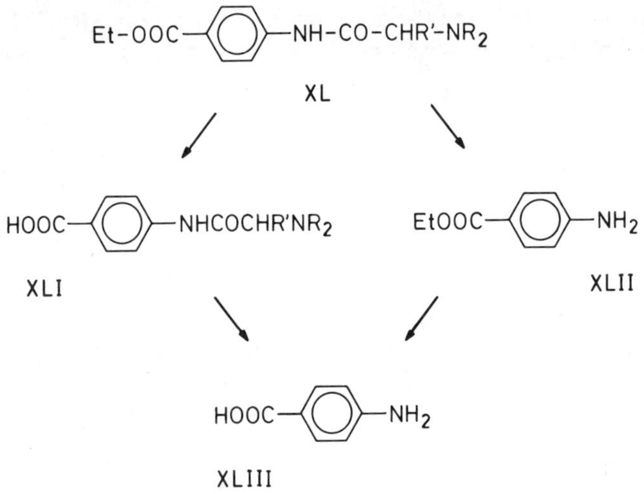

$$Et-OOC-\langle\bigcirc\rangle-NH-CO-CHR'-NR_2$$

XL

$$HOOC-\langle\bigcirc\rangle-NHCOCHR'NR_2 \qquad EtOOC-\langle\bigcirc\rangle-NH_2$$

XLI   XLII

$$HOOC-\langle\bigcirc\rangle-NH_2$$

XLIII

2.4.4 Peptidases

A number of peptidases and proteases exist in brain (Guroff, 1980, pp. 267–268). For the medicinal chemist and the neurochemist, the most interesting and promising ones may well be those involved in the metabolism of biologically active peptides acting in the central nervous system (for a review of peptidergic pathways in the CNS, see Brownstein, 1980).

A few peptide drugs are currently in regular therapeutic use, but their number can be expected to increase dramatically during the coming years. This will provide a better knowledge of their cerebral metabolism (activation or inactivation) under the influence of such enzymes as peptidylamino-acid hydrolases (EC 3.4.12.–) and peptidyldipeptide hydrolases (EC 3.4.15.–). For example, a synthetic opioid peptide, Met-enkephalin-Arg[6]-Phe[7], was shown to be converted to Met-enkephalin by brain and kidney dipeptidyl-peptide hydrolases (EC 3.4.14.–) (Benuck et al., 1981). Obviously a field of extraordinary importance lies in the extension of peptide investigations.

2.5 CONJUGATION REACTIONS

Conjugation reactions have for many decades been considered as purely detoxication processes. This concept, however, has had to be modified in view of the increasing evidence for pharmacologically active conjugates.

Such an activity may be of a pharmacological or toxicological nature (Caldwell, 1980). Pharmacologically active conjugates are exemplified by morphine 6-glucuronide and morphine 6-sulfate which have high affinity for the opiate receptor (Oguri, 1980). Examples of toxication through conjugation are numerous and have been extensively reviewed (Caldwell, 1980; Reichert, 1981).

2.5.1 Methyltransferases (EC 2.1.1.–)

Methyltransferases catalyse the transfer of a methyl group from the donor, generally S-adenosylmethionine, to an acceptor of suitable nucleophilic character such as a phenol, an amine or a thiol. The general mechanism of the transmethylation reaction can be postulated to involve a S_N2-like transition state, as proven for catechol O-methyltransferase (Hegazi et al., 1979) and as illustrated in Fig. 9.

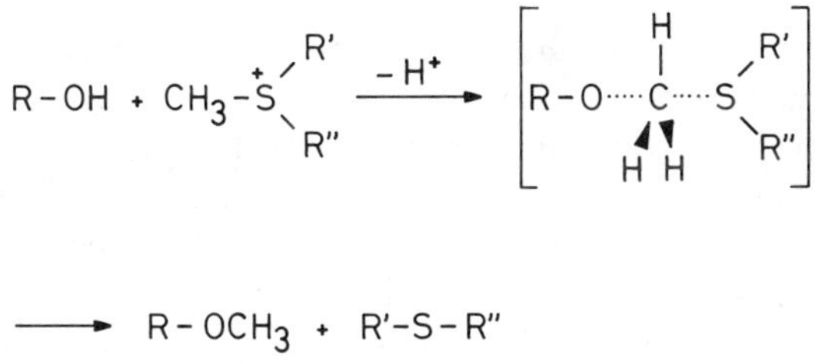

$$R-OH + CH_3-\overset{+}{\underset{R''}{\overset{R'}{S}}} \quad \xrightarrow{-H^+} \quad \left[R-O\cdots\overset{\overset{H}{|}}{\underset{\underset{H\ H}{\blacktriangle\blacktriangledown}}{C}}\cdots\overset{R'}{\underset{R''}{S}} \right]$$

$$\longrightarrow \quad R-OCH_3 + R'-S-R''$$

FIG. 9. Reaction mechanism of catechol O-methyltransferase, showing a S_N2-like transition state (Hegazi et al., 1979).

2.5.1.1 Catechol O-methyltransferase (EC 2.1.1.6)

Catechol O-methyltransferase (COMT) is predominantly located in the liver, but is also present in several other tissues and organs including the brain. In these tissues, the majority of the enzyme activity is found in the cytosol, although a membrane bound enzyme also exists (Testa and Jenner, 1976, p. 313; Borchardt, 1980). This appears to be the case in rat brain (Borchardt and Cheng, 1978) although not in pig liver and brain where only cytosolic COMT could be characterized (Goldberg and Tipton, 1978). In the human brain, membrane-bound COMT has been detected. Using norepinephrine and dopamine as substrates, the membrane-bound activity was 1–3.5-fold greater than the activity found in the cytosol (Roth, 1980).

The regional distribution of COMT in pig brain shows a relatively even pattern throughout the organ (Table 9).

TABLE 9

The regional distribution of COMT in pig brain (Goldberg and Tipton, 1978)

	Specific activity (mU mg^{-1})	Percentage of total activity
Cerebellum	0·016	10·9
Thalamus	0·016	13·5
Medulla and pons	ND[a]	—
Frontal lobe	0·017	17·0
Parietal lobe	0·020	19·4
Temporal lobe	0·013	15·3
Occipital lobe	0·019	17·0
Corpus callosum	0·010	2·8
Hypothalamus	0·010	0·5
Pituitary gland	ND	—

[a]Not detectable.

COMT shows high substrate selectivity for the catechol moiety (*ortho*-diphenol grouping), but a rather broad selectivity as regards other substituents of the aromatic ring (Borchardt, 1980). Physiological substrates are the catecholamines (dopamine, norepinephrine, epinephrine) as well as their metabolites (3,4-dihydroxymandelic acid and 3,4-dihydroxyphenylacetic acid, 3,4-dihydroxyphenylethyleneglycol). For these compounds, the methylation reaction shows a high product selectivity for the *meta*-hydroxyl group.

Other physiological substrates include catechol estrogens (see section 3.5) which competitively inhibit the *O*-methylation of catecholamines. This establishes a biochemical link in the CNS between estradiol and catecholamines (Fishman and Norton, 1975a, 1975b, and references therein).

1,2,3,4-Tetrahydroisoquinolines (TIQ) derivatives are a group of presumably non-physiological metabolites of catecholamines (see section 2.6). Examples are 6,7-dihydroxy-TIQ (XLIV) and salsolinol (XLV). These compounds are substrates for brain COMT, yielding the 7-*O*-methyl derivatives (Bail *et al.*, 1980; Origitano and Collins, 1980). Interestingly, this position corresponds to the *para*-OH group in the parent dopamine molecule, implying reversed regioselectivity.

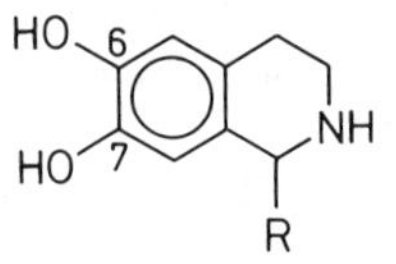

R = H   XLIV

R = Me   XLV

A number of xenobiotic catechols are methylated by COMT, with kinetic parameters and *meta/para* ratios strongly dependent upon the structure of substrate (Borchardt, 1980). Examples of drugs acting as substrates of COMT are α-methyl-DOPA and isoproterenol. Alpha-substitution of catecholamines modifies in a complex manner their affinity for, and rate of reaction with, COMT (Gordonsmith *et al.*, 1982). As early as 1965, Daly and colleagues (Daly *et al.*, 1965) showed that a considerable variety of phenols could be hydroxylated by rabbit liver preparation to catechols which were then *O*-methylated by COMT. Besides simple mono-, di- and tri-substituted phenols, drugs such as nalorphine, levorphanol, phenazocine, phentolamine, diethylstilbestrol and estradiol also act as substrates. COMT thus offers an interesting potential for the methylation of catechols within brain, be they xenobiotics or their metabolites.

Hydroxyindole O-*methyltransferase* (EC 2.1.1.4) is another *O*-methylating enzyme. Its restricted distribution to the pineal gland (Sikic, 1980; Morton and Potgieter, 1982) and its narrow substrate selectivity suggest this enzyme is of little apparent consequence to drug metabolism (Sikic, 1980).

2.5.1.2 Phenylethanolamine N-*methyltransferase* (*EC 2.1.1.28*)

Phenylethanolamine *N*-methyltransferase (PNMT) is located mainly in the adrenal medulla and in the brain, its physiological role being the *N*-methylation of norepinephrine to epinephrine (Sikic, 1980; Guroff, 1980, p. 182).

PNMT displays a rather narrow substrate selectivity, its activity being restricted to phenylethylamines and phenylisopropylamines having a β-hydroxy group, although these requirements are not absolute (Sikic, 1980, and references therein). In the rat, the K_m values of brain PNMT were determined to be in the 0.4–1.4 mM range using norepinephrine, octopamine and phenylethanolamine as substrates, whereas the affinities for adrenal PNMT were 10–40 times greater (Yu, 1978). These facts taken together suggest a limited role of PNMT in the cerebral metabolism of xenobiotics, particularly considering the high degree of similarity that exists among the brain PNMTs of various species (Fuller and Hemrick, 1979, and references therein). A number of properties of human brain PNMT, including regional distribution, have recently been described (Trocewicz *et al.*, 1982).

2.5.1.3 Other cerebral methyltransferases

Tryptamine N-*methyltransferase* (indoleamine *N*-methyltransferase (EC 2.1.1.49) is a relatively non-specific lung and brain enzyme which has been studied in humans (Borchardt, 1980, and references therein). This enzyme converts tryptamine (XLVI, R = H) and 5-hydroxytryptamine (XLVI, R = OH) to *N,N*-dimethyltryptamine (XLVII, R = H) and bufotenin (XLVII, R = OH), respectively (Barker *et al.*, 1980; Gomes *et al.*, 1981).

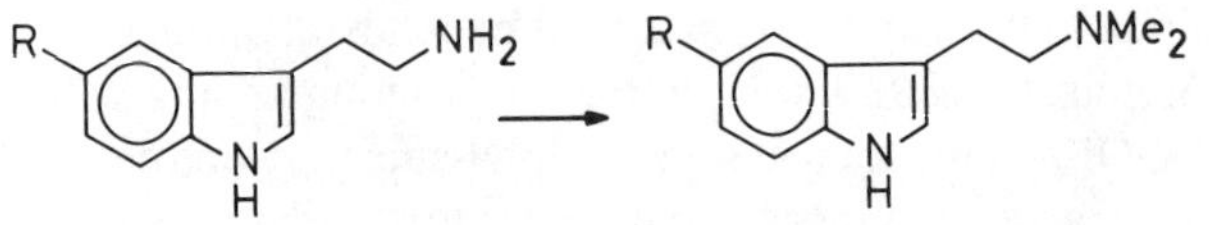

XLVI   XLVII

These two naturally occurring substances have been implicated in the aetiology of schizophrenia. But little appears known on the potential of cerebral tryptamine NMT for methylating xenobiotics.

Another cerebral enzyme is *histamine N-methyltransferase* (HNMT, EC 2.1.1.8), which methylates histamine (XLVIII) to yield N^τ-methylhistamine (XLIX). Enzyme activity is present in organs other than the brain, and it appears to have a rather narrow, but as yet poorly understood, substrate selectivity (Sikic, 1980; Borchardt, 1980). While a number of imidazole derivatives, in particular histidine and histamine metabolites, were not methylated, some other imidazole derivatives underwent methylation, e.g. 5-methyl- and N^α-methylhistamine (Borchardt, 1980). It would be interesting to know whether imidazole-containing histamine antagonists, and other heterocyclic systems, are substrates for the enzyme.

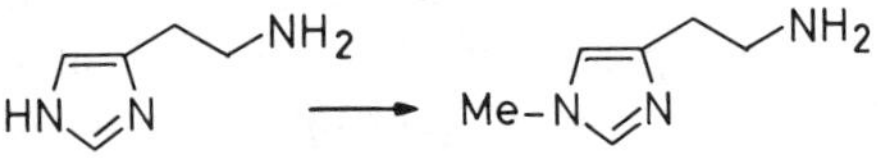

XLVIII   XLIX

The properties of *thiol S-methyltransferase* (EC 2.1.1.9) have been examined in rat brain, and its distribution investigated (Hiemke and Ghraf, 1983). This enzyme is known to play a role in the metabolism of thiol-containing xenobiotic metabolites, in particular breakdown products of glutathione conjugates (Mannervik, 1982) (see also section 2.5.6). A possible role in cerebral drug metabolism is thus suggested.

To conclude this section, it is worth mentioning the recent discovery in rat brain cytosol of *calmodulin N-methyltransferase* (Sitaramayya *et al.*, 1980), an enzyme of the group of protein *N*-methylases. With the development of synthetic peptide drugs, these enzymes may perhaps one day find a role in xenobiotic methylation.

2.5.2 Sulfotransferases (EC 2.8.2.–)

Sulfotransferases catalyse the transfer of a sulfate group from the donor, 3'-phosphoadenosine 5'-phosphosulfate (PAPS), to an acceptor which is either a phenol or an alcohol, an amine, or a hydroxylamine, so yielding sulfate esters, sulfamates, or N,O-sulfates, respectively (Fig. 10).

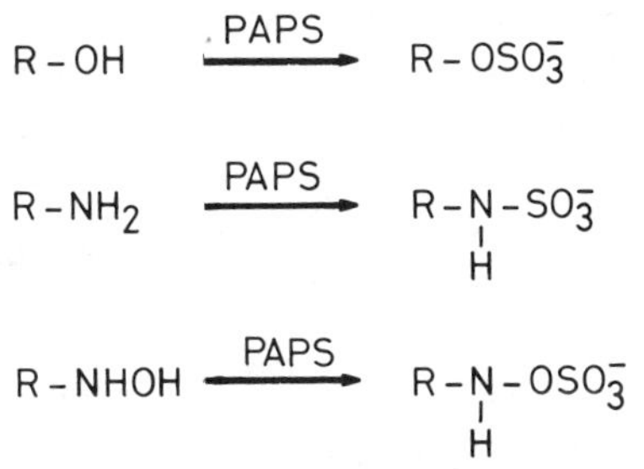

$$R-OH \xrightarrow{\text{PAPS}} R-OSO_3^-$$

$$R-NH_2 \xrightarrow{\text{PAPS}} R-\underset{H}{N}-SO_3^-$$

$$R-NHOH \xrightarrow{\text{PAPS}} R-\underset{H}{N}-OSO_3^-$$

FIG. 10. Reactions catalysed by sulfotransferases.

Sulfotransferases are involved in the metabolism of a number of endogenous classes of compounds, and their broad substrate selectivity permits the sulfation of many structurally different xenobiotics or their metabolites (Testa and Jenner, 1976, pp. 186–189; Jakoby et al., 1980; Powell and Roy, 1980).

Several forms of sulfotransferase have been characterized (Jakoby et al., 1980), e.g.

phenol sulfotransferase (aryl sulfotransferase, EC 2.8.2.1.), which acts on phenols, catecholamines, and organic hydroxylamines;
hydroxysteroid sulfotransferase (EC 2.8.2.2), which acts on primary and secondary alcohols in addition to the principal substrates;
arylamine sulfotransferase (EC 2.8.2.3.);
estrone sulfotransferase (EC 2.8.2.4) which reacts with the phenolic group of estrogens;
bile acid sulfotransferase (EC 2.8.2.14).

However, this classification is temporary and will probably have to be modified in the future as additional substrates emerge. Thus, the existence of at least eight mammalian sulfotransferases has been cited (Singer et al., 1982), the first seven of which are rat liver enzymes: phenol sulfotransferases 1 and 2, specific estradiol sulfotransferase, three forms designated I, II and III (broad-specificity sulfotransferase I, 3β-hydroxysteroid sulfotransferase II, and glucocorticoid-preferring sulfotransferase III), mineralcorticoid sulfotransferase, and bovine estrogen-A-ring sulfotransferase. In addition, bile acid and carcinogen (aromatic hydroxylamine) sulfotransferase activity may represent unique forms of the enzyme. This enumeration demonstrates the wide variety of sulfotransferase substrates.

The highest levels of sulfotransferase activity are found in the liver, but other organs including the brain show some activity (Powell and Roy, 1980). Sulfotransferases are found in the brain of several species including the rat (Meek and Neff, 1973), and man (Renskers et al., 1980). Thus, in man, the sulfation of dopamine, of other biogenic amines, and of structurally related products is mediated by brain sulfotransferase found in the cytosol (Renskers et al., 1980). Several forms of phenol sulfotransferases exist in human tissues, activity in the frontal cortex being smaller by 1 to 2–3 orders of magnitude than that found in the adrenals, blood platelets or jejunum (Rein et al., 1982).

Sulfate conjugation is one of the three main routes of inactivation of catecholamines, together with COMT and MAO. Up to 80% of dopamine metabolites are sulfated in Parkinsonian patients (Rutledge and Hoehn, 1973). This finding suggests that alteration in sulfation reactions may influence the turnover equilibrium of catecholamines, particularly since the sulfoconjugation is concentration-dependent (Renskers et al., 1980).

Virtually nothing is known of the conjugation of xenobiotics by brain sulfotransferases, although sulfation of phenol by human frontal cortex 30 000 g supernatant has been demonstrated (Rein et al., 1982). Some indirect evidence also exists through competition for sulfotransferase occurring between drugs and endogenous molecules. Thus, pyrogallol and morphine interfere with the cerebral sulfoconjugation of 4-hydroxy-3-methoxyphenylethyleneglycol, the major metabolite of norepinephrine in the mammalian brain (Powell and Roy, 1980). A direct sulfation of morphine occurring within brain would be of particular interest in view of the very high affinity of morphine 6-sulfate, but not morphine 3-sulfate, for the opiate receptor (Oguri, 1980).

2.5.3 UDP-Glucuronyltransferases (EC 2.4.1.17)

UDP-glucuronyltransferase (UDPG-T) transfers D-glucuronic acid from uridine diphosphoglucuronic acid (UDPGA) to a considerable number of exogenous and endogenous substrates of varying structure, forming O-, N-, S- and C-glucuronides (Kasper and Henton, 1980). UDPG-T activity has been measured in several rat organs (Table 10) showing a very low level to exist in brain (Aitio and Marniemi, 1980). These results, however, may not be applicable to all species or all substrates due to the functional heterogeneity of the enzyme (Bock et al., 1982).

As early as 1967, Benzi et al. (Benzi et al., 1967) reported the formation of small amounts of oxazepam glucuronide in the isolated monkey brain perfused with an oxazepam solution. In contrast, the glucuronide of acetaminophen (paracetamol) was not detected in the brain of mice receiving a toxic dose, although the drug was present in relatively high concentrations and even though glucuronidation is its major route of metabolism (Fischer *et al.*, 1981).

TABLE 10

UDP-Glucuronyltransferase activity in 10 000 g supernatant preparations from rat tissues using 4-methylumbelliferone as the substrate (Aitio and Marniemi, 1980)

Tissue	Activity	
	nmol g^{-1} tissue min^{-1}	nmol per whole organ min^{-1}
Liver	460	3200
Duodenal mucosa	260	96
Adrenal gland	170	6·3
Kidney	150	120
Spleen	30	35
Lung	28	34
Thymus	19	8·8
Diaphragm	4·2	3·4
Heart	1·4	1·1
Brain	0·8	1·3

UDP-Glucuronyltransferase activities have recently been examined in mice brain microsomes (Shigezane *et al.*, 1982), showing 4-nitrophenol and 4-hydroxybiphenyl to be conjugated at rates approximately 200 and 1000 times smaller, respectively, than those in mice liver microsomes. While the glucuronidation of 4-methylumbelliferone was measurable, that of *ortho*-aminophenol, bilirubin, and morphine was too low to be determined. Interestingly, 4-nitrophenylglucuronide formation was markedly increased by the parenteral administration of 3-methylcholanthrene-type inducers, but not by that of phenobarbital. The existence of multiple enzymatic forms is indicated in mice brain microsomes.

Taken globally, the above results indicate modest cerebral UDPG-T activity with relatively limited significance.

2.5.4 N-*Acetyltransferase* (*EC 2.3.1.5*)

The acetyl-coenzyme A (Ac-CoA) dependent *N*-acetyltransferase displays a two-step mechanism involving an initial transfer of the acetyl group from Ac-CoA to form an acetyl-enzyme intermediate, followed by acetylation of the substrate with regeneration of the enzyme (Weber and Glowinski, 1980).

The substrates of *N*-acetyltransferase are primary amino groups such as are found in aromatic amines, hydrazines and hydrazides of moderate to weak basicity. In addition, some basic arylalkylamines also act as substrates

(Testa and Jenner, 1976, pp. 180–186; Weber and Glowinski, 1980). One of the most interesting aspects of *N*-acetylation is the existence in the rabbit and man of a hereditary polymorphism in the rate of xenobiotic acetylation, a phenomenon related to enzyme multiplicity (Weber and Glowinski, 1980; Patterson *et al.*, 1980).

N-Acetyltransferase is a cytosolic enzyme found in a variety of tissues from many species, although particulate forms also have been described (Weber *et al.*, 1980). The pineal gland contains a *N*-acetyltransferase involved in the synthesis of melatonin (L), a metabolite of serotonin, and a pineal hormone (Cardinali, 1981). Evidence for the existence of melatonin in the human brain has been described (Kopp *et al.*, 1980). Pineal *N*-acetylation of a variety of endogenous compounds (e.g. tryptamine, serotonin, and the borderline case phenylethylamine) occurs and in addition xenobiotics such as *para*-aminobenzoic acid, sulfamethazine, and 3,4-dimethoxyphenylethylamine are also substrates (Weber *et al.*, 1980). However, *N*-acetyltransferase activity is far from being limited to the pineal gland, and in rat brain occurs in every region investigated, although activity varies (Table 11). A number of properties of this enzyme have been described (Yu and Boulton, 1979; Weber and Glowinski, 1980).

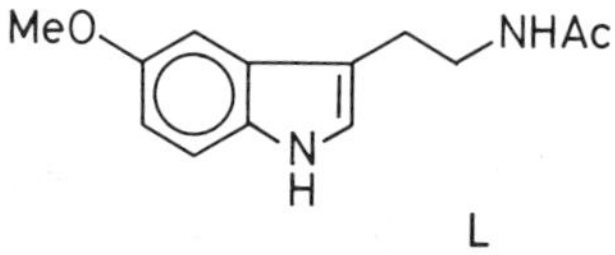

L

No systematic study for the acetylation of exogenous amines in brain has been conducted. Monkey brains perfused with a solution of aminopyrine produced small amounts of *N*-acetyl-4-aminoantipyrine (Benzi *et al.*, 1967). Similarly, rat brain preparations incubated with 3,4,5-trimethoxyphenyl-ethylamine (mescaline, LI) and Ac-CoA yielded the *N*-acetyl conjugate (Ho *et al.*, 1973). These two examples are of interest because they indicate acetylation of both a strongly and a moderately basic amine.

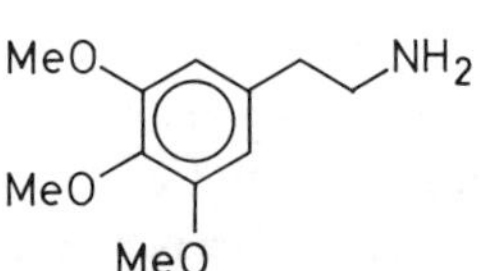

LI

Brain *N*-acetyltransferase therefore may play a role in the metabolism of exogenous bases crossing the blood-brain barrier. In addition, xenobiotics may inhibit the enzyme and thus interfere with its physiological function(s).

TABLE 11

Extrapineal N-acetylation in rat brain cytosol (Hsu *et al.*, 1976)

Region	Specific activity (nmol mg^{-1} protein h^{-1})	
	Tryptamine	Phenylethylamine
Whole brain	1·15 ± 0·14	1·98 ± 0·13
Cerebellum	1·64 ± 0·05	2·80 ± 0·30
Corpus callosum	1·04 ± 0·08	1·96 ± 0·11
Frontal cortex	1·02 ± 0·08	1·40 ± 0·15
Hippocampus	0·97 ± 0·03	1·60 ± 0·16
Parietal cortex	0·91 ± 0·10	1·29 ± 0·13
Pons/trapezoid	0·89 ± 0·08	1·34 ± 0·13
Cingulate cortex	0·86 ± 0·05	1·91 ± 0·17
Medulla	0·82 ± 0·06	1·57 ± 0·16
Midbrain	0·76 ± 0·09	1·47 ± 0·11
Septal nuclei	0·74 ± 0·06	1·03 ± 0·09
Lumbosacral cord	0·72 ± 0·06	1·69 ± 0·08
Hypothalamus	0·69 ± 0·10	1·18 ± 0·11
Corpus striatum	0·63 ± 0·06	1·32 ± 0·08
Cervical cord	0·59 ± 0·06	0·91 ± 0·13
Occipital cortex	0·57 ± 0·05	1·46 ± 0·14
Remainder of brain	0·88 ± 0·07	1·43 ± 0·12

That such interaction can occur is indicated by the study of Yang and Neff (1976) showing that β-carboline and indole derivatives (e.g. harmaline, harmine, harmane, harmol, melatonin) cause marked inhibition of rat brain N-acetyltransferase, but not of the pineal enzyme. The implications of these phenomena await a better understanding of the physiological role of brain N-acetyltransferase.

Choline acetyltransferase (EC 2.3.1.6), an O-acetyltransferase enzyme, will not be discussed here due to its very strict substrate specificity. Besides choline, only homocholine appears to be a substrate in rat brain preparations (Boksa and Collier, 1980).

2.5.5 Acylases

Conjugation with amino acids forms a major route for the metabolism of exogenous carboxylic acids. In this reaction, the acid is initially converted to acyl-CoA by enzymes known as acid:CoA ligases (EC 6.2.1.3, acyl-CoA synthetases, AMP-forming) which can activate C_4-C_{12} fatty acids and a range of aromatic acids. In the second step, the reactive acyl-CoA forms an amide derivative with an amino acid, e.g. glycine or glutamine, the reaction being catalysed by amino acid acylases such as glycine N-acyltransferase (EC 2.3.1.13) or glutamine N-acyltransferase (EC 2.3.1.14) (Caldwell *et al.*, 1980; Killenberg and Webster, 1980; Caldwell, 1982a).

It appears that glycine conjugation of exogenous acids does not occur in brain, as opposed to the liver and the kidney (Caldwell *et al.*, 1980).There is no data available on conjugation with other amino acids, such as glutamine. However, cerebral acylation reactions involving exogenous acids may not be as negligible as currently believed. We must consider that acyl-CoA intermediates not only result in the production of amino acid conjugates, but also in a pathway of chain elongation as exists in the anabolism of fatty acids.

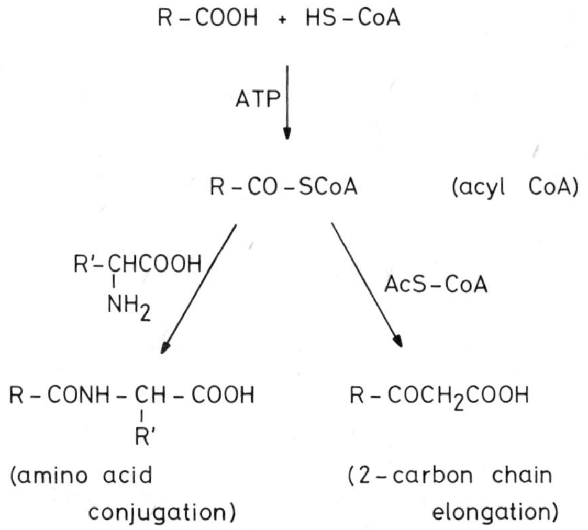

$$R - COOH + HS - CoA$$

ATP

$$R - CO - SCoA \qquad (acyl \quad CoA)$$

R'-CHCOOH
|
NH₂

AcS - CoA

R - CONH - CH - COOH
|
R'

R - COCH₂COOH

(amino acid conjugation)

(2 - carbon chain elongation)

FIG. 11. Acyl-CoA as a pivotal intermediate in the metabolism of carboxylic acids leading to amino acid conjugates or to chain elongation by a 2-carbon fragment (Marsh *et al.*, 1981; Caldwell, 1982b).

Figure 11 shows diagrammatically these aspects of carboxylic acid metabolism (Caldwell, 1982b). For example, the addition of a 2-carbon fragment to benzoic acid has been demonstrated in the horse (Marsh *et al.*, 1981). Also, of interest in the present context is the identification of phenylbutyric acid (LIII) as a cerebral metabolite in rats dosed with phenylacetic acid (LII) (Loo *et al.*, 1980). This suggests the cerebral formation of acyl-CoA from exogenous acids, followed by a second step such as chain elongation or mixed triglyceride formation (Caldwell, 1982b).

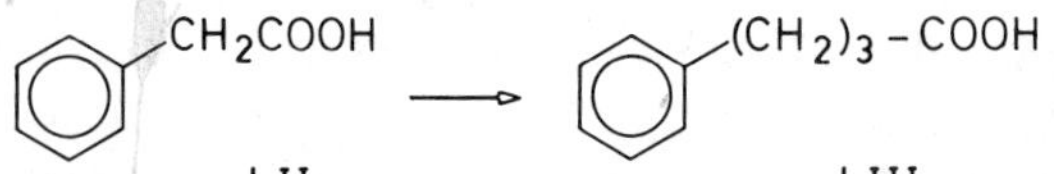

CH₂COOH

(CH₂)₃ - COOH

LII

LIII

Brain dysfunction induced by phenylacetic acid in experimental phenyl-ketonuria may be due to a reduced supply of CoA and acetyl-CoA affecting brain growth (Loo *et al.*, 1980).

2.5.6 Glutathione S-transferases (EC 2.5.1.18)

Glutathione is a tripeptide (L-γ-glutamyl-L-cysteinylglycine, GSH) found in all cells in concentrations ranging from 0·1 to 10 mM. For example, in rat organs, the concentration of glutathione ranges from 0·5 to 3 mM. However, these concentrations are subject to variation with respect to the growth, nutritional status and hormonal balance of the animal (Chasseaud, 1980).

GSH is a nucleophilic molecule reacting with a considerable variety of electrophilic structures in reactions catalysed by glutathione *S*-transferase (see, however, later for non-enzymatic reactions). The major classes of substrates include halogenonitrobenzenes and congeners, aryl nitro compounds, arylalkyl halides, aryl alkyl esters, alkyl and alicyclic halides and sulfates, alkyl methanesulfonates, allyl compounds, α,β-unsaturated carbonyls, organophosphorus compounds, and epoxides (Chasseaud, 1976; Testa and Jenner, 1976, pp. 205–214).

Several forms of GSH *S*-transferase exist; their classification according to chemical classes of substrates was an empirical one which became obsolete when the various isozymes were physically separated. Thus various trans-ferases designated AA, A, B, C, D and E have been isolated from rat liver cytosol (Testa and Jenner, 1976, pp. 325–328; Jakoby and Habig, 1980). Some of these forms are also microsomal, and differ in their inducibility from the soluble isozymes (Friedberg *et al.*, 1979; Mukhtar *et al.*, 1981a). Gluta-thione *S*-transferase B has been identified as the cytoplasmic binding protein ligandin (Jakoby and Habig, 1980).

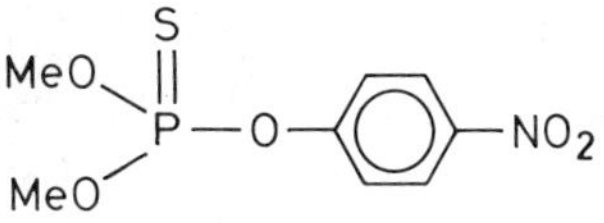

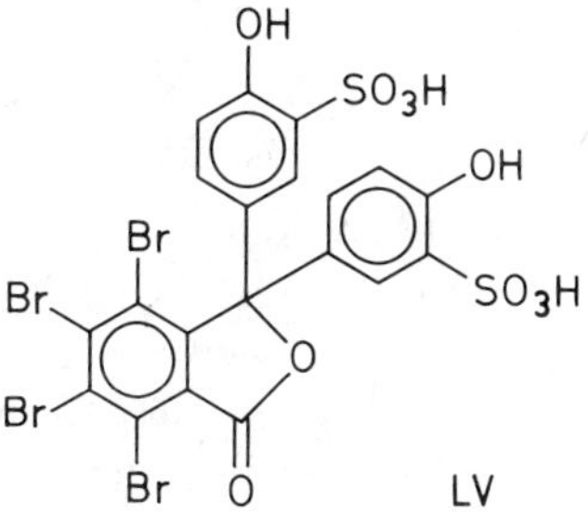

A number of reports document the presence of GSH *S*-transferase in brain, although ligandin appears to be absent from the central nervous system where it could provide protection from compounds such as bilirubin

(Arias *et al.*, 1976). Rat brain GSH *S*-transferase does not react detectably with methyl iodide, but metabolizes methyl parathion (LIV), diazinon and bromosulfophthalein (LV) at rates which are 5–10% of those found in the liver (Chasseaud, 1980). The GSH *S*-transferase activity towards 1-chloro-1, 4-dinitrobenzene and acrylamide in rat brain has been measured and compared to the hepatic activity (Dixit *et al.*, 1981). The results (Table 12) show relatively high activity in brain although the absence of standard deviations in this publication precludes a meaningful comparison. It must be noted that the results in Table 12 show enzymatic activity; the non-enzymatic reaction of glutathione with acrylamide was estimated at about half the rate of the enzymatic reaction in brain.

TABLE 12

Glutathione *S*-transferase activity in rat brain and liver (Dixit *et al.*, 1981)

Parameter	Liver	Brain
Enzymic activity towards		
CDNB[a]	4836	937
acrylamide[b]	0·243	0·081
K_m for CDNB	1·6 mM	2·5 mM
k_i of acrylamide towards		
CDNB[c]	4·0 mM	3·0 mM

[a]1-Chloro-2,4-dinitrobenzene, activity in nmol conjugate mg^{-1} protein min^{-1}.
[b]Activity in nmol GSH consumed per mg protein min^{-1}.
[c]Inhibition constants derived from Dixon plots.

Species, sex, strain and age variation in GSH *S*-transferase activity occur in brain and other organs (Das *et al.*, 1981a; Wheldrake *et al.*, 1981; Di Ilio *et al.*, 1982). In the rat, the ratio of cytosolic to microsomal activity shows considerable organ variation, its value being, e.g. 23 in the brain, 39 in the kidney, but only 5 in the lung (DePierre and Morgenstern, 1983).

In man, GSH *S*-transferase activity is quite marked, as shown by the investigation of Mukhtar *et al.* (1981b) using postmortem samples from 34 different organs of one or more of 132 individuals. The results for the activity in brain are quite comparable to those found in other tissues; the values (Table 13) show marked inter-individual variation over a ten-fold range, but not age-related differences. Noteworthy are the high fetal activities. The regulation of brain GSH *S*-transferase by sex hormones has been studied (Das *et al.*, 1982a), increasing our feeble understanding of metabolic regulations in connection with xenobiotic cerebral biotransformation.

An interesting aspect of GSH *S*-transferases is their inducibility, which has also been studied for the cerebral enzymes. Thus, 5 days' administration

TABLE 13

Postmortem glutathione S-transferase activity towards 1-chloro-2,4-dinitrobenzene
in human brain (Mukhtar et al., 1981b)

Individual	Activity (nmol conjugate mg^{-1} protein min^{-1})
Fetus	
12 weeks	132
13 weeks	127
16 weeks	23
24 weeks	55
Neonate	
3 weeks	55
Adult	
25 years	191
40 years	61
41 years	41
59 years	92
63 years	69

of 3-methylcholanthrene or benzo[a]pyrene to rats markedly induced brain
glutathione transferase activity towards 1-chloro-1,4-dinitrobenzene, while
phenobarbital was without effect (Das et al., 1981b). A recent study shows
that phenobarbital is a quite potent inducer of the brain enzyme under
identical animal and substrate conditions, but only after 21 days' administration (Chand and Clausen, 1982). Transplacental induction by 5,6-benzo-
flavone occurs in rats and mice (Table 7) (Rouet et al., 1981).

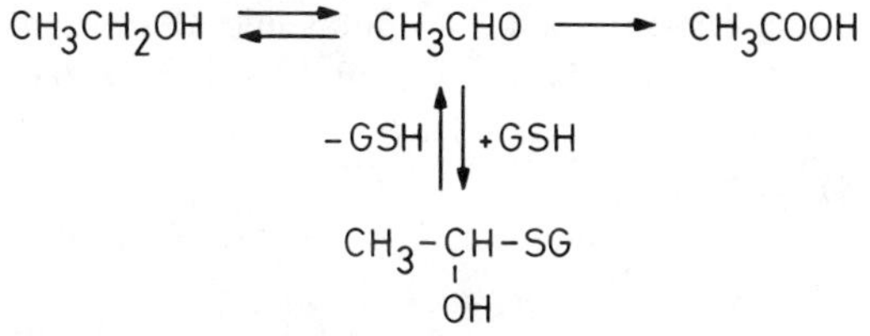

$$CH_3CH_2OH \rightleftharpoons CH_3CHO \longrightarrow CH_3COOH$$

$$-GSH \uparrow \downarrow +GSH$$

$$CH_3-\underset{\underset{OH}{|}}{CH}-SG$$

FIG. 12. Glutathione thiohemiacetal formation in the metabolism of ethanol
(from Ketterer, 1982).

For a number of electrophiles, non-enzymatic conjugation with GSH may
contribute significantly to the overall reaction. This topic has been extensively
discussed by Ketterer (1982), who showed that the relative importance of the
enzymatic versus non-enzymatic contributions depends both on the sus-
ceptibility of the electrophile to nucleophilic attack by GSH, and on the

catalytic effectiveness of the GSH transferases. The non-enzymatic contribution has to be taken into account in studies assessing cerebral GSH conjugation reactions. One example in which the non-enzymatic reaction may have clear toxicological implications is in the reversible formation of a glutathione thiohemiacetal from GSH and acetaldehyde (Fig. 12), as discussed by Ketterer (1982). This thiohemiacetal can provide a non-toxic reservoir of acetaldehyde, and it might be of interest to study it with respect to the cerebral metabolism of ethanol (see sections 2.2.1 and 2.2.2) as well as to the reaction of acetaldehyde with catecholamines (see next section).

Glutathione conjugation is classically considered as a detoxication process. Of particular relevance to the brain is the reaction of oxidized 6-hydroxydopamine (6-OHDA quinone, XXII in Fig. 6, see section 2.1.10) with GSH to yield the 2-S-glutathionyl derivative (LVI). This latter conjugate has been identified in the brain of rats and mice where 6-OHDA was injected into the hypothalamus (Liang et $al.$, 1977). Such a reaction certainly decreases the toxicity of 6-OHDA. But because so many compounds or their metabolites can react with GSH, competition for this thiol may result in increased toxicity of electrophiles.

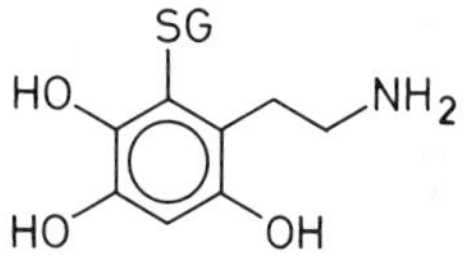

LVI

In other, although rare cases, GSH conjugation may directly lead to the synthesis of a reactive metabolite. Thus the glutathione conjugate (LVII) of 1,2-dibromoethane rearranges to a mutagenic thiiranium ion (LVIII) (van Bladeren et $al.$, 1980). The latter may bind covalently to cellular macromolecules, but may also be detoxified by hydration or by reaction with a second molecule of GSH.

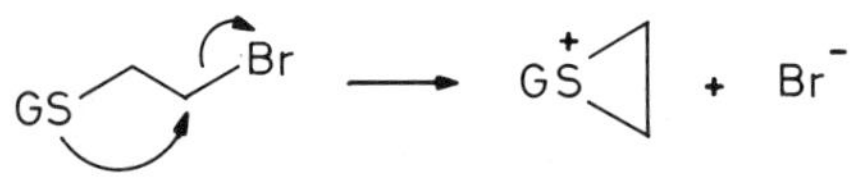

LVII   LVIII

In a number of cases, glutathione conjugates are excreted as such in the bile, but most are further degraded to mercapturic acids, which are conjugates of N-acetylcysteine (Tate, 1980). The brain has most, if not all, the enzymatic machinery necessary for the degradation of GSH conjugates (e.g. γ-glutamyl transpeptidase, EC 2.3.2.2, Reyes and Barela, 1980), although the cerebral formation of N-acetylcysteine conjugates (the term "mercapturic acids" is no longer appropriate in this case) has not been reported.

2.6 CONDENSATION REACTIONS TO ALKALOID-LIKE COMPOUNDS

Catecholamines such as epinephrine, norepinephrine or dopamine, and indolethylamines such as serotonin condense non-enzymatically with aldehydes such as acetaldehyde, formaldehyde or 3,4-dihydroxyphenyl-acetaldehyde, or with α-ketoacids, to yield basic bi- or polycyclic compounds. The first product of the reaction is a Schiff's base, which further undergoes a Pictet–Spengler reaction causing cyclization to tetrahydroisoquinoline (TIQ) or tetrahydro-β-carboline (THBC) derivatives (O'Donnell, 1982). A number of these condensation products have been detected *in vivo* in brain and other organs, or shown to be formed *in vitro*. Figures 13 and 14 display a selection of products formed from dopamine and tryptamines, respectively.

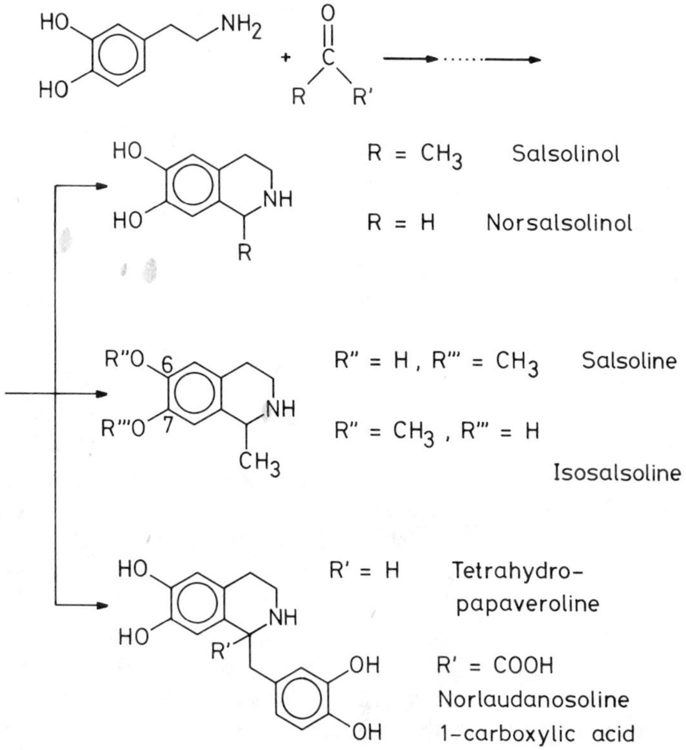

FIG. 13. Some condensation products of dopamine with aldehydes or α-ketoacids.

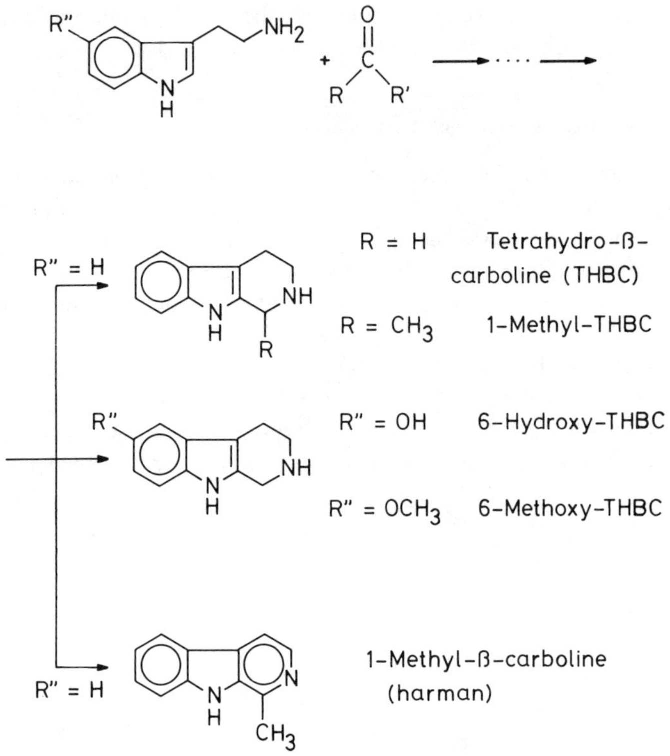

FIG. 14. Some condensation products of tryptamines with aldehydes.

Formation of condensation products occurs physiologically *in vivo*, but in some cases is markedly increased following ingestion of compounds such as alcohol or L-DOPA, or under pathological conditions such as phenylketonuria. Thus, the urinary excretion of salsolinol and (iso)salsoline is higher in alcoholics than in control subjects (Collins *et al.*, 1979).

These endogenous alkaloids exhibit a variety of biological actions of considerable importance and which have been extensively reviewed by Melchior and Collins (1982). Toxicity is apparent from the adrenergic nerve degeneration and hepatonecrosis induced by the condensation product of epinephrine with acetaldehyde (Azevedo and Osswald, 1977; Moura *et al.*, 1977). Some postulated neurological and psychiatric consequences of endogenous alkaloids will be considered in section 4.3.1.

3 Cerebral cytochrome P-450s and their reactions

General enzymatic and mechanistic aspects of cytochrome P-450s have already been considered in section 2.1.4, while the present section is specifically concerned with cerebral monooxygenases. To the best of our knowledge, this topic has never been reviewed. This is primarily due to the novelty of drug metabolism in this organ and despite a rapidly growing awareness of the physiological, pharmacological and toxicological implications. In an authoritative review published in 1980, Connelly and Bridges (Connelly and Bridges, 1980) examined the distribution and role of cytochrome P-450 in extrahepatic organs, giving due attention to the brain. Now, much more information is available.

3.1 SPECTRAL CHARACTERIZATION OF CEREBRAL CYTOCHROME P-450s

The characterization and quantification of cytochrome P-450 by the difference spectra of the CO-ferrocytochrome P-450 complex has become a standard technique following the studies of Omura and Sato (1962, 1964).

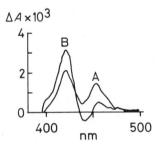

FIG. 15. Detection of cytochrome P-450 in rat brain microsomes. Sample cuvette: CO-dithionite reduced microsomes. Reference cuvette: dithionite-reduced microsomes. (A) Before, and (B) two minutes after addition of methylmercury chloride; protein concentration 1·75 mg ml^{-1}. (Cohn *et al.*, 1977. Reproduced with the permission of the Rockefeller University Press, New York.)

3.1.1 Subcellular and regional distribution of monooxygenase components

In dithionite-reduced microsomes from rat whole brain, Cohn *et al.* (1977) unambiguously identified cytochrome P-450 in the CO-difference spectrum (Fig. 15). Addition of methylmercury chloride resulted in degradation to inactive cytochrome P-420 (Fig. 15). However, it was not possible to quantify the concentration of the enzyme. In contrast, Sasame *et al.* (1977) succeeded in measuring the levels of cytochrome P-450 (and NADPH-cytochrome *c* reductase, see later) in both rat brain and liver microsomes. The levels in rat brain microsomes were 0.036 ± 0.004 nmol mg^{-1} protein as compared to 0.98 ± 0.06 nmol mg^{-1} protein in hepatic microsomes. The liver/brain ratio was thus determined as 27.

Guengerich and Mason (1979) found somewhat lower concentrations of cytochrome P-450 in rat brain (see section 3.1.2., Table 18), while Marietta *et al.* (1979) have confirmed the findings of Sasame *et al.* (1977) (Table 14). Microsomes from brain have an apparent lower content of cytochrome P-450 than the hepatic microsomes when compared on a gram of tissue basis than on a mg of protein basis, due to a poorer yield of microsomes. Interestingly, the brain has a relatively high content of cytochrome P-450 when the whole homogenate is considered. The losses of activity may according to Marietta *et al.* (1979) reflect the more lipidic and heterogenous composition of the brain, rendering the isolation of its microsomal hemoproteins more difficult. These losses also may reflect the relatively high levels of extra-microsomal cytochrome P-450 in brain, as discussed later.

TABLE 14

Comparison of the levels of cytochrome P-450 in rat brain and liver preparations (Marietta *et al.*, 1979)

	Cytochrome P-450		
	Microsomes		Homogenate
	(nmol mg^{-1} protein)	(nmol g^{-1} tissue)	(nmol g^{-1} tissue)
Brain	0.035 ± 0.003	0.160 ± 0.041	2.82 ± 0.30
Liver	1.19 ± 0.13	19.8 ± 3.8	32.6 ± 3.9
Liver/brain ratio	33.6	123	11.5

The spectral evidence for the presence of cytochrome P-450 in rat brain microsomes, as published by Sasame *et al.* (1977) and Marietta *et al.* (1979), is shown in Figs 16 and 17, respectively. Very similar spectra result from the reduction of microsomes with either NADPH (Fig. 16) or dithionite (Fig. 17). The larger peak in the 425 nm region is due to cytochrome b$_5$ (see later). Besides the CO-binding spectra of reduced cytochrome P-450, the oxidized enzyme yields type I binding spectra with substrates, and type II or reverse type I (also called modified type II) binding spectra with ligands. Very few such spectra have been reported for cerebral cytochrome P-450. Of particular interest is the reverse type I binding spectrum of 17β-estradiol (Fig. 18) as determined by Sasame *et al.* (1977). The fact that this steroid yields a typical type I spectrum with rat hepatic microsomes suggests binding to different isozymes in the brain and liver.

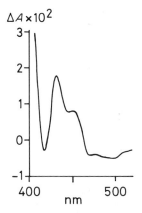

FIG. 16. Detection of cytochrome P-450 in rat brain microsomes. Sample cuvette: CO-NADPH reduced microsomes. Reference cuvette: CO-native (oxidized) microsomes; hemoprotein concentration 80 pmol ml^{-1}. (Sasame *et al.*, 1977.)

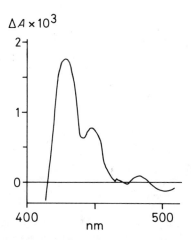

FIG. 17. Detection of cytochrome P-450 in rat brain microsomes. Sample cuvette: CO-dithionite reduced microsomes. Reference cuvette: CO-native (oxidized) microsomes. Protein concentration 2·5 mgml^{-1}. (Marietta *et al.*, 1979. Reproduced with the permission of the American Society for Pharmacology and Experimental Therapeutics.)

In mouse brain microsomes purified from haemoglobin, cytochrome P-450 levels (see section 3.1.2, Table 17) are lower than those found in rat brain (Nabeshima *et al.*, 1981). The methodology employed by Marietta *et al.* (1979) suggests the difference not to be due to haemoglobin contamination (see section 3.1.3) but to genuinely reflect a species difference. A

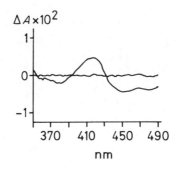

FIG. 18. Reverse type I (modified type II) binding spectrum of 17β-estradiol to native (oxidized) rat brain microsomes; hemoprotein concentration 80 pmol ml⁻¹, ligand concentration 0·3 mM (Sasame *et al.*, 1977).

considerable difference, over ten-fold, also exists in the levels of NADPH-cytochrome c reductase found in rat and mouse brain microsomes (Table 15, see also Table 17). Verification of this apparent difference is required.

TABLE 15

NADPH- and NADH-dependent reductase activities in microsomes of various rat brain regions (activities in nmol mg⁻¹ protein min⁻¹) (Takeshita *et al.*, 1982)

Region	NADPH-cyt c reductase	NADH-cyt b_5 reductase
Cerebral hemisphere	52·3 ± 2·9	13·9 ± 4·4
Midbrain	37·6 ± 2·6	10·5 ± 1·0
Cerebellum	20·5 ± 2·5	4·2 ± 2·3
Medulla oblongata	36·4 ± 0·1	14·8 ± 1·9

As mentioned above, cytochrome b_5 can be detected in rat brain microsomes (e.g. Figs 16 and 17). As early as 1965, Inouye and Shinagawa (1965) characterized this enzyme in rabbit brain microsomes, reporting amounts of 0.022 nmol mg⁻¹ protein. Practically no cytochrome b_5 was found in non-microsomal fractions.

Cytochrome P-450 can be demonstrated in the mitochondrial fraction of bovine brain (Oftebro *et al.*, 1979). Using methods devised to avoid interference by cytochrome oxidase, haemoglobin and methaemoglobin, a CO-binding spectrum similar to that of Fig. 16 was obtained. The amount of cytochrome P-450 was determined to be 0·57 nmol mg⁻¹ protein. Mito-chondrial cytochrome P-450 from the adrenal cortex, as opposed to the microsomal enzymes of various tissues, is not reduced directly by NADPH-cytochrome P-450 reductase (Fig. 3), but via an iron-sulfur protein known as ferredoxin. The presence of ferredoxin in bovine brain mitochondria (Oftebro *et al.*, 1979) indicates that mitochondrial cytochrome P-450-dependent hydroxylation systems are not limited to typically steroidogenic tissues such as the adrenal cortex, testis, ovaries and placenta, but also occur in brain next to organs such as the liver and kidneys.

In rat brain, mitochondrial cytochrome P-450 appears to predominate over that found in microsomes (25 ± 6 pmol mg^{-1} protein compared to 12 ± 6 pmol mg^{-1} protein) (Percy and Shanley, 1979). After administration of labelled 5-aminolaevulinic acid (a precursor of porphyrin) to rats, the radioactivity in brain mitochondria was approximately 5-times that measurable in brain microsomes, while in the liver the ratio was found to be the reverse (Percy and Shanley, 1979). These findings confirm the importance of mitochondrial cytochrome P-450 in brain.

Very little is known of the regional localization of cerebral cytochrome P-450 as investigated by spectral methods. In rat pups, the amount of cytochrome P-450 in the cerebrum was $0 \cdot 015$–$0 \cdot 029$ nmol mg^{-1} microsomal protein compared to $0 \cdot 030$–$0 \cdot 045$ nmol mg^{-1} microsomal protein in the cerebellum (Holtzman *et al.*, 1981). The corresponding values for cytochrome b_5 were $0 \cdot 041$–$0 \cdot 051$ and $0 \cdot 039$–$0 \cdot 066$ nmol mg^{-1} microsomal protein, respectively (Holtzman *et al.*, 1981). In the bovine brain, cytochrome b_5 (in nmol mg^{-1} microsomal protein) ranked in the order cortex $0 \cdot 012$, subcortical areas $0 \cdot 011$, midbrain $0 \cdot 007$, spinal cord and cerebellum $0 \cdot 005$, brainstem $0 \cdot 004$ (Inouye and Shinagawa, 1965). Rather large species differences occur between rabbit, cow and guinea pig (Inouye and Shinagawa, 1965). Corresponding results for cytochrome P-450 have been obtained by monitoring biotransformation reactions and will be considered later.

The two flavoproteins reductases (see Fig. 3) involved in the transfer of electrons to cytochrome P-450 can also be detected in brain microsomes by spectrally monitoring their activity. In rat brain microsomes, NADPH-cytochrome c (P-450) reductase activity was found to be $38 \cdot 9 \pm 4 \cdot 1$ nmol mg^{-1} protein min^{-1}, as compared to $121 \cdot 0 \pm 9 \cdot 0$ nmol mg^{-1} protein min^{-1} in rat hepatic microsomes (Sasame *et al.*, 1977). The liver/brain ratio is thus $3 \cdot 1$, i.e. ten-fold smaller than the corresponding ratio for cytochrome P-450 (see earlier). Why the NADPH reductase/cytochrome P-450 ratio should be ten-fold larger in rat brain than liver microsomes is not known but may be linked to the particular physiological function of the reductase in brain, or to organ differences in the turnover rate of the two enzymes.

NADH-cytochrome b_5 reductase was also characterized in rat brain (Takeshita *et al.*, 1982). The two reductases show a 2–3 fold variation in activity in various rat brain regions (Table 15) but the significance of these findings remains to be determined.

In conclusion, all four components (the two cytochromes and the two reductases) of cytochrome P-450 dependent monooxygenases exist in brain preparations, at least in the rat.

3.1.2 Influence of age and inducers

Brain cytochrome P-450 and b_5 levels in the rat vary as a function of age (Holtzman and Desautel, 1980). The cytochrome b_5 content increases between 30 days of age and maturity in both cerebrum and cerebellum, and this increase occurs independently of any change in cytochrome P-450 content (Table 16). Cytochrome P-450 levels increase between 5 days of age and maturity in the cerebrum, while in the cerebellum adult levels (identical to the cerebral ones) already exist in the pup.

TABLE 16

Variation with age of the amount of cytochromes P-450 and b_5 in rat brain (results in nmol mg^{-1} microsomal protein) (Holtzman and Desautel, 1980)

Age (days)	Cerebrum		Cerebellum	
	b_5	P-450	b_5	P-450
5	0·048 ± 0·004	0·019 ± 0·002	0·042 ± 0·013	0·036 ± 0·004
10	0·049 ± 0·004	0·027 ± 0·003	0·044 ± 0·016	0·030 ± 0·006
15	0·043 ± 0·004	0·021 ± 0·003	0·056 ± 0·006	0·039 ± 0·004
20	0·050 ± 0·005	0·028 ± 0·003	0·050 ± 0·006	0·034 ± 0·003
30	0·056 ± 0·005	0·027 ± 0·002	0·067 ± 0·004	0·029 ± 0·003
Adults	0·087 ± 0·011	0·035 ± 0·004	0·114 ± 0·021	0·033 ± 0·003

One of the most striking observations consistently made is the very high b_5/P-450 ratio found in brain as opposed to liver and most other tissues. This suggests that in brain cytochrome b_5 may exist both as an independent reductase and in association with cytochrome P-450.

Induction of cytochrome P-450 in brain has been monitored using marker substrates and hence will be considered later. Spectral determinations are of interest as an index of change in the entire population of cytochrome P-450s rather than ill-defined isozymes. Spectral and biochemical determinations thus are complementary, and it is regrettable that so few spectrally monitored induction studies have been published.

Tolerance to pentobarbital and morphine in mice was accompanied by changes in both cytochrome P-450 levels and NADPH-cytochrome c reductase activity in the liver (Nabeshima et al., 1981). Pentobarbital acted as an inducer of both enzymes, while morphine markedly decreased hepatic cytochrome P-450 levels without affecting reductase activity (Table 17). In contrast, neither drug had any clear effect on either cytochrome P-450 or NADPH-cytochrome c reductase in the brain.

TABLE 17

Effect of pentobarbital and morphine on liver and brain levels of cytochrome P-450 and NADPH-cytochrome c reductase in mice (Nabeshima *et al.*, 1981)

	Placebo[a]	Pentobarbital[a]	Morphine[a]
Cytochrome P-450			
Liver			
nmol mg^{-1} protein	0·525 ± 0·039	0·867 ± 0·039	0·367 ± 0·029
nmol g^{-1} tissue	23·9 ± 1·2	37·1 ± 0·7	14·9 ± 0·2
Brain			
nmol mg^{-1} protein	0·0107 ± 0·0002	0·0109 ± 0·0003	0·0097 ± 0·0004
nmol g^{-1} tissue	0·108 ± 0·010	0·112 ± 0·010	0·093 ± 0·010
NADPH-cytochrome c reductase (nmol mg^{-1} protein min^{-1})			
Liver	63·9 ± 1·0	101·2 ± 1·2	67·1 ± 1·7
Brain	3·01 ± 0·18	2·88 ± 0·10	2·28 ± 0·33

[a]Mice were implanted for 3 days with a pellet (placebo, 75 mg pentobarbital, or 75 mg morphine).

A comprehensive study by Guengerich and Mason (1979) compared the levels of cytochrome P-450 in a number of rat organs following 5 days' treatment with phenobarbital or 3 days' treatment with 3-methylcholanthrene (Table 18). The liver, testes, lungs and spleen responded to the inducers with a 2–3-fold increase in cytochrome P-450 levels. The heart, kidneys, stomach, colon and small intestine showed no increase. The brain responded to the inducers with a moderate but presumably genuine increase in cytochrome P-450 levels. However, the number of determinations ($n = 2$) does not allow statistical treatment. Indeed, these results may conflict with the lack of induction of cytochrome P-450 in mouse brain following pentobarbital treatment (Table 17) (Nabeshima *et al.*, 1981).

A number of enzymes are involved in the synthesis of cytochrome P-450 (for a general scheme see Testa and Jenner, 1981). The rate-limiting enzyme is 5-aminolaevulinate synthetase (ALA-synthetase, EC 2.3.1.37). In rat brain, homogenates of cerebellum showed the highest activity (56 pmol mg^{-1} protein h^{-1}) followed by midbrain and cortex (35 pmol mg^{-1} protein h^{-1}) while other brain regions were less active (Maines, 1980). Activity in whole homogenates from rat liver was 75 pmol mg^{-1} protein h^{-1}, indicating similar levels of this enzyme in brain as compared to liver. Such a finding contrasts with the fact that other enzymes of haem biosynthesis, namely

TABLE 18

Induction of cytochrome P-450 in microsomes from various rat tissues (results in nmol mg^{-1} protein) (Guengerich and Mason, 1979)

Tissue	Control	Phenobarbital	3-Methylcholanthrene
Liver	0·96 ± 0·05	2·02 ± 0·14	1·66 ± 0·35
Heart	0·12 ± 0·01	0·18 ± 0·004	0·12 ± 0·06
Kidney	0·064 ± 0·003	0·076 ± 0·008	0·076 ± 0·001
Stomach	0·030 ± 0·011	0·015 ± 0·002	0·025 ± 0·006
Testis	0·019 ± 0·004	0·066 ± 0·010	0·062 ± 0·007
Brain	0·017 ± 0·007	0·028 ± 0·001	0·024 ± 0·007
Lung	0·009 ± 0·003	0·027 ± 0·005	0·034 ± 0·009
Colon	< 0·008	< 0·006	< 0·007
Spleen	< 0·005	0·016 ± 0·002	0·014 ± 0·010
Small intestine	< 0·004	< 0·002	< 0·008

ALA-dehydratase (EC 4.2.1.24), uroporphyrinogen I (EC 4.3.1.8), uroporphyrinogen decarboxylase (EC 4.1.1.37) and ferrochelatase (EC 4.99.1.1), have activities in rat brain which range between 12% and 0·2% of those found in rat liver (Percy and Shanley, 1979). Futhermore, the cerebral enzymes involved in haem biosynthesis appear unaffected by treatments (e.g. starvation, phenobarbital) which influence the same enzymes in the liver. This may suggest that cellular demand for haem in brain would not be expected to fluctuate significantly, hence the absence of sensitive control mechanisms. This interpretation, however, must be considered with great care since marked induction of cytochrome P-450 is detectable in brain when marker substrates are assayed (see later). Obviously many more studies (e.g. De Matteis and Ray, 1982) are required before the brain biochemistry of haem in general and cytochrome P-450 in particular are sufficiently understood.

3.1.3 Experimental difficulties

The measurement of cytochrome P-450 levels in brain preparations is rendered difficult by the low amounts and by the presence of haemoglobin. Haemoglobin forms with CO a complex which interferes with the spectral determination of the CO-cytochrome P-450 complex. This leads to an exaggerated estimation of cytochrome P-450 levels, especially in tissues where they are low. The method of killing influences the blood content of the brain. Rinsing of the brain removes only a proportion of the blood, but perfusion is more effective. Furthermore, particulate fractions (mitochondria, microsomes, etc.) should be repeatedly washed by resuspension and centrifugation.

However, despite these precautions, the manner in which the difference spectra are recorded is of considerable importance. One of the best methods to eliminate haemoglobin interferences appears to be to introduce CO into both cuvettes, and to reduce with an appropriate reducing agent the microsomes in the sample cuvette (e.g. Figs 16 and 17). One paper describing such a method is that of Johannesen and DePierre (1978).

3.2 OXIDATIVE DESULFURATION

The cytochrome P-450 dependent oxidative metabolism of parathion is shown in Fig. 19. Monooxygenation leads to the formation of an intermediate oxathiaphosphirane derivative which breaks down to two metabolites. By expulsion of a sulfur atom, paraoxon is formed which is the oxygenated analogue of parathion and extremely toxic. The released sulfur atom binds to apocytochrome P-450, which is thus destroyed, and to other proteins (see Testa and Jenner, 1978, 1981). In addition, the oxathiaphosphirane intermediate can decompose by an initial hydrolytic cleavage to para-nitrophenol and diethyl phosphorothioic acid. These latter metabolites are relatively non-toxic, in contrast to paraoxon and to the activated sulfur atom. Thus parathion metabolism can have considerable toxicological importance.

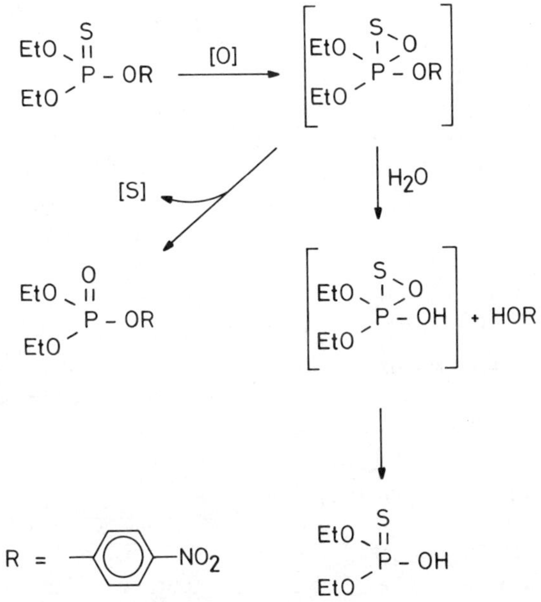

FIG. 19. The oxidative metabolism of parathion (from Testa and Jenner, 1976, p. 113).

The oxidative desulfuration of parathion was one of the first cytochrome P-450 mediated reactions extensively investigated in brain. Using a rat brain microsomal preparation Norman and Neal (1976) found the following K_m (in μM) and V_{max} (in pmol mg^{-1} protein min^{-1}) values: ^{35}S binding, $K_m = 30 \pm 3$, $V_{max} = 40 \pm 2$; paraoxon formation, $K_m = 24 \pm 3$, $V_{max} = 41 \pm 7$; diethyl phosphorothioic acid formation, $K_m = 59 \pm 9$, $V_{max} = 6 \pm 1$. These values demonstrate that the brain is capable of activiting parathion to toxic products, and in particular that covalent binding of sulfur does occur. The involvement of cytochrome P-450 was proven by the inhibitory effects of CO, SKF-525A and piperonyl butoxide.

As found with rat lung but in contrast to the liver, phenobarbital and 3-methylcholanthrene did not induce parathion metabolism in brain. NADPH was required for optimal activity, but in its absence the brain reaction, but not that in lung, proceeded to a significant extent. This might suggest both NADH- and NADPH-dependent activities, a point which will be discussed again below.

3.3 ARYL HYDROCARBON HYDROXYLASE ACTIVITY

3.3.1 Properties, distribution, species differences

Aryl hydrocarbon hydroxylase (AHH) is a cytochrome P-450 dependent activity oxidizing aromatic substrates, essentially polycyclic aromatic hydrocarbons (PAHs). AHH activity is induced by many compounds including PAHs and polyhalogenated aromatic hydrocarbons.

AHH is of interest in relation to the metabolic activation of PAHs to potent mutagens and carcinogens. Cohn et al. (1977) apparently were the first to detect AHH activity in rat brain. Using benzo[a]pyrene (BP, LIX) as substrate and 8-hydroxy-BP as the fluorescence standard, they reported reaction rates of 5 ± 1 pmol hydroxy-BP mg^{-1} protein h^{-1} in whole homogenates and 30 pmol hydroxy-BP mg^{-1} protein h^{-1} in whole homogenates and 30 pmol hydroxy-BP mg^{-1} protein h^{-1} in microsomes. However, since the main metabolite is 3-hydroxy-BP rather than the 8-hydroxy derivatives, the data may not be comparable with that of other studies reported below, which use 3-hydroxy-BP as the fluorescence standard. Thus, Guengerich and Mason (1979) report AHH activity in brain microsomes from uninduced rats of 24 ± 2 pmol 3-hydroxy-BP nmol^{-1} P-450 min^{-1} (see Table 24 in the next section). This value is in relative agreement with that published by Marietta et al. (1979), namely 9·5 pmol 3-hydroxy-BP nmol^{-1} P-450 min^{-1}.

Das and colleagues have extensively studied brain AHH. Brain microsomal AHH (Das et al., 1981c) showed a higher affinity for BP than liver microsomal AHH (K_m values 5·0–6·7 versus 40·0–46·5 μM, respectively), but with a

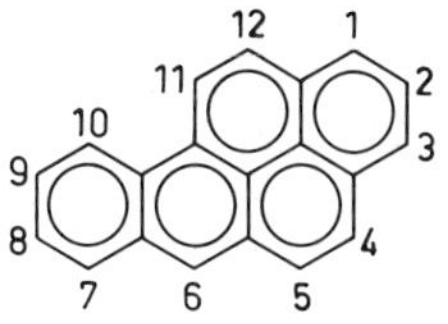

LIX

considerably lower rate of reaction (V_{max} 1·5–1·6 versus 400–415 pmol 3-hydroxy-BP mg^{-1} protein min^{-1}, respectively). These differences reflected the much lower AHH activity in brain than in liver, and also differences in the nature of the cytochrome P-450 isozymes involved. Further differences will become apparent in the next section where inhibition and induction experiments are discussed.

Specific AHH activity in brain is lower than in other organs, especially the liver (Table 19). When values are calculated in terms of whole organ activity, brain represents 0·025%, 0·9% and 27% of liver, kidney and lung activity respectively (Das *et al.*, 1981c). Only small regional differences in AHH exist in rat brain (Table 19). The subcellular distribution of brain AHH (Table 19) shows equal specific activity in microsomes and mitochondria, confirming the conclusion reached in section 3.1.1. Cytosolic activity (Table 19) appears due to contamination, while activity in the nuclear fraction may be partly genuine.

TABLE 19

Organ region and fraction distribution of aryl hydrocarbon hydroxylase activity in adult rat (Das *et al.*, 1981c)

Organ, region or fraction	Specific activity[a]	Total organ activity[b]
Liver[c]	101·3 ± 8·6	14 000 ± 1420
Lung[c]	1·77 ± 0·32	13·5 ± 1·6
Kidney[c]	22·2 ± 1·7	408 ± 28
Brain[c]	0·79 ± 0·08	3·65 ± 0·24
cerebrum[c]	1·03 ± 0·05	2·14 ± 0·26
cerebellum[c]	1·35 ± 0·05	0·72 ± 0·05
brain stem[c]	0·87 ± 0·08	0·76 ± 0·05
homogenate	0·27 — 0·28	
nuclei	0·13 — 0·17	
mitochondria	0·68 — 0·71	
14 000 g supernatant	0·28 — 0.34	
microsomes	0·70	
cytosol	0·06 — 0·08	

[a]in pmol 3-hydroxy-BP mg^{-1} protein min^{-1}.
[b]in pmol 3-hydroxy-BP per organ min^{-1}.
[c]Microsomes.

TABLE 20

Microsomal aryl hydrocarbon hydroxylase activity in rodent and avian brain
(Das *et al.*, 1981c)

Animals	Specific activity[a]	Total organ activity[b]
Rodent		
Rat		
male	0·75 ± 0·02	2·35 ± 0·06
female	0·73 ± 0·05	2·03 ± 0·20
Mouse		
male	0·37 ± 0·02	0·39 ± 0·02
female	0·43 ± 0·02	0·38 ± 0·02
Guinea pig		
male	0·26 ± 0·03	1·82 ± 0·20
female	0·40 ± 0·04	1·82 ± 0·20
Avians		
Pigeon		
male	0·15 ± 0·02	0·50 ± 0·11
female	0·11 ± 0·02	0·39 ± 0·10
Crow		
male	0·15 ± 0·04	0·75 ± 0·20
female	0·26 ± 0·05	1·45 ± 0·29
Kite		
male	0·27 ± 0·02	1·58 ± 0·01
female	0·32 ± 0·14	1·83 ± 0·60
Vulture		
male	0·14 ± 0·03	0·52 ± 0·10

[a]in pmol 3-hydroxy-BP mg^{-1} protein min^{-1}.
[b]in pmol 3-hydroxy-BP per organ min^{-1}.

TABLE 21

Mitochondrial and microsomal AHH activities in rodent brain (results in pmol
3-hydroxy-BP mg^{-1} protein min^{-1}) (Das *et al.*, 1982b)

Animals	Mitochondrial, NADH-dependent	Mitochondrial, NADPH-dependent	Microsomal, NADPH-dependent
Rat			
male	12·16 ± 0·48	4·66 ± 0·53	1·09 ± 0·04
female	11·26 ± 0·77	3·40 ± 0·43	1·07 ± 0·06
Mouse			
male	20·75 ± 0·41	6·67 ± 0·32	0·42 ± 0·06
female	17·55 ± 1·84	5·52 ± 0·66	0·44 ± 0·03
Guinea pig			
male	20·75 ± 0·91	6·89 ± 0·56	0·61 ± 0·04
female	15·99 ± 1·18	6·21 ± 0·39	0·55 ± 0·02

Microsomal and mitochondrial rat brain AHH activity differ in a number of ways. In particular, both contain NADPH and NADH-dependent activity, but the ratios vary (Das et al., 1981d). In rat brain microsomes, the NADH/NADPH ratio of activities is 0·5, while it is 2·8 in mitochondria. Indeed, most of the NADH-dependent AHH activity is concentrated in the mitochondria. Mitochondrial AHH activity has a higher affinity (K_m = 1·2 μM) for BP than microsomal NADPH-dependent activity; the V_{max} is ten-fold higher (Das et al., 1982b). Mitochondrial NADH-dependent AHH has a specific activity of 12·5–18·5 pmol 3-hydroxy-BP mg^{-1} protein min^{-1} in most regions of rat brain (cerebellum, medulla and pons, corpus striatum, hypothalamus, midbrain, hippocampus and cortex), with the exception of the olfactory lobes which have a two-fold higher activity (Das et al., 1982b).

AHH activity in brain occurs in a number of species besides the rat. In rabbit brain 9000 g supernatant preparations, AHH activity is 29·5 pmol polar metabolites mg^{-1} protein per 2 h (Omiecinski et al., 1980). In this study, all polar metabolites (phenols, dihydrodiols, etc.) of BP were quantified by a radiometric technique after aqueous partitioning; hence the results cannot be compared with those obtained using a fluorimetric technique.

Brain microsomal AHH activity found in a number of species is reported in Table 20 (Das et al., 1981c). Clearly, rodents have higher activity than birds. No marked sex differences were observed among the species investigated with the exception of the guinea pig and the crow in which females showed higher activity than males.

Clear species, but not sex, differences are observed when mitochondrial AHH activity is considered (Table 21). Thus the rat, which has a higher microsomal AHH activity than the mouse and guinea pig (see also Table 20), has the lowest mitochondrial activity (both NADH- and NADPH-dependent).

The metabolism of benzo[a]pyrene in brain microsomes from pregnant rats and mice and their fetuses was measured by the formation of a number of oxygenated metabolites (Rouet et al., 1981). In both species 19-day-old fetuses displayed an overall AHH activity 3–4 times that found in pregnant dams (see later Table 24). Although brain AHH activity is much lower than lung and liver activity, the capacity of fetal brain to metabolize BP is of toxicological significance. In particular it would appear important to investigate brain AHH activity in the fetuses of other mammals.

3.3.2 Induction and inhibition

The action of compounds to inhibit or induce a given enzyme system may be a key element to understanding the regulation of that system. A number of studies relevant to cerebral AHH have been undertaken.

Rat brain microsomal AHH activity is inhibited by carbon monoxide

(Das *et al.*, 1981c). However, brain microsomal AHH is considerably less sensitive to the formation of the ferrocytochrome P-450 ligand than liver AHH (Table 22). Again differences in the nature of the liver and brain enzymes appear indicated.

TABLE 22

Effect of carbon monoxide on rat microsomal AHH activity (control = room air = 100%) (Das *et al.*, 1981c)

Atmosphere	Brain	Liver
O_2 (100%)	111·9	103·9
CO/O_2 (50/50)	71·2	45·9
CO/O_2 (80/20)	67·7	15·3
CO (100%)	21·0	1·2

AHH activity is classically induced by polycyclic aromatic hydrocarbons (e.g. 3-methylcholanthrene, 3MC) and structurally related planar molecules. Following 6 days' treatment with 3MC, Cohn *et al.* (1977) reported a four-fold increase in rat brain microsomal AHH activity. Guengerich and Mason (1979) investigated the inducibility of AHH in various rat tissues. While a 5-day treatment with phenobarbital (PB) only induced liver and testis AHH activity, 3MC increased AHH activity in all organs examined except testis, small intestine and brain. The results for brain contradict those of others (Table 23). Thus, Cohn *et al.* (1977) and Das *et al.* (1981c) found that rat brain microsomal AHH activity was induced 70% following 5-day PB treatment, and 130–140% following 5-day treatment with BP or 3MC. Strain differences may explain this discrepancy but it is more probable that differences in the duration and regimen of inducer administration are responsible.

TABLE 23

Induction of microsomal AHH activity in various rat tissues (results in nmol 3-hydroxy-BP $nmol^{-1}$ P-450 min^{-1}) (Guengerich and Mason, 1979)

	Control	Phenobarbital	3-Methylcholanthrene
Lung	0·35 ± 0·04	0·48 ± 0·04	1·98 ± 0·14
Liver	0·22 ± 0·01	0·52 ± 0·04	1·62 ± 0·30
Testis	0·19 ± 0·01	0·44 ± 0·03	0·14 ± 0·03
Kidney	0·082 ± 0·005	0·070 ± 0·017	1·86 ± 0·22
Small intestine	≥0·070 ± 0·014	≥0·10 ± 0·01	≥0·070 ± 0·010
Spleen	≥0·060 ± 0·003	—[a]	0·11 ± 0·03
Heart	0·024 ± 0·009	0·026 ± 0·001	0·060 ± 0·010
Brain	0·024 ± 0·002	0·028 ± 0·002	0·036 ± 0·004
Stomach	0·011 ± 0·004	0·013 ± 0·001	0·043 ± 0·015

[a]Not reported.

The inducibility of brain microsomal AHH also has been investigated in rodent fetuses and compared to that of pregnant animals (Table 24) (Rouet et al, 1981). 5,6-Benzoflavone is particularly active in pregnant mice and rat fetuses, where it induces a 5–10 fold increase in the metabolism of BP. In pregnant rats and in mouse fetuses induction by 5,6-benzoflavone is moderate (1·5–2 fold). The relevance to man is unknown but studies in other species, particularly primates, may help to elucidate the toxicological importance of AHH induction.

The inducing effect of Aroclor 1254, a mixture of polychlorinated biphenyls, on AHH activity in brains of pregnant and fetal rats and mice has been studied using another polycyclic aromatic substrate, namely 7,12-dimethyl-benz[a]anthracene (LX) (Juchau et al., 1979). While AHH activity in pregnant mice and rats (Table 25) are comparable with respect to both total metabolism and regioselectivity of oxidation, it is clear that the mouse fetus displays a much higher activity than the rat fetus. This contrasts with data obtained when benzo[a]pyrene was the substrate (Table 24). Aroclor 1254 caused marked induction of AHH in pregnant rats, less so in pregnant and fetal mice, and moderate to no induction in fetal rats. Again, these results are at variance with those obtained using benzo[a]pyrene as substrate and 5,6-benzoflavone as inducer (Table 24).

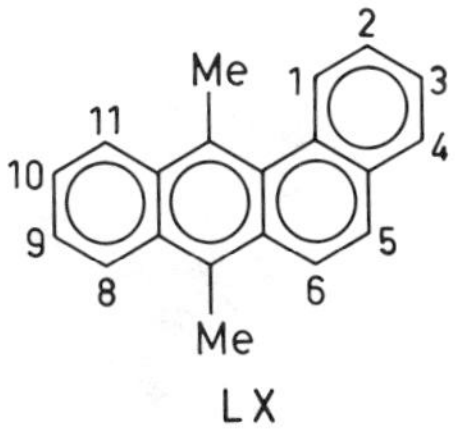

LX

Taken together, the results for the two substrates and the two inducers indicate that species and developmental variations in cerebral AHH activity are themselves substrate- and inducer-dependent, making it all the more difficult if not impossible at present to extrapolate to man.

Induction of mitochondrial AHH has also been investigated (Das et al., 1982b). In the brain of male rats treated for 5 days with BP, both NADH- and NADPH-dependent AHH showed a 90% increase in BP 3-hydroxylation. A 5-day treatment with 3MC caused a 60–70% increase of both NADH- and NADPH-dependent forms, while phenobarbital (5 days) was without effect. This suggests some interesting differences between the mitochondrial and microsomal forms of AHH.

TABLE 24

Effect of 5,6-benzoflavone (BF) on benzo[a]pyrene metabolism in brain microsomes from pregnant dams and fetuses (19 days old) of mouse and rat (results in pmol metabolite mg^{-1} protein min^{-1}) (Rouet et al., 1981)

| | Metabolites | | | | | | |
	9,10-diol	4,5-diol	7,8-diol	quinones	9-hydroxy	3-hydroxy	Total
Mice							
Pregnant dams							
control	0·5	0·2	0·3	0·6	0·3	0·5	2·4
BF	5·8	2·7	2·9	5·8	3·9	3·9	25
Fetuses							
control	1	0·7	0·9	1·6	1·2	3·2	8·6
BF	2·7	1·7	2·3	4·1	2·6	3·7	17·1
Rats							
Pregnant dams							
control	0·4	0·3	0·2	2·6	0·3	0·4	4·2
BF	0·7	0·8	0·4	2·3	0·7	1·3	6·2
Fetuses							
control	1·5	2	0·4	6·8	1·6	3·2	15·5
BF	10	7·2	4·4	41	6·9	9·6	79

TABLE 25

Effect of Aroclor 1254, a mixture of polychlorinated biphenyls (PCB) on 7,12-dimethylbenz[a]anthracene (DMBA) metabolism in brain 9000 g supernatant preparations from pregnant dams and fetuses of mouse and rats (results in pmol metabolite mg^{-1} protein min^{-1}) (Juchau et al, 1979)

	Metabolites						
	Phenols[a]	12-OHM[b]	7-OHM[c]	7,12-diOHM[d]	8,9-diol[e]	7-OHM-5,6-diol[f]	DCA[g]
Mice							
Pregnant dams							
control	4·4	11·6	10·9	23·9	19·2	12·3	30·7
PCB	9·0	15·3	14·9	39·7	25·9	17·3	49·6
Fetuses (17 days old)							
control	8·4	19·4	18·6	53·5	35·4	25·2	50·0
PCB	21·7	28·0	21·3	65·5	43·0	23·2	84·3
Rats							
Pregnant dams							
control	11·1	9·0	6·3	18·2	8·9	6·5	20·5
PCB	21·5	19·8	15·1	55·9	28·5	8·5	61·2
Fetuses (19 days old)							
control	3·0	3·6	3·1	2·3	8·2	6·5	10·1
PCB	2·9	5·2	5·6	12·6	4·2	5·3	15·1

[a]Total of 3-, 4- and 5-hydroxy metabolites.
[b]12-Hydroxymethyl-7-MBA.
[c]7-Hydroxymethyl-12-MBA.
[d]7,12-Dihydroxymethyl-BA.
[e]DMBA-*trans*-8,9-diol.
[f]7-Hydroxymethyl-12-MBA-*trans*-5,6-diol.
[g]1,4-Dimethyl-2-phenylnaphthalene-3,2'-dicarboxaldehyde.

163

Further differences between mitochondrial and microsomal AHH are seen in CO inhibition experiments. Rat brain microsomal NADPH-dependent AHH activity was inhibited by 60% (in atmospheres of 80 and 100% CO), while NADH-dependent activity was only depressed by 10%. In contrast, mitochondrial NADPH-dependent AHH activity was inhibited by only 10%, while NADH-dependent activity was inhibited by 40-50% (Das et al., 1982b). The weak inhibition of some forms of AHH was quite unexpected (compare also with Table 22) and requires confirmation using different experimental conditions.

Selective inhibitors (Table 26) also emphasize differences between brain microsomal and mitochondrial forms of AHH. The results obtained for brain microsomal AHH are in good agreement with the general properties of these inhibitors, namely the non-selective activity of benzylimidazole, the selectivity of metyrapone and SKF-525A for native (and PB-inducible) forms of cytochrome P-450 and the selectivity of α-naphthoflavone for the 3MC-inducible forms of cytochrome P-450 (Testa and Jenner, 1981). In mitochondria, however, SKF-525A shows marked activity, especially following 3MC induction (Das et al., 1982b).

TABLE 26

Inhibition of control and 3MC-stimulated rat brain microsomal and mitochondrial aryl hydrocarbon hydroxylase (no inhibitor: specific activity in pmol 3-hydroxy-BP mg^{-1} protein min^{-1}; inhibitor present: residual activity in %) (from Das et al., 1981c, 1982b)

	Microsomal		Mitochondrial,NADH-stimulated	
Inhibitor	Control	3MC	Control	3MC
None	0·45-0·48	0·98-1·05	8·53	16·32
1-Benzylimidazole				
1 mM	7	8	14	25
Metyrapone				
1 mM	52	76	38	51
SKF-525A				
0·01 mM	83	95	66	50
0·1 mM	73	90	40	37
1 mM	62	81	33	26
α-Naphthoflavone				
0·001 mM	83	46	72	44
0·01 mM	58	31	62	29
0·1 mM	21	14	37	13

The induction and inhibition effects discussed above are fundamentally different from the activating action of a number of haemoproteins on AHH activity when added to the incubation medium. Thus, haematin added to rabbit brain 9000 g supernatant preparations increased AHH activity 70-fold (7000%). Haemoglobin caused an eight-fold increase, protoporphyrin IX a two-fold increase, while biliverdin, myoglobin and catalase were inactive (Omiecinski et al., 1980). These effects observed over a 2-h incubation period developed only progressively, resulting in a parabolic-like increase in activity with time. While the activating effect of haemoprotein was greatest in rabbit tissues, it occurred in every extrahepatic tissue in every species examined (Omiecinski et al., 1980 and references therein). It was postulated that in these tissues, pools of free apocytochrome exist that have a low affinity for the haem prosthetic group. Haematin would then by an unknown mechanism cause an increase in affinity. Because the haematin-mediated increase in AHH activity is not spectrally detectable, it is believed to involve only a limited population of cytochrome P-450s with high turnover numbers.

3.3.3 Experimental difficulties

The comments made in section 3.1.3 with respect to the perturbating effect of blood constituents are also valid here. The activating effect of haemoglobin mentioned in the previous section may give artificially high values for AHH activity. Similarly, the presence of AHH activity in lymphocytes (e.g. Børresen et al., 1981) may be affected in a similar manner.

Another problem in the determination of AHH activity is covalent binding of metabolites to macromolecules which may prevent their detection. But the manner of defining and assessing AHH activity are many, and covalent binding should only influence the results if an estimation of total metabolic products is undertaken.

These remarks should not hide the fact that biotransformation data such as AHH activity provide a more reliable and discriminative means of assessing the properties of cytochrome P-450 than is provided by spectral studies.

3.4 AMPHETAMINE RING HYDROXYLATION

Amphetamine (V) undergoes biotransformation in brain to para-hydroxy-amphetamine (VI), norephedrine (VII) and para-hydroxynorephedrine (VIII) (see section 2.1.3.1). All three compounds were isolated from rat brain following intracisternal administration of amphetamine, but not after intraperitoneal administration. Since the polar metabolites VI-VIII cannot readily cross the blood–brain barrier, this would suggest their formation within brain tissue (Kuhn *et al.*, 1978). Brain slices incubated with amphetamine also produced the three metabolites; after 30-min incubation, 0·6–0·8 % of the substrate had undergone *para*-hydroxylation. This reaction was also characterized by Cho *et al.* (1977) in synaptosomal preparations from striatum and cortex.

The involvement of cytochrome P-450 in the cerebral *para*-hydroxylation of amphetamine is indicated by the effect of iprindole, an inhibitor of this reaction in the liver. Pretreatment of rats with iprindole markedly depressed *para*-hydroxylation of intracisternally administered amphetamine. β-Hydroxylation mediated by dopamine β-hydroxylase was not affected (section 2.1.3.1). These results are not, however, definitive proof of cerebral cytochrome P-450 involvement.

para-Hydroxyamphetamine is further hydroxylated in rat brain to yield alpha-methyldopamine (XXVIII, catecholamphetamine). For this reaction, clear proof exists for the involvement of cytochrome P-450, although brain microsomes may have been contaminated with haemoglobin (Hoffman *et al.*, 1979). As shown in Table 27, the reaction is to some extent NADPH-dependent, and also partly NADPH-independent. This latter activity is probably NADH-dependent (see section 3.3.). The classical cytochrome P-450 inhibitors CO and SKF-525A caused a marked decrease in α-methyldopamine formation, providing hard evidence for the involvement of cytochrome P-450.

TABLE 27

Effect of inhibitors on the formation of catecholamphetamine from *para*-hydroxyamphetamine by rat brain microsomes (specific activity in pmol product mg^{-1} protein per 15 min) (Hoffman *et al.*, 1979)

Conditions	Specific activity
Control	1·35 (100%)
Without NADPH	0·87 (64%)
CO/O$_2$ (80/20)	0·30 (22%)
N$_2$ (100%)	0·75 (56%)
SKF-525A (1 mM)	0·39 (29%)

It would be interesting to know the effects of selective inducers, and whether mitochondrial cytochrome P-450 can also mediate phenyl hydroxylation. To the best of our knowledge these data are not available. However, the ring hydroxylation of amphetamine is an indication that many drugs bearing a phenyl ring are potential precursors of phenols in brain.

3.5 FORMATION OF CATECHOL ESTROGENS AND ANALOGUES

Aromatic ring hydroxylation of endogenous estrogens such as estradiol (LXI, 17β-estradiol) to yield catechols such as 2-hydroxyestradiol is recognized as being an important metabolic route of these steroids. In humans, for

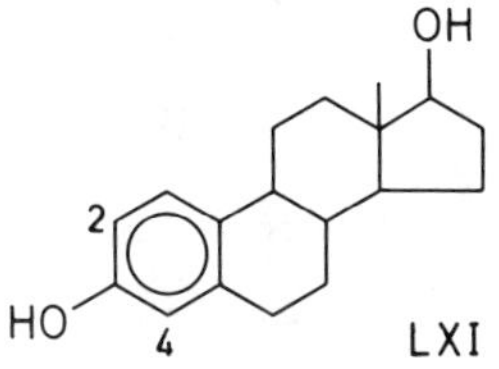

example, 2-hydroxylation was shown to account for 33% of a dose of estradiol, with only two-thirds of the resulting metabolites being excreted in urine (Fishman *et al.*, 1970). In rats the organ distribution of estrogen 2-hydroxylase showed that the liver was the most active organ with the brain second in specific activity (Table 28). The data do not incorporate the hypothalamus; this organ shows several-fold higher activity than that of the liver in terms of weight of tissue. The ratio is somewhat dependant on condition but in homogenates from female rats the hypothalamus was 3 times as active as the liver on the basis of mg of tissue (Fig. 20); the cerebral cortex and anterior pituitary had a lower activity (Fishman and Norton, 1975a, 1975b).

TABLE 28

Distribution of estrogen 2-hydroxylase in 8- to 10-week old rats (results in pmol product mg^{-1} microsomal protein per 10 min) (Paul *et al.*, 1980)

Organ	Male	Female
Liver	9900 ± 300	1500 ± 200
Brain	15·1 ± 1·7	8·7 ± 1·6
Kidney	8·1 ± 1·0	
Testis	5·7 ± 0·1	
Adrenal	4·2 ± 0·8	
Lung	2·7 ± 0·6	
Pituitary	0·7 ± 0·1	
Heart	0·5 ± 0·3	
Placenta (17 days)		0·5 ± 0·04
Uterus		ND[a]
Ovary		ND
Pineal	ND	

[a]Not detectable.

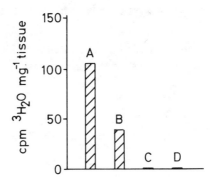

FIG. 20. Estradiol 2-hydroxylation per weight of tissue in homogenates of female rat tissues after 25 min incubation. A, hypothalamus; B, liver; C, cerebral cortex; D, anterior pituitary. (Fishman and Norton, 1975a.)

There are marked differences between male and female rats in estrogen 2-hydroxylase activity (Table 28). This sexual dimorphism is hormonally controlled, since ovariectomy considerably increases estradiol 2-hydroxylation in female rat brain and hypothalamus (Fishman and Norton, 1975a, 1975b), while castration results in a profound decrease in activity in male rats (Pau et al., 1980).

Subcellular distribution studies in rat brain indicate estrogen 2-hydroxylase activity to be essentially microsomal (3/4 of total activity); 13% of total activity was found in mitochondria, and less than 10% in nuclei and cell debris (Paul et al., 1977). The pattern of distribution is indicative of a monooxygenase system. Proof of the involvement of cytochrome P-450 in catechol estrogen forming activity comes from the inhibitor studies (Paul et al., 1977). SKF-525A and CO strongly depress the catechol formation (Table 29). In addition, enzyme activity is essentially NADPH-dependent (Table 29). However, in contrast to most other cytochrome P-450 mediated reactions, neither brain nor liver catechol estrogen formation is induced by phenobarbital or 3-methylcholanthrene (Paul et al., 1980). This rather unexpected result indicates the involvement of cytochrome P-450 isozymes with special properties.

Most studies of catechol estrogen formation have used estradiol as substrate. Although not hydroxylated as rapidly as estradiol, other estrogens such as estrone are also good substrates. In contrast, testosterone, progesterone and cholesterol, which lack an aromatic ring, do not yield catechol metabolites. Synthetic estrogens such as diethylstilbestrol and 17α-ethynylestradiol, on the other hand, are good substrates (Paul et al. 1977).

TABLE 29

Effect of incubation conditions and inhibitors on catechol estrogen forming activity of hypothalamic microsomes from female rats (specific activity in pmol product mg^{-1} protein per 10 min) (Paul et al., 1977)

Conditions	Specific activity	(%)
Control (NADPH + regenerating system)	122 ± 14	(100)
NADPH, no regenerating system	107 ± 12	(89)
NADH, no regenerating system	33 ± 2	(27)
SKF-525A (1 mM)	35 ± 6	(29)
CO/O_2 (80/20)	63 ± 7	(51)
CO/O_2 (90/10)	44 ± 4	(36)

Most results presented so far were obtained using analytical techniques thought selective for 2-hydroxyestradiol. However, a discriminative technique showed that both 2- and 4-hydroxyestrogens are produced when estradiol is incubated with rat brain slices or homogenates (Ball et al., 1978). Interestingly, although the amount of 4-hydroxyestrogen formed is quite small, the relative formation of this metabolite by brain exceeds that of the liver.

More recent studies (Hersey et al., 1981a, 1981b) suggest that the extent of 4-hydroxylation may have been underestimated. However, before discussing this point, it is necessary to comment on the increase in specific activity casued by the non-ionic detergent Tween-80, when added to various fractions obtained from rabbit hypothalamus (Hersey et al., 1981a). The 17 500 g and the 100 000 g cytosol supernatant preparations were particularly active, but the 17 500 g and the 100 000 g (microsomal) pellets were also active. This localization was unexpected and contrasts with that found in rat brain (see above). If this difference is genuine it may indicate the presence in the rabbit hypothalamus of soluble cytochrome P-450 isozymes. This would be a spectacular finding since up to now, soluble forms of cytochrome P-450 have been found only in bacteria. Rigorous confirmation of these data is required. The activating effect of Tween-80 in rabbit hypothalamus was not seen in rat liver fractions; on the contrary, the detergent virtually abolished activity (Hersey et al., 1981a).

Using an improved analytical technique, Hersey et al. (1981b) measured estradiol 2- and 4-hydroxylase activity in rabbit hypothalamus fractions activated with Tween-80. The results (Fig. 21) show that the two metabolites are produced in comparable amounts with enzyme activity, as stressed above, being maximal in the 17 500 g and 100 000 g supernatant fractions. The involvement of cytochrome P-450 is shown by the almost complete inhibition of enzyme activity by SKF-525A (IC_{50} c. 1 mM). Similarly, in a

CO/O_2 80/20 atmosphere, approximately 75% inhibition of 2- and 4-hydroxylation is observed (Hersey *et al.*, 1981b). It thus appears that some rather unusual properties are associated with the brain and hypothalamic catechol estrogen forming cytochrome P-450s.

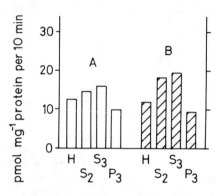

FIG. 21. The formation of 2- and 4-hydroxyestradiol (panels A and B, respectively) in subcellular fractions of fresh female rabbit hypothalamus, in the presence of Tween-80 (0·1%). H, homogenate; S_2, 17 500 g supernatant; S_3 and P_3, 100 000 g supernatant and pellet, respectively. (Hersey *et al.*, 1981b. Reproduced with the permission of The Endocrine Society.)

In humans, estradiol 2- and 4-hydroxylase have been studied in a number of tissues (Paul *et al.*, 1980), but data for brain are only available from fetuses. The brain from human fetuses is very active in hydroxylating estradiol, with specific activities comparable to those found in the hypothalamus of adult rats. In the human fetus, the highest activity was found in the pituitary and the lowest in the limbic areas, with intermediate activity in the cortex and hypothalamus (Fishman *et al.*, 1976a). This regional distribution contrasts with that found in animals, and its significance is not understood.

The formation of catechol estrogens has important physiological implications which are slowly being unravelled (e.g. Paul *et al.*, 1980; Foreman and Porter, 1980) (see section 4.2.1). Of relevance here is the fact that xenobiotic phenols such as synthetic estrogens are also substrates (see above). Catechol estrogen forming cytochrome P-450s can thus metabolize some xenobiotics, and they may represent a site of metabolic interaction between endogenous substrates and exogenous compounds affecting estrogen metabolism.

Furthermore, the formation of catechol estrogens may have toxicological significance. Indeed, 2-hydroxyestradiol incubated with rat brain microsomes was activated by superoxide to chemically reactive metabolites binding covalently to proteins (Sasame *et al.*, 1977). Binding rates of 2 nmol mg^{-1} protein min^{-1} were observed; other catechols such as catecholamines also resulted in covalent binding, but at lower rates. These results suggest that *in vivo*, covalent binding of catechol estrogens may occur resulting in toxic effects should protective mechanisms lose efficiency through saturation or degeneration.

3.6 AROMATASE

Aromatase is an enzyme system involved in the synthesis of estrogens from precursor steroids which are themselves androgens. The sequence of reactions is complex and can be summarized for androstenedione (LXII) as follows: two consecutive hydroxylation reactions occur at the C-19 methyl group which following loss of H$_2$O is oxidized to a formyl group. A 2β-hydroxylation reaction yields an intermediate (LXIII) which is unstable and breaks down to estrone (LXIV) (Goto and Fishman, 1977; Fishman and Goto, 1981). This sequence has been elucidated in human placenta microsomes, and there is convincing evidence (Connelly and Bridges, 1980), also from recent inhibition studies, that the enzyme system is cytochrome P-450 dependent (Metcalf *et al.*, 1981).

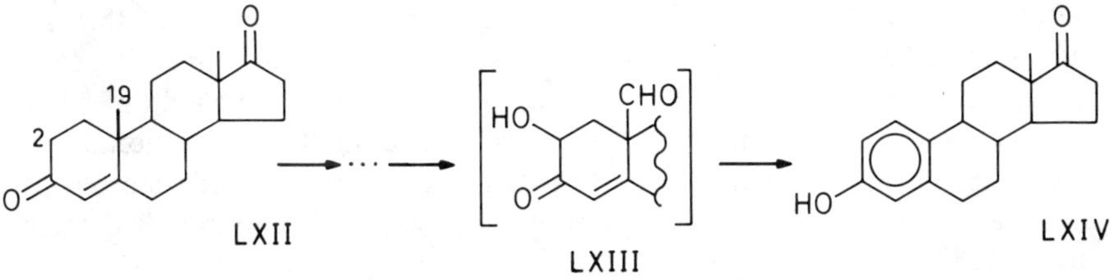

Aromatization of androgens is an important metabolic reaction in brain tissues. The biochemical, endocrinological and anatomical aspects of this topic have been exhaustively reviewed by Naftolin *et al.* (1975a, 1975b). In human fetal brain tissue most aromatase activity is localized in the hypothalamus (anterior > posterior), with moderate activity in the limbic area, and low activity in the pituitary and cortex. These findings correlate with the role of the hypothalamus in the control of sexual functions.

The subcellular distribution of aromatase activity in the hypothalamus of the ovariectomized rhesus monkey showed a predominantly mitochondrial localization (Table 30) (Billiar *et al.*, 1981). Some activity was also present in nuclei, microsomes and in the cytosol. The latter may represent contamination of fractions and/or partial solubilization of the enzyme. Also, the values in Table 30 ignore the fact that estrogens themselves can be further metabolized, in particular to catechols as described above.

TABLE 30

The aromatization of androstenedione to estrone in hypothalamus fractions of ovariectomized rhesus monkeys (results in % of substrate metabolized to product) (Billiar *et al.*, 1981)

Fraction	% conversion
Homogenate	12·2
crude nuclear pellet	20·2
nuclei	7·7
supernatant of nuclei	13·1
Mitochondria	33·1
Microsomes	10·5
Cytosol	6·1

Androstenedione is not the only substrate for brain aromatase and there are some investigations on the aromatization of testosterone. Thus, cultured turtle brain cells appear more efficient in metabolizing androstenedione than testosterone. As can be seen in Fig. 22, there is very little oxidation of estradiol to estrone following aromatization. In contrast, older cell cultures acquire the capacity to reduce to estradiol most of the estrone formed from androstenedione (Callard *et al.*, 1980). The difference in the aromatization of the two substrates, and particularly its variation with the age of the culture, suggests the involvement of distinct isozymes, but more probably differences with age in the membrane and other properties of cells affecting the penetration of the substrates into the enzyme compartment. The aromatization of testosterone to estradiol has also been investigated in adult male mice brain (Weidenfeld *et al.*, 1983).

That the active site(s) of aromatase display affinity for additional compounds is suggested by the strong inhibitory effect produced by androsta-1,4,6-triene-3,17-dione (LXV) on androstenedione aromatization (Billiar *et al.*, 1981). The kinetic type of inhibition occurring (e.g. competitive or non-competitive) is unknown so limiting the understanding of the inhibitory mechanism of LXV. It would also be of considerable interest to know whether LXV can itself undergo aromatization.

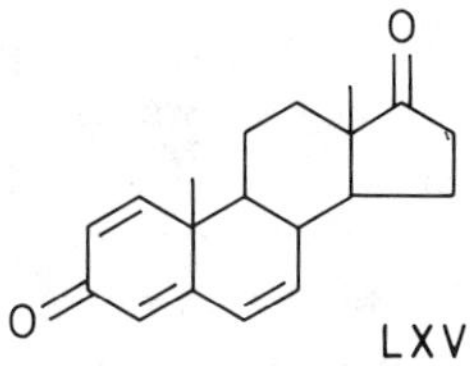

LXV

An entirely different type of aromatization occurs with dihydropyridine

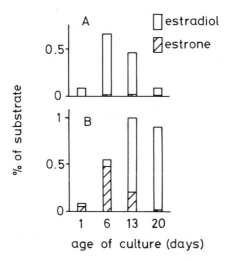

FIG. 22. The aromatization of testosterone (panel A) and androstenedione (panel B) to estrone and estradiol in cultured turtle brain cells. The cells were cultured for 1, 6, 13 or 20 days, and the substrates added 24 h prior to collection. (Callard *et al.*, 1980. Reproduced with the permission of Elsevier Biomedical Press, Amsterdam.)

derivatives (e.g. LXVI) which can be oxidized to the corresponding pyridinium derivative (LXVII). For R = methyl or benzyl, the rate constant of aromatization are in the range $2–8 \times 10^{-4}$ s^{-1} in rat brain or liver homogenates or in whole blood (Bodor *et al.*, 1981). The reaction is most probably not mediated by cytochrome P-450, but rather by a dehydrogenase, or another redox enzyme system. Interest in this reaction lies in the fact that lipophilic dihydropyridine derivatives easily cross the blood–brain barrier, while the *in situ* formed pyridinium cation is not readily eliminated from the brain. These derivatives are thus considered as drugs for site-specific, sustained release to the brain (Bodor *et al.*, 1981) (see section 4.4.2 and Bodor's contribution in this volume)

LXVI   LXVII

3.7 REACTIONS OF N- AND O-DEALKYLATION

The possibility of dealkylation occurring in brain was first raised in the 1960s in relation to the analgesic effect of, and the development of tolerance to, morphine and other opiates. Using these drugs and a few model substrates, cerebral dealkylation reactions together with some properties of the relevant enzymes (distribution, inducibility) have been investigated. For a good understanding of the following pages, let us briefly recall that with a few possible exceptions (role of N-oxides?) dealkylation reactions proceed in two steps: a cytochrome P-450 mediated hydroxylation of the carbon atom (C_α) adjacent to the heteroatom X, followed by a non-enzymatic cleavage of the C_α-X bond (Testa and Jenner, 1976; pp. 82–103).

3.7.1 Substrates for cerebral dealkylation; distribution of enzyme activity

Indirect evidence for the dealkylation of morphine (LXVIII, R = methyl), and nalorphine (LXVIII, R = allyl) in rat brain was obtained by Milthers as early as 1962 (Milthers, 1962). As expected, the brain levels of both drugs were higher in hepatectomized than in normal rats (Table 31). However, the brain concentrations of the common metabolite normorphine (LXVIII, R = H) were also higher in hepatectomized than in normal rats (Table 31).

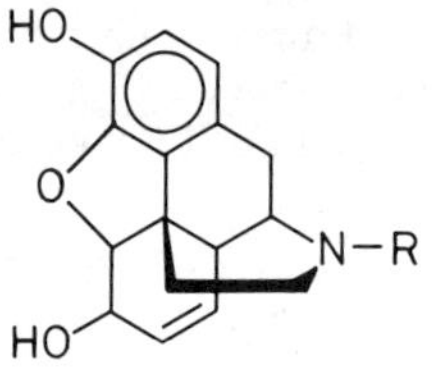

LXVIII

Were the liver the only site of N-dealkylation, no normorphine should be found in the brain of hepatectomized animals. The fact that this is not the case suggests the occurrence of extrahepatic N-dealkylation, and the increased levels of normorphine relative to normal may indicate an *in situ* generation.

TABLE 31

Concentration of total morphine or nalorphine and their metabolite normorphine in the brain of normal or hepatectomized rats 15 min after an i.v. dose of 100 mg kg^{-1} of either drug (brain concentrations in µg g^{-1}) (Milthers, 1962)

	Normal rats	Hepatectomized rats
Morphine (n = 8)	7·1 ± 1·6	26 ± 4
Normorphine	<0·6	1·3 ± 0·3
Nalorphine (n = 4)	27 ± 7	257 ± 26
Normorphine	1·2 ± 0·1	4·9 ± 2·4

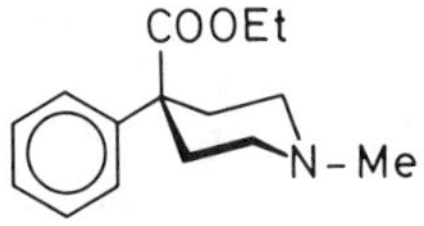

$$\text{LXIX}$$

LXIX

Direct evidence for demethylation reactions occurring in brain was obtained by Elison and Elliott (1963). Using rat brain slices, morphine, codeine and meperidine (LXIX) were demethylated (Table 32). Codeine and meperidine, which are more lipophilic than morphine, were better substrates. Codeine contains two non-equivalent methyl groups and N-demethylation is considerably faster than O-demethylation, a regioselectivity also observed in the liver. But despite these qualitative similarities hepatic demethylation is far more extensive than the cerebral reaction.

TABLE 32

Demethylation of opiates by rat brain slices, as monitored by $^{14}CO_2$ formation (results are in % of incubated amounts) (Elison and Elliott, 1963)

Substrate	Source of brain slices		
	Male	Female	Tolerant male
[N-$^{14}CH_3$]Morphine	$1 \cdot 80 \pm 0 \cdot 35$	$0 \cdot 55 \pm 0 \cdot 27$	$1 \cdot 95 \pm 0 \cdot 94$
[N-$^{14}CH_3$]Codeine	$3 \cdot 53 \pm 0 \cdot 93$	—	—
[O-$^{14}CH_3$]Codeine	$0 \cdot 72 \pm 0 \cdot 26$	—	—
[N-$^{14}CH_3$]Meperidine	$5 \cdot 06 \pm 1 \cdot 50$	—	—

Demethylase activity in the brain of female rats was lower than that in the brain of male rats, a sex difference also shown using rat liver. In contrast to hepatic demethylation, brain demethylase activity was not altered in rats tolerant to morphine. The comparatively lower levels of N-demethylase activity in brain correspond to the much lower levels of cytochrome P-450 and AHH activities in brain as compared to liver, as illustrated by the studies of Marietta et al. (1979).

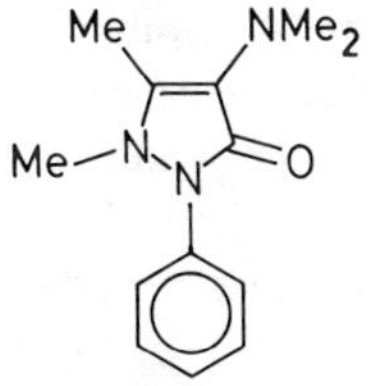

LXX

There are a number of differences in the kinetics of aminopyrine (LXX) demethylation in rat liver and brain microsomes (Table 33). While the reaction in brain displays apparent linear kinetics, that in liver shows bi-exponential kinetics. The affinity of aminopyrine is lower for cerebral than hepatic cytochrome P-450, and the specific activity is lower even expressed per nanomole of cytochrome P-450 (in the latter case, $c.$ 17% of hepatic activity, see Table 33).

TABLE 33

A comparison of rat brain and liver microsomal N-demethylase activities
(Marietta et $al.$, 1979)

Reaction	Brain	Liver
Aminopyrine N-*demethylation*		
K_m (mM)	$3·39 \pm 1·07$	$0·18 + 0·03$
		$1·13 \pm 0·32$
V_{max}		
nmol HCHO mg^{-1} protein per 10 min	$0·261 \pm 0·033$	$29·4 \pm 6·2$
		$54·9 \pm 14·7$
nmol HCHO nmol^{-1} P450 per 10 min	$6·98 \pm 0·67$	$21·3 \pm 1·8$
		$39·4 \pm 3·2$
Meperidine N-*demethylation* (0·40 mM)		
rate in nmol mg^{-1} protein per 10 min	$0·0236$	$68·3$
rate in nmol nmol^{-1} P450 per 10 min	$0·695$	$58·6$

Meperidine (LXIX) N-demethylation in brain is again lower than in liver, since it represents 1·2% of the latter when expressed per nanomole cytochrome P-450. The examples given provide some indication of differences between hepatic and cerebral monooxygenases. Why the brain N-demethylase enzymes are less efficient than the hepatic forms in metabolizing xenobiotics is unclear. It may be, however, that the optimal experimental conditions for *in vitro* studies vary widely for these tissues, and that currently available results from incubations with brain fractions have been obtained under far from optimal conditions. In particular, the synergistic effect of NADH may have been overlooked.

Previously we have repeatedly noted the NADH-mediated contributions to brain monooxygenase reactions. A similar involvement of a NADH-dependent compound exists for aminopyrine demethylase (Marietta et $al.$, 1979). As shown in Fig. 23, brain demethylase activity has a NADH-mediated component of greater proportion than observed in the liver. The results in Fig. 23 are strikingly similar to those reported in Table 29 for hypothalamic catechol estrogen-forming activity.

To obtain an *in vivo* assessment of the regional localization of morphine N-demethylase in rat brain, Fishman et $al.$ (1976b) administered a mixture

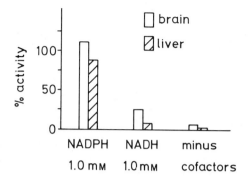

FIG. 23. Rat brain and liver microsomal aminopyrine N-demethylase activity expressed as a percentage of the NADPH-regenerating system activity (Marietta *et al.*, 1979. Reproduced with the permission of the American Society for Pharmacology and Experimental Therapeutics).

TABLE 34

Rat tissue $^3H/^{14}C$ isotope ratio after administration of $[6\text{-}^3H]$- plus $[N\text{-}^{14}C]$morphine (normalized to dose ratio = 1) (Fishman *et al.*, 1976b)

Tissue	Experiment[a]		
	1	2	3
Blood	0.89 ± 0.02	1.02 ± 0.07	0.92 ± 0.02
Cerebral cortex	0.82 ± 0.03	0.85 ± 0.11	0.89 ± 0.04
Hypothalamus	1.04 ± 0.07^b	1.22 ± 0.13^b	1.00 ± 0.07^b
Medial thalamus	1.24 ± 0.25^b	1.40 ± 0.23^b	0.98 ± 0.07
Corpus striatum	1.15 ± 0.08^b	1.20 ± 0.07^b	0.99 ± 0.06^b
Midbrain	0.83 ± 0.04	0.86 ± 0.10	0.91 ± 0.07
Cerebellum	0.82 ± 0.06	0.93 ± 0.08	0.88 ± 0.04
Medulla	0.88 ± 0.04	0.97 ± 0.11	0.97 ± 0.07
Liver	1.20 ± 0.07^b	1.21 ± 0.05^b	1.25 ± 0.09^b

[a]The dose was 2.5 mg morphine per animal, plus 0.1 mg naloxone in experiment 2; the animals were killed 30 min (experiments 1 and 2) or 60 min (experiment 3) after dosing.
[b] $p < 0.02$ or better, relative to blood.

of $[6\text{-}^3H]$- and $[N\text{-}^{14}CH_3]$morphine, and after a given time interval measured the $^3H/^{14}C$ ratio in various tissues. This technique is based on the hypothesis that the ^{14}C-containing fragments formed from the methyl group by demethylation disappear from the site of reaction much more rapidly than the ^3H-containing compounds. Thus demethylation in a tissue should as a first approximation result in a $^3H/^{14}C$ ratio higher than that found in the blood. The results, some of which are presented in Table 34, indeed indicated the liver as a site of N-demethylation. In brain, demethylation appeared to occur only in the hypothalamus, medial thalamus, and corpus striatum. The opiate antagonist naloxone did not influence the results. Such an experimental approach certainly has some drawbacks (in particular, no brain demethylation was detectable after tracer doses of morphine), but it is nevertheless valuable. That the hypothalamus contains both N-demethylating and catechol-forming cytochrome P-450s is *per se* of interest.

Using *para*-chloro-N-methylaniline as substrate, N-demethylase activity was also demonstrated in the brain of human fetuses. In whole homogenates from brain, activity was 8·8 nmol product g^{-1} tissue h^{-1}, representing the 1%, 1·6% and 29% of the activity in the liver, adrenals and lungs respectively (Rifkind and Petschke, 1981).

3.7.2 Inhibition and induction

Evidence for the involvement of cytochrome P-450 in brain dealkylation comes from inhibition and induction experiments. In the presence of CO or SKF-525A, rat brain microsomal aminopyrine N-demethylase activity is inhibited (Table 35), but less so than the liver enzyme. In fact, the data for the CO inhibitory effects markedly resemble those for the inhibition of brain and liver AHH activity (Table 22). Inhibition of demethylase activity by SKF-525A is also in close agreement with those for brain AHH activity (Table 26).

TABLE 35

Effect of inhibitors on rat microsomal aminopyrine N-demethylase activity (control = room air = 100%) (Marietta *et al.*, 1979)

Conditions	Brain	Liver
O_2 (100%)	109·8	100·7
CO/O_2 (50/50)	69·7	43·1
CO/O_2 (80/20)	53·2	18·4
CO (100%)	19·5	0·6
SKF-525A (0·01 mM)	76·3	35·6
SKF-525A (0·1 mM)	60·2	21·6

The differences in the sensitivity of brain and liver demethylase to inhibitors suggests that different cytochrome P-450 isozymes mediate the reaction in the two organs, and/or that their biological environment is sufficiently different to modify the activity of inhibitors.

Brain dealkylase activity is altered by enzyme inducers. Using *para*-chloro-N-methylaniline as a marker substrate, the induction of N-demethylase activity was compared in brain and liver (Table 36) (Chand and Clausen,

TABLE 36

Effect of phenobarbital (PB) and sodium salicylate (SS) on rat brain and liver microsomal para-chloro-N-methylaniline N-demethylase activity (activities in nmol product mg^{-1} protein min^{-1}) (Chand and Clausen, 1982)

Inducer	Brain	Liver
A. *Short-term studies* (3 days)		
Control	0·029 ± 0·001	0·635 ± 0·072
PB 75 mg kg^{-1} day^{-1}	0·040 ± 0·001	1·112 ± 0·035
SS 500 mg kg^{-1} day^{-1}	0·038 ± 0·001	1·042 ± 0·068
B. *Longer-term studies* (21 days)		
Control	0·029 ± 0·001	0·656 ± 0·024
PB 10 mg kg^{-1} day^{-1}	0·034 ± 0·002	0·759 ± 0·063
SS 50 mg kg^{-1} day^{-1}	0·034 ± 0·002	0·756 ± 0·050

1982). In short-term studies, acute doses of phenobarbital and sodium salicylate induced the activity in both organs. Phenobarbital was the more active inducer, and the liver more responsive (75% and 64% increases) than the brain (38% and 31% increases). In prolonged "therapeutic" experiments, the two organs responded moderately (15–17% increases). Thus, in brain a PB-inducible cytochrome P-450 isozyme mediating N-dealkylation exists.

TABLE 37

Effect of cytochrome P-448 inducers on 7-ethoxycoumarin O-deethylase activity in rat brain and liver microsomes (Guengerich and Mason, 1979; Rouet et al., 1981)

Animals	Brain	Liver
A. *Males*[a]		
Control	0·10 ± 0·02	1·12 ± 0·43
3MC	1·90 ± 0·74	8·55 ± 0·99
B. *Pregnant females*[b]		
Control	0·17 ± 0·03	3·10 ± 0·01
BF	0·38 ± 0·03	4·60 ± 0·31

[a]Induction: 3-day treatment with 3-methylcholanthrene (3MC); activities in nmol product nmol^{-1} P-450 min^{-1}.
[b]Induction: single dose of 5,6-benzoflavone (BF); activities in nmol product mg^{-1} protein min^{-1}.

In contrast to aminopyrine and para-chloro-N-methylaniline which are substrates for PB-inducible cytochrome P-450s, the hepatic O-dealkylation of 7-ethoxycoumarin (LXXI) is mediated by cytochrome P-448. Studies by Guengerich and Mason (1979) and Rouet et al. (1981) (Table 37) have

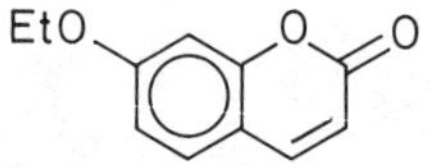

LXXI

established that O-dealkylation of 7-ethoxycoumarin is also inducible in rat brain microsomes. The increase of activity in brain following 3 days' treatment with 3MC is particularly impressive. A single dose of BF 24 h before sacrifice doubles the activity in the brain of pregnant rats. These studies demonstrate significant 7-ethoxycoumarin O-deethylase activity in rat brain, and its induction by inducers of cytochrome P-488.

3.8 OUTLOOK

We have demonstrated the considerable body of evidence already available on the properties of, and the reactions mediated by, cerebral cytochrome P-450 linked enzymes. This topic, which has not previously been reviewed, raises speculations as to the toxicological and pharmacological implications of brain monooxygenases and this will be dealt with in section 4.

To conclude this section, it is apparent that the metabolic reactions characterized so far as being mediated by brain cytochrome P-450 consist essentially of carbon monooxygenation (sp^3 and sp^2 carbon atoms). The reactions we have reviewed are: oxidative desulfuration, oxidation of aromatic rings, aromatization, N- and O-dealkylation. The hydroxylation of hexobarbital, which proceeds mainly by attack at the allylic position, has also been characterized in rat brain (Marietta et al., 1979).

Reactions not so far investigated are N-oxidation to form hydroxylamines or N-oxides, and reductive reactions, particularly the reduction of aromatic nitro derivatives and haloalkanes. The latter may have particular importance in relation to the metabolic activation of halogenated solvents (e.g. CCl_4, $CHCl_3$, see Anders, 1982) and volatile anaesthetics such as halothane. There remains an enormous research potential in this field.

This section also has indicated the differences that exist between hepatic and cerebral monooxygenases. These include the ratio of the terminal oxidase, cytochrome P-450, to other components such as NADPH-cytochrome c reductase and cytochrome b_5. Differential responses to inducers and inhibitors, the presence of marked NADH-activities, the presence of mitochondrial monooxygenases, are all findings which raise a multitude of questions as to their biological significance. Here again, the possibilities of future research are immense.

4 Roles of cytochrome P-450 in brain, and the consequences of xenobiotic interactions with these and other cerebral enzymes

In the previous sections of this chapter, we have examined in great detail the manner in which a range of cerebral enzyme systems are actually or potentially able to metabolize xenobiotics. Particular attention was paid to cytochrome P-450s and to the reactions they mediate. These enzyme systems are of pharmacological or toxicological relevance for a number of reasons. Indeed, drugs and other xenobiotics might interfere with their functioning and regulation, e.g. as inducers or inhibitors, thus upsetting their physiological role. In addition, biotransformation in brain inactivates xenobiotics or generates active metabolites, thus influencing the pharmacological or toxicological response kinetically or qualitatively. A particular case is represented by an abnormal functioning of cerebral enzymes resulting in the formation of active but unphysiological metabolites of endogenous compounds.

The object of this final section is to provide examples of where the metabolism of xenobiotics may influence the normal functioning of the brain, or where cytochrome P-450 dependent enzyme systems may themselves be involved in normal or aberrant brain function. This topic is approached from a pharmacological or biochemical viewpoint rather than from the chemical stance of earlier sections. We do not intend to provide a complete picture of present knowledge in this area since much remains speculation. However, sufficient examples should be provided to illustrate the previously underrated importance of such processes occurring within the central nervous system. We do not, for example, intend to deal with the manner in which many xenobiotic compounds can act as enzyme inhibitors through their actions as alternate substrates or by enzyme inactivation. Similarly, little attention will be given to the many cases of where covalent binding can lead, for example, to the inactivation of receptor systems, such as is shown by the irreversible binding of phenoxybenzamine to a variety of neurotransmitter receptors in brain. Rather, we will be concerned with illustrations of areas of pharmacology, biochemistry, toxicology and medicine which in the future may have to be reconsidered in the light of cerebral xenobiotic metabolism.

Firstly, however, we must consider one major issue, namely, the central role attributed to cytochrome P-450. In particular we wish to stress one aspect of the action of cytochrome P-450 which is of central importance to our understanding of xenobiotic metabolism in brain, that is its physiological role in brain function.

4.1 THE CENTRAL ROLE AND POTENTIAL PHYSIOLOGICAL SIGNIFICANCE OF
CEREBRAL CYTOCHROME P-450

In section 3 we have discussed at length the wide variety of transformations of xenobiotic molecules carried out by monooxygenases. The crucial role of cytochrome P-450 is a corollary of this wide substrate selectivity and of the large number of reactions it mediates. As such, cytochrome P-450 provides a critical link in the transformation of both exogenous and endogenous molecules. It is this central role which makes the enzyme of such importance when considering xenobiotic metabolism in brain. Indeed, cerebral cytochrome P-450 not only transforms xenobiotics and mediates physiological reactions, but, in combination with other enzyme systems, may take part in complex metabolic pathways controlling neuronal function. It is in this latter role that cytochrome P-450 may possess its greatest potential since it will contribute to normal brain function as well as providing a point of impact on which foreign compounds may interfere with cerebral processes. Some examples of the potential significance of cytochrome P-450 systems in this role will be presented in the following sections.

Before proceeding to examine the potential of cerebral xenobiotic transformation it seems important to comment on the classical differentiation of xenobiotic-metabolizing enzymes and those involved in the anabolism and catabolism of physiological compounds. Thus it has become apparent that endobiotic-metabolizing enzymes can also metabolize drugs and other foreign compounds, and that the so-called xenobiotic-metabolizing enzymes play a role in normal endogenous metabolism.

Cytochrome P-450 linked monooxygenase systems act on a variety of endogenous substrates in a physiologically significant manner. For example, cytochrome P-450s present in hepatic endoplasmic reticulum are the main enzymes responsible for the biosynthesis and metabolism of bile acids. They also hydroxylate steroid hormones such as testosterone and prostaglandins. The immediate question, however, is whether the forms of cytochrome P-450 mediating the biotransformation of endogenous substrates are the same or distinct from those forms of the enzyme responsible for the metabolism of xenobiotic compounds. The same situation would appear to apply to the cytochrome P-450 systems found in steroidogenic tissues such as the adrenals, placenta and testes. Steroidogenic cytochrome P-450s do not exhibit the low substrate selectivity usually associated with drug-metabolizing activity; these enzymes show high substrate and product selectivity. However, the same enzymes are also capable of binding and metabolizing xenobiotics so showing overlapping substrate selectivity although actually appearing involved in purely physiological processes.

This difference becomes even more complex when considering the same endobiotic-metabolizing system in different organs. Thus, estrogen 2-hydroxylase activity in liver and brain are both mediated by cytochrome P-450 dependent monooxygenases but these appear to differ from each other and from xenobiotic-metabolizing enzymes in general in a number of respects. For example, in the rat the hepatic enzyme has a higher affinity for estradiol than does the cerebral enzyme. Although the liver enzyme is sensitive to changes in thyroid function this is not reflected in the brain form (Paul et al., 1980).

The object of this brief discussion of the physiological importance of cytochrome P-450 is to merely emphasize that in organs such as the brain it is difficult, if not impossible, to differentiate the roles this enzyme might play in both endogenous metabolism and in the metabolism of foreign compounds. As such the cerebral effects of a xenobiotic might be interpreted as being due to either a disruption of the normal physiological action of cytochrome P-450 or by acting as a substrate for this enzyme so producing some active metabolite. To illustrate how complex the interaction between cytochrome P-450, xenobiotics, and normal physiological metabolism can be, we will now consider a number of situations relevant to neurology, pharmacology and toxicology.

4.2 INVOLVEMENT OF CYTOCHROME P-450 IN CEREBRAL NEUROTRANSMISSION AND HORMONAL REGULATION

4.2.1 Formation of estrogens and catechol estrogens

Perhaps the most important role for cerebral cytochrome P-450 demonstrated to date is the transformation of androgens to estrogens by aromatization, and of the latter to catechol estrogens by 2-hydroxylation. The evidence for the involvement of cytochrome P-450 in these processes is strong and has been reviewed in detail in sections 3.5 and 3.6.

The aromatization of androgens occurring in the diencephalon and limbic system is seen as an essential step in brain sex differentiation in neonatal rodents (Lieberburg et al., 1977; McEwen et al., 1977). Aromatase activity in the forebrain of human fetuses is potentially vital as a source of estrogens during embryogenesis; this mechanism further plays a role in triggering components of sexual behaviour in a variety of animal species of both sexes from fish to mammals (Naftolin et al., 1975a, 1795b; Callard et al., 1978).

The physiological significance of the formation of catechol estrogens in brain may be considerable and their detection may have provided evidence for the existence of a novel neuromodulatory system. Indeed, the metabolism of hormonal substrates by neuroendocrine target tissues is critical to the expression of the physiological action of these hormones as pointed out by Axelrod and his colleagues (Paul *et al.*, 1980). Previously no such activating metabolic pathway had been demonstrated for estrogen and all physiological action had been attributed to effects of estradiol. The fact that the brain has the highest estrogen 2-hydroxylase activity of any tissue other than liver suggests that it is a particular target for this substance. The significant quantities of catechol estrogens that are found in specific areas of brain, including the pituitary and hypothalamus, and the fact that formation of these compounds occurs under normal circumstances, strongly suggests that they may play a physiological role within the brain. At present catechol estrogens are thought to act by occupying estrogen receptors as weak agonists or antagonists but other interactions in the brain are also likely. How catechol estrogens interact with other neuronal systems is unclear but they may have actions of relevance to catecholamine transmission in brain. Thus, 2-hydroxy-estradiol inhibits tyrosine hydroxylase by competing for its pterine co-factor so leading to inhibition of synthesis (Lloyd and Weisz, 1978). In addition, catechol estrogens may potentiate adrenergic function by inhibiting catechol *O*-methyltransferase activity (Lloyd *et al.*, 1978). Rather than having a direct neurotransmitter role it is likely that estrogens or catechol estrogens exert a modulatory role on the activity of other transmitter systems. For example, it is known that the peripheral administration of estrogens to animals can alone increase the number of dopamine receptors present in brain, but can also reverse the ability of neuroleptic drugs to increase the number of striatal dopamine receptors (Hruska and Silbergeld, 1980; Fields and Gordon, 1982). Although not proven the suspicion is that such compounds are first converted to catechol estrogens before acting on dopaminergic pathways, in agreement with the dopamine receptor affinity of 2-hydroxyestradiol in rat anterior pituitary (Schaeffer and Hsueh, 1980).

Much remains to be done to establish the role played by catechol estrogens and indeed estrogens in general within the brain. However, it would seem that a role for cytochrome P-450 is well established and that this may represent one of the first examples of the involvement of this enzyme system in brain neuromodulation. This implies an important step forward in our understanding of how cytochrome P-450 can modulate body functions and how xenobiotics interfering with its actions may alter physiological processes.

Indeed, any interference of xenobiotic with the cytochrome P-450 mediated processes described above would have profound sexual, reproductive, and/or neurological influences. Preliminary results strongly support this hypothesis. For example, 2,4,5,2′,4′,5′-hexachlorobiphenyl strongly induces hepatic steroid 16α-hydroxylase (Dieringer *et al.*, 1979). This suggests comparable effects in brain and other steroid-metabolizing tissues, with easily envisioned consequences. Even more alarming is the recent report (Gupta *et al.*, 1982) that prenatal exposure of rats to phenobarbital causes a decrease in plasmatic and cerebral levels of testosterone which appears life-lasting. One is thus led to wonder about the magnitude of the toxicological hazards linked to unmetabolizable lipid-soluble compounds such as polyhalogenated biphenyls and dibenzodioxins, which are strong inducers of cytochrome P-450 (Jondorf, 1981).

4.2.2 Possible involvement of cytochrome P-450 in the formation of β-carbolines

In the understanding of the mode of action of anxiolytic benzodiazepine drugs a major step forward was the discovery that these substances act at a specific benzodiazepine receptor which forms part of the GABA receptor complex (see Usdin et al., 1982). The action of benzodiazepines at this site is to facilitate GABA transmission. More recently, the search for an endogenous ligand for these benzodiazepine receptors has centred on the discovery that β-carbolines can potently displace ^{3}H-benzodiazepines from their specific binding sites to the GABA receptor complex (Lippke et al., 1983). The present hypothesis is based on the idea that a β-carboline, e.g. methyl β-carboline-3-carboxylate (LXXII), is the natural transmitter at this site. In this respect it is interesting that a pathway has been demonstrated involving the transformation of indolethylamines to β-carbolines (Barker et al., 1980) (see section 2.6). At least one of the steps in this transformation may be mediated by cytochrome P-450. So it may be that this enzyme also functions in the formation of an endogenous ligand for benzodiazepine receptors and again exerts a role in normal endogenous physiological transmission. If such β-carbolines do not function within the GABA complex then they may alter 5HT action in man since there is recent evidence to suggest effects on this system in brain.

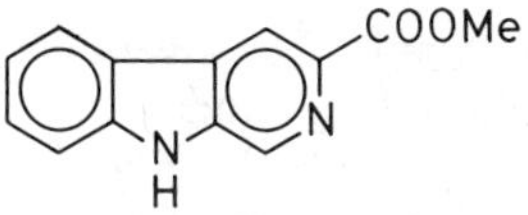

LXXII

4.2.3 Other potential involvements of cytochrome P-450 in brain

With the recognition that cytochrome P-450 plays a functional role within brain other examples of its involvement become apparent. To illustrate this point we will refer to some topics of current interest in which cytochrome P-450 is known, or is postulated, to be involved.

The brain contains the enzymatic machinery for the synthesis of *prostaglandins and analogues*, and PGE, PGF and thromboxanes are present in this organ (Nutgeren and Hazelhof, 1973; Wolfe et al., 1976). The functions of these compounds within brain are only partly known, for example synthetic derivatives have been shown to activate adenylate cyclase. Of relevance here is the fact that prostaglandins are substrates of cytochrome P-450 monooxygenases, resulting in the formation of a number of oxidized metabolites (Kupfer, 1980). Furthermore, prostacyclin synthase and thromboxane synthase are cytochrome P-450 enzymes (Graf et al., 1983; Ullrich and Haurand, 1983). Thus interference with these cytochrome P-450 dependent systems could affect whatever functions prostaglandins and analogues exert in the central nervous system.

There has been much recent interest in *adenosine* as a potential neuro-modulator. The ability of adenosine to increase cyclic AMP formation in intact cells was first demonstrated in slices of cerebral cortex (Sattin and Rall, 1970) and have since been demonstrated in several tissues and in numerous cells in tissue culture (see Bruns, 1980). There are two major types of adenosine receptors which stimulate and inhibit adenylate cyclase, respectively, and are located on the cell surface (Londos et al., 1980; Daly, 1982). Interest in adenosine receptors and adenosine effects in brain centre on the fact that both types of adenosine receptors are blocked by methyl-xanthines such as theophylline or caffeine. Cerebral metabolism of these substances may act to limit their action at adenosine receptors; it may also be that adenosine in itself, or whatever the naturally occurring ligand at these sites is, undergoes cytochrome P-450 mediated metabolism.

Lastly, mention must be made of the role that *morphine* N-demethylation in brain may play in the action of the drug at opiate sites. The close linkage of this action to areas of the brain in which opiate receptors are detected might imply some physiological role (Fishman et al., 1976b). Although the part played by this cytochrome P-450 dependent system is not known, any environmental factor which could alter the level of enzyme activity and so influence the interaction of opiate drugs with this receptor might also exert an effect on opiate transmission in brain and so modulate brain function.

Clearly, the examples which we are able to give at this stage are hypothetical in the main. The potential for neuromodulation via cytochrome P-450 dependent monooxygenases is apparent as is the ability of the brain to transform xenobiotics, so as to interfere with ongoing neurotransmission. It is only through an awareness that this possibility exists and by taking it into account in various hypotheses and experimental designs that we will be able to verify or falsify it.

4.3 POTENTIAL ROLE OF METABOLIC REACTIONS IN NEUROLOGICAL AND PSYCHIATRIC DISORDERS

There is no known cause for the majority of psychiatric and neurological cases affecting brain function but many theories exist as to how disruption of brain function might lead to the symptomatology of such disorders. The possibility exists that the clinical and biochemical interaction of xenobiotics to alter brain function may be important. In some cases there is evidence suggesting the involvement of cytochrome P-450 mediated reactions. In this section we will consider various possibilities but from the outset it must be said that these are highly speculative and in no way must they be considered as being directly related to the cause of any disorder.

4.3.1 Formation of endogenous tetrahydroisoquinoline derivatives

Metabolism of alcohol to acetaldehyde may induce the formation of pharmacologically active alkaloids from monoamines in brain (Cohen, 1976). In addition, amines also react with other endogenous carbonyl derivatives such as aldehydes produced by the deamination of catecholamines (section 2.6). As a result of such reaction a variety of alkaloid-like substances may be derived (Figs 13 and 14).

The structural similarity between alkaloids derived from catecholamine neurotransmitters has led to a variety of evidence suggesting actions which would alter or disrupt neurotransmission (see for example Meyerson and Clement-Cormier, 1980). These alkaloids may share uptake and storage mechanisms with catecholamines and so act as false neurotransmitters. They may show stereoselective agonist or antagonist actions at α- and β-adreno-receptors, and may inhibit enzymatic processes related to neuronal function such as catechol O-methyltransferase, monoamine oxidase, dopamine sensitive adenylate cyclase, Na^+,K^+-ATPase and phosphodiesterase.

The ingestion of large quantities of L-DOPA, by increasing available monoamines and their metabolites, results in greater alkaloid formation. Thus, tetrahydroisoquinoline (TIQ) alkaloids and salsolinol formed in Parkinsonian patients taking L-DOPA (Sandler et al., 1973) have been implicated in the "on-off" phenomenon and in nigrostriatal neuronal loss. However, as concluded by Melchior and Collins (1982), "there is still no compelling evidence that they are either beneficial or detrimental in the therapy of Parkinson's disease".

Abnormal condensation products also have been implicated in the aetiology of schizophrenia. Tetrahydro-β-carbolines are formed from the endogenous hallucinogen N,N-dimethyltryptamine (I) and increase central serotonin levels by inhibiting MAO and neuronal reuptake (Melchior and Collins, 1982).

The chemical formation in brain of TIQ alkaloids or their oxidative metabolites may account for some of the neuropharmacological effects of alcohol and for a part of the neuropathology of chronic alcoholism (Collins, 1982). To date, however, only small amounts of condensation products have been detected in brain tissue, but the possibility exists that these alkaloids, in certain circumstances, may be produced in higher concentrations in discrete brain structures. Chronic infusion of tetrahydropapaveroline or other isoquinoline alkaloids into the lateral ventricle of the rat results in an increase of ethanol preference in this species (Melchior and Myers, 1977), so it is possible that neuroamine condensation products as well as their further metabolites may participate in the biochemical or pharmacological processes involved in the dependence, withdrawal or maintenance of excessive alcohol consumption.

The interesting point of this particular example is how a metabolite of a relatively small xenobiotic molecule can by chemical reaction result in the production of complex alkaloid-type molecules which exert considerable effects on normal brain functioning.

4.3.2 Formation of N,N-dimethyltryptamine in brain

One of the many theories of the biochemical basis of schizophrenia is the trans-methylation hypothesis. In 1952 Osmond and Smythies proposed that the *in vivo* synthesis of mescaline-like hallucinogens was a factor contributing to the aetiology of schizophrenia. Following the discovery of enzymes which catalyse the *O*- and *N*-methylation of catecholamines as well an indoleamines (Axelrod, 1961), this endogenous hallucinogen hypothesis was extended to include *in vivo* formation of indole derivatives such a N,N-dimethyltryptamine (DMT, I) (Brune and Himwich, 1962). Indole *N*-methyltransferase utilizing *S*-adenosylmethionine (SAM) as a methyl donor has since been identified in human lung, brain, blood and CSF (Rosengarten and Friedhoff, 1976) and subsequent analyses have led to the identification of DMT in man. There is at the present time considerable controversy as to the role a substance such as DMT might play in the aetiology of schizophrenia. However, consideration of the synthetic and degradative pathways for DMT would indicate ideal opportunities for the involvement of cytochrome P-450 and other enzyme systems in a collaborative manner (see section 2.1.1).

4.3.3 Production of reactive species as a cause of cell death in Parkinson's disease

There are two major theories of how reactive intermediates might act to produce the loss of pigmented dopamine-containing neurones characterizing Parkinson's disease. Firstly it is possible that the pathway leading to the formation of melanin from dopamine is disrupted in some way so as to produce toxic amounts of reactive quinones or radical intermediates. Secondly, it is possible that the presence of monooxygenases within the brain could lead to the production of toxic amounts of activated oxygen species which result in cell death. Evidence can be presented to support both these hypotheses.

The presence of the NADPH-cytochrome c(P-450) reductase and cytochrome P-450 system in brain results in the production of superoxide radical anions some of which may be available to react with cellular components rather than being detoxified (see sections 2.1.9 and 2.1.10) (Uemura *et al.*, 1980; Trager, 1982). Radicals formed from such enzymatic reactions might in some circumstances accumulate to a level at which they exert toxicity on dopamine cell bodies found in the substantia nigra. Normally, a variety of scavenger systems would act to prevent the accumulation of potentially toxic oxygen species. Among the mechanisms involved are superoxide dismutase and catalase. In addition there is the glutathione peroxidase system in which the enzymatic oxidation of glutathione to its disulfide oxidized form is linked to the inactivation of hydrogen peroxide and other peroxides, notably those derived from the oxidation of membrane phospholipids. So it would be necessary to explain why these normal protective mechanisms were no longer effective in those patients developing Parkinson's disease.

The alternative explanation is that during the oxidative degradation of L-DOPA or dopamine in brain, reactive oxygen species (hydrogen peroxide, superoxide, hydroxyl radical, or singlet oxygen) are formed which can damage neuronal membranes and other cellular components (see sections 2.1.9 and 2.1.10). This would occur as part of the oxidative mechanism responsible for the formation of melanin in brain. Again it would be necessary to explain why toxic amounts of such reactive species accumulate in individuals developing Parkinson's disease. A possibility also involving the pathway leading to melanin formation is the production of aberrant reactive species resembling the known neurotoxin 6-hydroxydopamine. Such compounds are capable of undergoing cyclic one-electron redox reactions, probably via semiquinone radical intermediates. Under these conditions oxygen undergoes reductive conversion to hydrogen peroxide and other reactive oxygenated species which would be the primary mediators of neuronal destruction. But again, one is left with the problem that under normal circumstances physiological scavenging mechanisms should ensure the inactivation of even these aberrant active species.

It may be, therefore, that while such potentially toxic materials are continually formed, there are disruptions of the mechanisms normally responsible for the inactivation of reactive species that lead to cellular toxicity. In this light changes in the nigral content of glutathione in Parkinson's disease may be of importance (Perry *et al.*, 1982). In control subjects the mean content of total glutathione and of reduced glutathione was significantly lower in the substantia nigra than in other brain regions, but in Parkinson's disease the nigral reduced glutathione content was still lower, and significantly so. Such a relative deficiency of total glutathione and reduced glutathione was not observed in the caudate of the Parkinsonian brain. So the data suggests that the amount of glutathione available for scavenging reactive oxygen radicals is relatively low in the substantia nigra compared to other human brain regions and that the nigral deficiency of reduced glutathione is particularly severe in Parkinson's disease. Also persuasive in this argument is the fact that epidemiological studies have shown Parkinson's disease is less common among persons who smoke cigarettes for many years than among normal smokers (Godwin-Austen et al., 1982). Heavy smokers have chronically elevated blood levels of carboxyhaemoglobin and presumably increased partial pressures of carbon monoxide in brain cells. This might provide a reducing environment which could partially protect nigrostriatal neurones from oxygen damage.

Although in this section we have stressed the potential role of oxidative species in the production of nigral cell damage resulting in Parkinson's disease, there are a considerable number of other brain degenerative disorders. It is quite feasible that other forms of involvement of reactive oxygen species produced either directly or indirectly by monooxygenases or by other pathways might also be involved in some instances.

4.4 CEREBRAL BIOTRANSFORMATION OF DRUGS AND PRODRUGS TO PHARMACOLOGICALLY ACTIVE METABOLITES

A frequent consequence of xenobiotic biotransformation in any tissue is the formation of pharmacologically or toxicologically active metabolites, and of course the brain is no exception to this rule. In this section we will consider how a drug molecule might be altered in brain so as to account for at least some of its pharmacological actions, and especially how prodrugs have been designed for delivery of active molecules to the brain.

4.4.1 Metabolism of amphetamine

Amphetamine (V) is an indirectly acting sympathomimetic agent causing release of catecholamines from sympathetic nerve endings. In addition, amphetamine can be hydroxylated to active metabolites by biotransformation pathways also occurring in brain, as discussed in sections 2.1.3.1 and 2.4. The metabolites norephedrine (VII) and para-hydroxynorephedrine (VIII) may act as false neurotransmitter substances causing the release of catecholamines from nerve endings. In addition, the catechol metabolite α-methyldopamine (XXVIII) may in turn be further metabolized to α-methylnoradrenaline. The latter compound is a pharmacologically active central hypertensive metabolite and may also function as a false neurotransmitter. Because the K_m value of the catechol-forming enzyme probably exceeds the concentration of para-hydroxyamphetamine it is unlikely that substantial amounts of α-methyldopamine are normally formed (Hoffman *et al.*, 1979). With chronic use, however, it may be possible for this metabolite to accumulate and perhaps play a role in the development of tolerance to amphetamine.

4.4.2 Prodrugs of dopamine agonists

One area in which prodrugs have been employed in an attempt to improve the central actions of drug molecules is in the production of dopamine agonist compounds. Two major areas of effort can be identified. Firstly, there are dopamine agonists such as 6,7-ADTN or dopamine itself which do not pass the blood–brain barrier on peripheral administration. Secondly, there are those dopamine agonist compounds which have a short effective half-life and are poorly available on oral administration and these include the classical dopamine agonist compound, apomorphine. Attempts have been made to improve the central action of such compounds by the production of prodrug derivatives.

6,7-ADTN is a potent dopamine agonist compound when injected directly into dopamine-containing areas of the brain and also acts on dopamine receptors when incorporated into *in vitro* receptor ligand binding assays. However, on peripheral administration it does not produce changes in motor behaviour associated with a central action on dopamine receptors. Attempts have been made to introduce 6,7-ADTN into the brain by producing diester prodrugs (XXXVI) (Horn *et al.*, 1982) (see section 2.4.2). In comparison to 6,7-ADTN itself, a rapid elevation of 6,7-ADTN levels was observed in brain in the first 5–15 minutes following administration of diacetyl or diisobutyl derivatives. Administration of dibenzoyl or dipivaloyl analogues resulted in high brain concentrations of 6,7-ADTN lasting for several hours.

N-Propylnorapomorphine (NPA) is a potent dopamine agonist of short duration. A prodrug derivative of NPA has been produced by synthesizing (—)-10,11-methylenedioxy-*N*-propylnorapomorphine (LXXIII) (Baldessarini *et al.*, 1982). It was found that the prodrug of NPA itself was virtually inactive *in vitro* compared to NPA in stimulating cyclic AMP synthesis and much

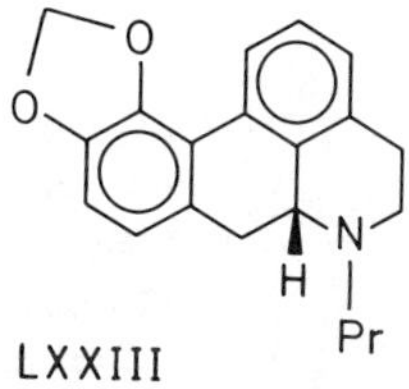

LXXIII

weaker than NPA in competing for dopamine receptor binding sites labelled by ^{3}H-apomorphine. Yet the prodrug was very much more active in inducing stereotype behaviour *in vivo* and was of longer duration of action than NPA. Analysis revealed that NPA could be detected in brain after the peripheral administration of the prodrug. The findings were used to support the proposal that the prodrug of NPA is an orally effective and relatively long-acting dopamine agonist and its action may be due to removal of the methylene group to liberate NPA, possibly by enzymatic oxidation. It is not clear whether NPA production occurs in the periphery or in the brain. However, the longer duration of the compound might suggest that the methylenedioxy bridge is cleaved close to the site of action rather than in peripheral tissues.

The dihydropyridine-pyridinium approach (see section 3.6) has also been applied by Bodor (Bodor and Farag, 1983) to the design of dopamine prodrugs such as acetyl and pivaloyl esters LXXIV. The results so far are consistent with (a) delivery of the dihydropyridine derivative LXXIV to the brain by passive diffusion through the blood–brain barrier; (b) rapid oxidation in brain of the dihydropyridine carrier to the corresponding quaternary pyridinium LXXV; (c) selective concentration in brain of the LXXV precursor through a slowdown of its efflux; (d) slow release of dopamine by amide and ester hydrolytic cleavage. A significant central dopaminergic activity was sustained for hours in rats administered a single i.v. dose of the dipivaloyl ester LXXIV (see Bodor's chapter in this volume).

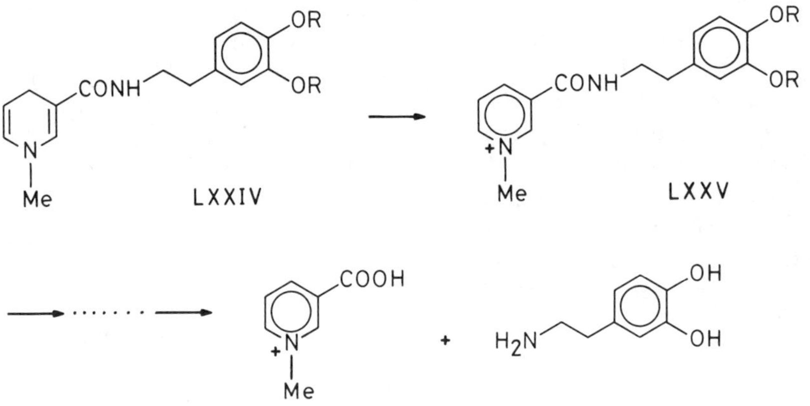

Taken globally, the above three examples stress the interest of the prodrug approach in increasing brain delivery as well as duration of action of centrally acting drugs. However, a good understanding of physiological and biochemical properties of the brain as compared to other tissues and organs is indispensable to the successful design of such prodrugs.

4.5 TOXICOLOGICAL IMPLICATIONS OF CEREBRAL XENOBIOTIC METABOLISM

The ability to metabolize xenobiotics in brain provides not only the potential for pharmacological activation but has also the same implications for toxicity as observed in peripheral tissues. This means that a number of xenobiotics are potentially toxic to the brain if undergoing bioactivation. At the present time there is only indirect evidence to implicate such mechanisms in cerebral toxicity but it is interesting to explore this possibility by reference to three examples.

4.5.1 Covalent binding of morphine

In section 2.1.3.2, we discussed the formation of morphine 2,3-quinone (XVIII) and indicated that this metabolite might be retained in brain by covalent binding. Indeed, irreversible binding of morphine or more probably its metabolites was observed in rat brain and other organs (Mullis *et al.*, 1979). Recent evidence, however, suggests morphinone (LXXVI) to be responsible for the main retention of radioactivity following administration of labelled morphine to mice (Nagamatsu *et al.*, 1983). The oxidation of morphine (LXVIII, R = Me) to morphinone appears to be mediated by a cytosolic dehydrogenase and to occur in such organs as the liver, the lungs, the kidneys and the brain. Of interest is the reactivity of morphinone towards thiol groups, resulting in the formation of a glutathione conjugate (LXXVII, R = glutathionyl) or in covalent binding to proteins (LXXVII, R = protein).

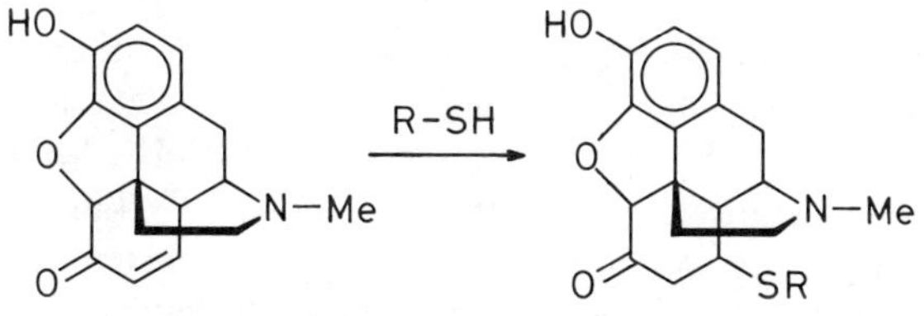

LXXVI   LXXVII

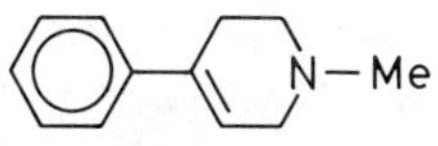

LXXVIII

Such a mechanism of covalent binding may have toxicological and pharmacological implications. Indeed, thiol blocking agents inactivate opiate receptors, and it is suggested (Nagamatsu *et al.*, 1983) that covalent binding of morphinone to thiol groups of opiate receptors, if occurring, may be related to protracted morphine effects such as tolerance and withdrawal symptoms.

4.5.2 Activation of carcinogens in brain

As pointed out in section 3.3 there is good evidence for the presence of aryl hydrocarbon hydroxylase activity in brain. This ability to transform polycyclic hydrocarbons provides the brain with the potential to form procarcinogens. The enzyme activity would appear inducible and so may be altered by the administration of other xenobiotics. There is some evidence to suggest that this may be a mechanism of importance at least in animal species since some hamster fetal brain cells become malignant when incubated with benzpyrene *in vitro* (Markovits *et al.*, 1976). In addition, treatment of pregnant rats with polycyclic aromatic hydrocarbons yielded a high percentage of brain tumours in the newborn animals (Rice *et al.*, 1978). Species differences in the extent of activity also may be of importance since it would appear that mouse fetal brain tissue is very active in metabolizing polycyclic aromatic hydrocarbons to mutagenic metabolites in comparison to rat tissue (Juchau *et al.*, 1979). What happens in man is unknown but this potential route for the formation of carcinogens should not be overlooked when investigating the mechanism by which cerebral tumours are initiated.

4.5.3 Toxic effects of N-methyl-4-phenyl-1,2,5,6-tetrahydropyridine

A recent example where brain metabolism might be intimately involved in toxicity (or indeed in the pathology of disease states) is apparent with *N*-methyl-4-phenyl-1,2,5,6-tetrahydropyridine (LXXVIII, MPTP). This compound, an illicit drug related to pethidine, caused Parkinsonian-like states in drug addicts (Langston *et al.*, 1983). On post mortem examination the brain from one user of this material was shown to have a lesion of the substantia nigra which had been accompanied in life by Parkinsonian symptoms (Davis *et al.*, 1979). Subsequent study has revealed that the administration of MPTP to primates again produces the cardinal symptoms of Parkinson's disease and that this is accompanied by a selective lesion of those dopamine cell bodies found in the zona compacta of substantia nigra (Burns *et al.*, 1983). There appears to be no damage to dopamine cells adjacent to this region in the ventral tegmental area and no damage to cells of the noradrenaline system arising in the locus coeruleus or of the 5HT neurones arising from the raphe system. Interestingly, MPTP does not produce destruction of dopamine cell bodies when administered to guinea pigs or rats (Chiueh *et al.*, 1983). This latter fact would suggest either that human or primate substantia nigra is more susceptible to the actions of MPTP or that the compound itself is not the active moiety but rather is converted to some active metabolite *in vivo*. Also of interest is the fact that MPTP produces such a selective lesion of one group of dopamine-containing cell bodies in brain. This would suggest that whatever moiety is responsible for the destruction of these cells it is not formed systemically since this would be expected to produce widespread cell loss but rather that it is produced by local action within the area of the substantia nigra. While there are only preliminary reports on the metabolism of MPTP in the periphery or in brain, it would seem that this example may provide firstly a classical case of how xenobiotic-metabolizing enzymes can cause toxic effects within brain and secondly it would provide one of the few clues as to the cause of idiopathic Parkinson's disease. The demonstration that xenobiotic-metabolizing enzymes may be involved in this manner may shed a whole new light on their actions within the central nervous system.

5 Conclusion

The human brain is the most wonderful achievement of biological evolution on our planet, since depending on one's philosophical attitude it can be considered as the physical support of the mind, or as the material door to the spiritual world.

An enormous amount of scientific knowledge has accumulated on brain functions and functioning. However, this entire knowledge is but a drop of water in the sea of our ignorance, and it is futile for a proper understanding of the extraordinary levels of complexity at which this organ operates.

Nevertheless, comprehending the brain's functioning begins at the molecular level. Such a reductionistic approach cannot be dispensed with, since it is an irreplaceable facet of any scientific inquiry. The present review is devoted to one topic of cerebral chemistry among many, namely the biotransformation of xenobiotics, the enzyme systems which mediate these reactions, and some pharmacodynamic consequences thereof.

Xenobiotic biotransformation in brain is just one aspect of the manifold interactions between xenobiotics and cerebral enzymes. From a pharmacological viewpoint, the most important among these interactions are those which trigger the therapeutic response, for example the inhibition of MAO by some antidepressant drugs, or those which may contribute to the desired effect, for example the inhibition of aldehyde reductase by some anticonvulsants (Javors and Erwin, 1980). Such types of interactions are not considered here since they obviously fall outside the scope of this review.

In addition, xenobiotics may interact with cerebral enzymes to produce side effects which to the organism can be detrimental, beneficial, or silent. Such is the case for enzyme induction or inhibition, which are effects of particular significance in our context when the enzymes involved also recognize xenobiotics as their substrates. A number of relevant examples are discussed in the text in connection with cytochrome P-450.

The first conclusion to emerge from this review is that cerebral metabolism is an important and reasonably well-documented phenomenon with the potential for marked pharmacological and toxicological consequences. The second and perhaps less apparent conclusion is that modification of enzyme activity by xenobiotics acting as, e.g. inducers or inhibitors, may have far-reaching consequences. This should be obvious considering that the brain fulfils the most central control and coordinating functions, not to mention the brain–mind connection. The number of xenobiotics potentially able to play such a role in the brain is considerable, while our present understanding of induction and inhibition of cerebral enzymes, and the consequences thereof, is negligible, to say the least. Such a discrepancy is intolerable and can only be corrected if an adequate awareness grows among biologists.

References

Ahmed, N. K., Felsted, R. L. and Bachur, N. R. (1979). *J. Pharmacol. Exp. Ther.* **209**, 12–19.

Aitio, A. and Marniemi, J. (1980). *In* "Extrahepatic Metabolism of Drugs and Other Foreign Compounds" (T. E. Gram, ed.), pp. 365–387. MTP Press, Lancaster, UK.

Alexander, L. S. and Goff, H. M. (1982). *J. Chem. Educ.* **59**, 179–182.

Alvares, A. P. (1981). *Drug Metab. Rev.* **12**, 431–436.

Alvares, K. and Balasubramanian, A. S. (1982). *Biochem. Biophys. Acta* **692**, 124–133.

Anders, M. W. (1982). *Trends Pharmacol. Sci.* **3**, 356–357.

Arias, I. M., Fleischner, G., Kirsch, R., Mishkin, S. and Gatmaitan, Z. (1976). *In* "Glutathione: Metabolism and Function" (I. M. Arias and W. B. Jakoby, eds), pp. 175–188. Raven Press, New York.

Axelrod, J. (1961). *Science* **134**, 343.

Azevedo, I. and Osswald, W. (1977). *Naunyn-Schmied. Arch. Pharmacol.* **300**, 139–144.

Bail, M., Miller, S. and Cohen, G. (1980). *Life Sci.* **26**, 2051–2061.

Baldessarini, R. J., Neumeyer, J. L., Campbell, A., Sperk, G., Ram, V., Arana, G. W. and Kula, N. S. (1982). *Eur. J. Pharmacol.* **77**, 87–88.

Ball, P., Haupt, M. and Knuppen, R. (1978). *Acta Endocrinol.* **87**, 1–11.

Barker, S. A., Monti, J. A. and Christian, S. T. (1980). *Biochem. Pharmacol.* **29**, 1049–1057.

Barrass, B. C. and Coult, D. B. (1973). *Biochem. Pharmacol.* **22**, 2897–2904.

Barrass, B. C., Coult, D. B., Rich, P. and Tutt, K. J. (1974). *Biochem. Pharmacol.* **23**, 47–56.

Battersby, A. R., Sheldrake, P. W., Staunton, J. and Williams, D. C. (1976). *J. Chem. Soc. P.T.I.*, 1056–1062.

Battie, C. and Verity, M. A. (1981). *J. Neurochem.* **36**, 1308–1310.

Becker, A. R. and Sternson, L. A. (1980). *Bioorg. Chem.* **9**, 305–312.

Bellucci, G., Berti, G., Ferretti, M., Marioni, F. and Re, F. (1981). *Biochem. Biophys. Res. Commun.* **102**, 838–844.

Benuck, M., Berg, M. J. and Marks, N. (1981). *Biochem. Biophys. Res. Commun.* **99**, 630–636.

Benzi, G., Berte, F., Crema, A. and Frigo, G. M. (1967). *J. Pharm. Sci.* **56**, 1349–1351.

Billiar, R. B., Takaoka, Y., Johnson, W., White, R. J. and Little, B. (1981). *Neuroendocrinology* **32**, 355–363

Black, S. D. and Coon, M. J. (1982). *J. Biol. Chem.* **257**, 5929–5938.

Bock, K. W., Lilienblum, W. and Pfeil, H. (1982). *Biochem. Pharmacol.* **31**, 1273–1277.

Bodor, N. and Farag, H. H. (1983). *J. Med. Chem.* **26**, 528–534.

Bodor, N., Farag, H. H. and Brewster, M. E. (1981). *Science* **214**, 1370–1372.

Boksa, P. and Collier, B. (1980). *J. Neurochem.* **34**, 1470–1482.

Bolcsak, L. E. and Nerland, D. E. (1983). *J. Biol. Chem.* **258**, 7252–7256.

Bonfils, C., Balny, C. and Maurel, P. (1981). *J. Biol. Chem.* **256**, 9457–9465.

Borchardt, R. T. (1980). *In* "Enzymatic Basis of Detoxication" (W. B. Jakoby, ed.) Vol. II, pp. 43–62. Academic Press, Orlando, New York and London.

Borchardt, R. T. and Cheng, C. F. (1978). *Biochim. Biophys. Acta* **522**, 49–62.

Børresen, A.-L., Berg, K. and Magnus, P. (1981). *Clin. Genetics* **19**, 281–289.

Bosron, W. F. and Li, T. K. (1980). *In* "Enzymatic Basis of Detoxication" (W. B. Jakoby, ed.), Vol I, pp. 231–248. Academic Press, Orlando, New York and London.

Boulton, A. A. and Juorio, A. V. (1983). *Experientia* **39**, 130–134.

Boyd, J. A. and Eling, T. E. (1981). *J. Pharmacol. Exp. Ther.* **219**, 659–664.

Brannan, T. S., Maker, H. S., Weiss, C. and Cohen, G. (1980). *J. Neurochem.* **35**, 1013–1014.

Brownstein, M. J. (1980). *Proc. R. Soc. London, Ser. B* **210**, 79–90.

Brune, G. G. and Himwich, H. E. (1962). *J. Nerv. Ment. Dis.* **134**, 447–450.

Bruns, R. F. (1980). *Can. J. Physiol. Pharmacol.* **58**, 673–691.

Burns, R. S., Chiueh, C. C., Markey, S. P., Ebert, M. H., Jacobowitz, D. M. and Kopin, I. J. (1983). *Proc. Natl. Acad. Sci. USA* **80**, 4546–4551.

Cahill, A. L. and Ehret, C. F. (1981). *J. Neurochem.* **37**, 1109–1115.

Caldwell, J. (1980). *In* "Concepts in Drug Metabolism" (P. Jenner and B. Testa, eds), Part A, pp. 211–250. Dekker, New York.

Caldwell, J. (1982a). *In* "Metabolic Basis of Detoxication" (W. B. Jakoby, J. R. Bend and J. Caldwell, eds), pp. 271–290. Academic Press, Orlando, New York and London.

Caldwell, J. (1982b). Lecture presented at the Eighth European Workshop on Drug Metabolism, University of Liège, September 5–9. Abstracts, p. 72.

Caldwell, J., Idle, J. R. and Smith, R. L. (1980). *In* "Extrahepatic Metabolism of Drugs and Other Foreign Compounds" (T. E. Gram, ed.), pp. 453–492. MTP Press, Lancaster, UK.

Callard, G. V., Petro, Z. and Ryan, K. J. (1978). *Am. Zool.* **18**, 511–523.

Callard, G. V., Petro, Z. and Ryan, K. J. (1980). *Brain Res.* **202**, 117–130.
Callery, P. S., Stogniew, M. and Geelhaar, L. A. (1979). *Biomed. Mass Spectrosc.* **6**, 23–26.
Callery, P. S., Geelhaar, L. A., Nayar, M. S. B., Stogniew, M. and Rao, K. G. (1982). *J. Neurochem.* **38**, 1063–1067.
Cánovas, F. G., García-Carmona, F., Sánchez, J. V., Iborra Pastor, J. L. and Lozano Teruel, J. A. (1982). *J. Biol. Chem.* **257**, 8738–8744.
Cardinali, D. P. (1981). *Endocr. Rev.* **2**, 327–346.
Cash, C. D., Maitre, M. and Mandel, P. (1979). *J. Neurochem.* **33**, 1169–1175.
Cawthon, R. M., Pintar, J. E., Haseltine, F. P. and Breakfield, X. O. (1981). *J. Neurochem.* **37**, 363–372.
Chand, P. and Clausen, J. (1982). *Chem.-Biol. Interact.* **40**, 357–363.
Chasseaud, L. F. (1976). *In* "Glutathione: Metabolism and Function" (I. M. Arias and W. B. Jakoby, eds), pp. 77–114. Raven Press, New York.
Chasseaud, L. F. (1980). *In* "Extrahepatic Metabolism of Drugs and Other Foreign Compounds" (T. E. Gram, ed.), pp. 427–452. MTP Press, Lancaster, UK.
Chemnitius, J. M., Haselmeyer, K. H. and Zech, R. (1983). *Arch. Toxicol.* **53**, 235–244.
Chiueh, C. C., Burns, R. S., Markey, S. P., Jacobowitz, D. M., Ebert, M. H. and Kopin, I. J. (1983). Presented at 5th Catecholamine Symposium, Göteborg, Sweden.
Cho, A. K., Fischer, J. F. and Schaeffer, J. C. (1977). *Biochem. Pharmacol.* **26**, 1367–1372.
Christophersen, B. O. (1968). *Biochim. Biophys. Acta* **164**, 35–46.
Cohn, J. A., Alvares, A. P. and Kappas, A. (1977). *J. Exp. Med.* **145**, 1607–1611.
Cohen, G. (1976). *Biochem. Pharmacol.* **25**, 1123–1128.
Collins, M. A. (1982). *Trends Pharmacol. Sci.* **3**, 373–375.
Collins, M. A., Nijm, W. P., Borge, G. F., Teas, G. and Goldfarb, C. (1979). *Science* **206**, 1184–1186.
Connelly, J. C. and Bridges, J. W. (1980). *In* "Progress in Drug Metabolism' (J. W. Bridges and L. F. Chasseaud, eds), Vol. 5, pp. 1–111. Wiley, Chichester, UK.
Coon, M. J. and Persson, A. V. (1980). *In* "Enzymatic Basis of Detoxication" (W. B. Jakoby, ed.), Vol. I, pp. 117–134. Academic Press, Orlando, New York and London.
Crespi, F., Buda., M., McRae Degueurce, A. and Pujol, J. F. (1980). *Brain Res.* **191**, 501–509.
Daly, J. W. (1982). *J. Med. Chem.* **25**, 197–207.
Daly, J., Inscoe, J. K. and Axelrod, J. (1965). *J. Med. Chem.* **8**, 153–157.
Das, M., Dixit, R., Seth, P. K. and Mukhtar, H. (1981a). *J. Neurochem.* **36**, 1439–1442.
Das, M., Seth, P. K. and Mukhtar, H. (1981b). *Res. Commun. Chem. Pathol. Pharmacol.* **33**, 377–380.
Das, M., Seth, P. K. and Mukhtar, H. (1981c). *J. Pharmacol. Exp. Ther.* **216**, 156–161.
Das, M., Seth, P. K. and Mukhtar, H. (1981d). *Drug Metab. Disp.* **9**, 69–70.
Das, M., Agarwal, A. K. and Seth, P. K. (1982a). *Biochem. Pharmacol.* **31**, 3927–3930.
Das, M., Seth, P. K., Dixit, R. and Mukhtar, H. (1982b). *Arch. Biochem. Biophys.* **217**, 205–215.

Davis, G. C., Williams, A. C., Markey, S. P., Ebert, M. H., Caine, E. D., Reichert, C. M. and Kopin, I. J. (1979). *Psychiatry Res.* 1, 249–254.

Degtiar, V. G., Loseva, L. A. and Isatchenkov, B. A. (1981). *Endocrinol. Experim.* 15, 181–190.

DeLuca, H. F., Zile, M. and Sietsema, W. K. (1981). *Ann. N. Y. Acad. Sci.* 359, 25–36.

De Matteis, F. and Ray, D. E. (1982). *J. Neurochem.* 39, 551–556.

DePierre, J. W. and Morgenstern, R. (1983). *Biochem. Pharmacol.* 32, 721–723.

Dieringer, C. S., Lamartiniere, C. A., Schiller, C. M. and Lucier, G. W. (1979). *Biochem. Pharmacol.* 28, 2511–2514.

Di Ilio, C., Polidoro, G., Arduini, A. and Federici, G. (1982). *Gen. Pharmacol.* 13, 485–490.

Diliberto, E. J. Jr. and Allen, P. L. (1980). *Molec. Pharmacol.* 17, 421–426.

Dixit, R., Mukhtar, H., Seth, P. K. and Murti, C. R. K. (1981). *Biochem. Pharmacol.* 30, 1739–1745.

Donaldson, J., LaBella, F. S. and Gesser, D. (1980). *Neurotoxicology* 2, 53–64.

Doshi, P. S. and Edwards, D. J. (1981). *J. Chromat.* 210, 505–511.

Elbaum, D. and Nagel, R. L. (1981). *J. Biol. Chem.* 256, 2280–2283.

Elison, C. and Elliott, H. W. (1963). *Biochem. Pharmacol.* 12, 1363–1366.

Felsted, R. L. and Bachur, N. R. (1980). *In* "Enzymatic Basis of Detoxication" (W. B. Jakoby, ed.), Vol. I, pp. 281–293. Academic Press, Orlando, New York and London.

Fields, J. Z. and Gordon, J. H. (1982). *Life Sci.* 30, 229–234.

Fischer, L. J., Green, M. D. and Harman, A. W. (1981). *J. Pharmacol. Exp. Ther.* 219, 281–286.

Fishman, J. and Goto, J. (1981). *J. Biol. Chem.* 256, 4466–4471.

Fishman, J. and Norton, B. (1975a). *Adv. Biosci.* 15, 123–131.

Fishman, J. and Norton, B. (1975b). *Endocrinology* 96, 1054–1059.

Fishman, J., Guzik, H. and Hellman, L. (1970). *Biochemistry* 9, 1593–1598.

Fishman, J., Naftolin, F., Davies, I. J., Ryan, K. J. and Petro, Z. (1976a). *J. Clin. Endocrinol. Metab.* 42, 177–180.

Fishman, J., Hahn, E. F. and Norton, B. I. (1976b). *Nature* 261, 64–65.

Foreman, M. M. and Porter, J. C. (1980). *J. Neurochem.* 34, 1175–1183.

Friedberg, T., Bentley, P., Stasiecki, P., Glatt, H. R., Raphael, D. and Oesch, F. (1979). *J. Biol. Chem.* 254, 12028–12033.

Fuller, R. W. and Hemrick, S. K. (1979). *Comp. Biochem. Biophys.* 62, 243–245.

Gander, J. E. and Mannering, G. J. (1980). *Pharmacol. Ther.* 10, 191–221.

Garattini, E., Gazzotti, G. and Salmona, M. (1981). *Experientia* 37, 230–231.

Gaunt, G. L. and de Duve, C. (1976). *J. Neurochem.* 26, 749–759.

Glatt, H. R., Cooper, C. S., Grover, P. L., Sims, P., Bentley, P., Merdes, M., Waechter, F., Vogel, K., Guenthner, T. M. and Oesch, F. (1982). *Science* 215, 1507–1509.

Godwin-Austen, R. B., Lee, P. N., Marmot, M. G. and Stern, G. M. (1982). *J. Neurol. Neurosurg. Psych.* 45, 577–581.

Goldberg, R. and Tipton, K. F. (1978). Biochem. Pharmacol. 27, 2623–2629.

Gomes, U. C. R., McCarthy, B. W. and Shanley, B. C. (1981). *Biochem. Pharmacol.* 30, 571–577.

Goodwin, B. L. (1979). *In* "Aromatic Amino Acid Hydroxylases and Mental Disease" (M. B. H. Youdim, ed.), pp. 5–76. Wiley, Chichester, U. K.

Gordonsmith, R. H., Raxworthy, M. J. and Gulliver, P. A. (1982). *Biochem. Pharmacol.* 31, 433–437.

200   M. MESNIL, B. TESTA AND P. JENNER

Gorman, A. A. and Rodgers, M. A. J. (1981). *Chem. Soc. Rev.* **10**, 205–231.
Goto, J. and Fishman, J. (1977). *Science* **195**, 80–81.
Graf, H., Ruf, H. H. and Ullrich, V. (1983). *Ang. Chem. Int. Ed.* **22**, 487–488.
Grimes, J. D. (1982). *Can. Med. Ass. J.* **126**, 468.
Guengerich, F. P. and Mason, P. S. (1979). *Molec. Pharmacol.* **15**, 154–164.
Guenthner, T. M., Hammock, B. D., Vogel, U. and Oesch, F. (1981). *J. Biol. Chem.* **256**, 3163–3166.
Guenthner, T. M., Vogel-Bindel, U. and Oesch, F. (1982), *Arch. Toxicol. Suppl.* **5**, 365–367.
Gunsalus, I. C., Pederson, T. C. and Sligar, S. G. (1975). *Ann. Rev. Biochem.* **44**, 377–407.
Gupta, C., Yaffe, S. J. and Shapiro, B. H. (1982). *Science* **216**, 640–643.
Guroff, G. (1980). "Molecular Neurobiology". Dekker, New York.
Gutteridge, J. M. C., Rowley, D. A. and Halliwell, B. (1982). *Biochem. J.* **206**, 605–609.
Hamon, M., Bourgoin, S. and Youdim, M. B. H. (1979). *In* "Aromatic Amino Acid Hydroxylases and Mental Disease" (M. B. H. Youdim, ed.), pp. 233–297. Wiley, Chichester, U.K.
Hanzlik, R. P., Edelman, M., Michaely, W. J. and Scott, G. (1976). *J. Am. Chem. Soc.* **98**, 1952–1955.
Hassan, H. M. and Fridovich, I. (1980). *In* "Enzymatic Basis of Detoxication" W. B. Jakoby, ed.), Vol. I, pp. 311–332. Academic Press, Orlando, New York and London.
Hefti, F. and Melamed, E. (1980). *Trends Neurol. Sci.* **3**, 229–231.
Hegazi, M. F., Borchardt, R. T. and Schowen, R. L. (1979). *J. Am. Chem. Soc.* **101**, 4359–4365.
Hersey, R. M., Gunsalus, P., Lloyd, T. and Weisz, J. (1981a). *Endocrinology* **109**, 1902–1911.
Hersey, R. M., Williams, K. I. H. and Weisz, J. (1981b). *Endocrinology* **109**, 1912–1920.
Heymann, E. (1980). *In* "Enzymatic Basis of Detoxication" (W. B. Jakoby, ed.), Vol. II, pp. 291–323. Academic Press, Orlando, New York and London.
Hiemke, C. and Ghraf, R. (1983). *J. Neurochem.* **40**, 592–594.
Ho, B. T., Pong, S. F., Browne, R. G. and Walker, K. E. (1973). *Experientia* **29**, 275–277.
Hoffman, A. R., Sastry, B. V. R. and Axelrod, J. (1979). *Pharmacology* **19**, 257–260.
Holtzman, D. and Desautel, M. (1980). *J. Neurochem.* **34**, 1535–1538.
Holtzman, D., Hsu, J. S. and Desautel, M. (1981). *Toxicol. Appl. Pharmacol.* **58**, 48–56.
Horn, A. S., Griever-Kazemier, H. and Dijkstra, D. (1982). *J. Med. Chem.* **25**, 993–996.
Howard, P. C. and Beland, F. A. (1982). *Biochem. Biophys. Res. Commun.* **104**, 727–732.
Hruska, R. E. and Silbergeld, E. K. (1980). *Eur. J. Pharmacol.* **61**, 397–400.
Hsu, L. L., Geyer, M. A. and Mandell, A. J. (1976). *Biochem. Pharmacol.* **25**, 815–819.
Hsu, L. L., Halaris, A. E. and Freedman, D. X. (1982). *Int. J. Biochem.* **14**, 581–584.
Ichikawa, Y. and Yamano, T. (1967). *Arch. Biochem. Biophys.* **121**, 742–749.
Inoue, K. and Lindros, K. O. (1982). *J. Neurochem.* **38**, 884–888.
Inouye, A. and Shinagawa, Y. (1965). *J. Neurochem.* **12**, 803–813.
Ishimitsu, S., Fujimoto, S. and Ohara, A. (1980). *Chem. Pharm. Bull.* **28**, 1653–1655.

Jakoby, W. B. and Habig, W. H. (1980). In "Enzymatic Basis of Detoxication" (W. B. Jakoby, ed.), Vol. II, pp 63–94. Academic Press, Orlando, New York and London.

Jakoby, W. B., Sekura, R. D., Lyon, E. S., Marcus, C. J. and Wang, J.-L. (1980). In "Enzymatic Basis of Detoxication" (W. B. Jakoby, ed.) Vol. II, pp. 199–228. Academic Press, Orlando, New York and London.

Javors, M. and Erwin, V. G. (1980). Biochem. Pharmacol. 29, 1703–1708.

Jenner, P., Testa, B. and Di Carlo, F. J. (1981). Trends Pharmacol. Sci. 2, 135–137.

Johannesen, K. A. M. and DePierre, J. W. (1978). Analyt. Biochem. 86, 725–732.

Johnson, M. K. (1975). Arch. Toxicol. 34, 259–288.

Johnson, R. C. and Shah, S. N. (1981). J. Neurochem. 37, 594–596.

Johnston, J. P. (1968). Biochem. Pharmacol. 17, 1285–1297.

Jondorf, W. R. (1981). In "Concepts in Drug Metabolism" (P. Jenner and B. Testa, eds), Part B, pp. 307–376. Dekker, New York.

Jonsson, G. (1980). Ann. Rev. Neurosci. 3, 169–187.

Juchau, M. R., DiGiovanni, J., Namkung, M. J. and Jones, A. H. (1979). Toxicol. Appl. Pharmacol. 49, 171–178.

Kamyshanskaya, N. S. and Moskovitina, T. A. (1981). Voprosy Meditsinskoi Khimii, USSR 27, 261–265.

Kasper, C. B. and Henton, D. (1980). In "Enzymatic Basis of Detoxication" (W. B. Jakoby, ed.), Vol. II, pp. 3–36. Academic Press, Orlando, New York and London.

Kellogg, E. W. III and Fridovich, I. (1975). J. Biol. Chem. 250, 8812–8817.

Ketterer, B. (1982). Drug Metab. Rev. 13, 161–187.

Killenberg, P. G. and Webster, L. T. Jr. (1980). In "Enzymatic Basis of Detoxication" (W. B. Jakoby, ed.), Vol. II, pp. 141–167. Academic Press, Orlando, New York and London.

Klingenberg, M. (1958). Arch. Biochem. Biophys. 75, 376–386.

Köchli, H. W., Wermuth, B. and von Wartburg, J.-P. (1980). Biochim. Biophys. Acta 616, 133–143.

Kopp, N., Claustrat, B. and Tappaz, M. (1980). Neurosci. Lett. 19, 237–242.

Kornbrust, D. J. and Mavis, R. D. (1980a). Molec. Pharmacol. 17, 408–414.

Kornbrust, D. J. and Mavis, R. D. (1980b). Molec. Pharmacol. 17, 400–407.

Kovachich, G. B. and Mishra, O. P. (1980). J. Neurochem. 35, 1449–1453.

Kuhn, C. M., Schanberg, S. M. and Breese, G. R. (1978). Biochem. Pharmacol. 27, 343–351.

Kupfer, D. (1980). Pharmacol. Ther. 11, 469–496.

Kurono, Y., Maki, T., Yotsuyanagi, T. and Ikeda, K. (1979). Chem. Pharm. Bull. 27, 2781–2786.

Langston, J. W., Ballard, P., Tetrud, J. W. and Irwin, I. (1983). Science 219, 979–980.

Lasker, J. M., Sivarajah, K., Mason, R. P., Kalyanaraman, B., Abou-Donia, M. B. and Eling, T. E. (1981). J. Biol. Chem. 256, 7764–7767.

Ledig, M., Fried, R., Ziessel, M. and Mandel, P. (1982). Develop. Brain Res. 4, 333–337.

Leung, T. K. C., Lai, J. C. K. and Lim, L. (1982). Comp. Biochem. Physiol. Part C 71, 219–222.

Lewis, M. H., Widerlöv, E., Knight, D. L., Kilts, C. D. and Mailman, R. B. (1983). J. Pharmacol. Exp. Ther. 225, 539–545.

Liang, Y.-O., Plotzky, P. M. and Adams, R. N. (1977). J. Med. Chem. 20, 581–583.

Lieberburg, I., Wallach, G. and McEwen, B. S. (1977). Brain Res. 128, 176–186.

Lind, C., Hochstein, P. and Ernster, L. (1982). *Arch. Biochem. Biophys.* **216**, 178–185.

Lippke, K. P., Schunack, W. G., Wenning, W. and Müller, W. E. (1983). *J. Med. Chem.* **26**, 499–503.

Little, C. and O'Brien, P. J. (1968). *Biochem. Biophys. Res. Commun.* **31**, 145–150.

Lloyd, T. and Weisz, J. (1978). *J. Biol. Chem.* **253**, 4841–4843.

Lloyd, T., Weisz, J. and Breakefield, X. O. (1978). *J. Neurochem.* **31**, 245–250.

Londos, C., Cooper, D. M. F. and Wolff, J. (1980). *Proc. Natl Acad. Sci. USA* **77**, 2551–2554.

Loo, Y. H., Miller, K. A., Nowlin, J. and Horning, M. G. (1980). *Life Sci.* **26**, 657–663.

Lotti, M. and Johnson, M. K. (1980). *Arch. Toxicol.* **45**, 263–271.

Løvstad, R. A. (1979). *Experientia* **35**, 1642–1644.

Lysz, T. W. and Needleman, P. (1982). *J. Neurochem.* **38**, 1111–1117.

Maguire, M. E., Goldmann, P. H. and Gilman, A. G. (1974). *Molec. Pharmacol.* **10**, 563–581.

Maker, H. S., Weiss, C., Silides, D. J. and Cohen, G. (1981). *J. Neurochem.* **36**, 589–593.

Maksay, G., Kardos, J., Simonyi, M., Tegyey, Zs. and Ötvös, L. (1981). *Arzneim.-Forsch.* **31**, 979–981.

Maines, M. D. (1980). *Biochem. J.* **190**, 315–321.

Malmström, B. G. (1982). *Ann. Rev. Biochem.* **51**, 21–60.

Mann, S. P. and Gordon, J. I. (1979). *J. Neurochem.* **33**, 133–138.

Mannering, G. J. (1981). *In* "Concepts in Drug Metabolism" (P. Jenner and B. Testa, eds), Part B, pp. 53–166. Dekker, New York.

Mannervik, B. (1982). *In* "Metabolic Basis of Detoxication" (W. B. Jakoby, J. R. Bend and J. Caldwell, eds), pp. 185–206. Academic Press, Orlando, New York and London.

Marietta, M. P., Vesell, E. S., Hartman, R. D., Weisz, J. and Dvorchik, B. H. (1979). *J. Pharmacol. Exp. Ther.* **208**, 271–279.

Markovits, P., Levy, S., Nocentini, S., Mazabraud, A., Velizarou, A., Sebharvel, P. and Benda, P. (1976). *C.r. Séanc. Acad. Sci. Paris* **282**, 2015–2020.

Marnett, L. J. (1981). *Life Sci.* **29**, 531–546.

Marsh, M. V., Hutt, A. J., Caldwell, J., Smith, R. L., Horner, M. W., Houghton, F. and Moss, M. S. (1981). *Biochem. Pharmacol.* **30**, 1879–1882.

Marshall, K. S. and Castagnoli, N. Jr. (1973). *J. Med. Chem.* **16**, 266–270.

Masters, B. S. S. and Okita, R. T. (1980). *Pharmacol. Ther.* **9**, 227–244.

Mavelli, I., Rigo, A., Federico, R., Ciriolo, M. R. and Rotilio, G. (1982). *Biochem. J.* **204**, 535–540.

May, S. W. and Phillips, R. S. (1980). *J. Am. Chem. Soc.* **102**, 5981–5983.

May, S. W., Phillips, R. S., Mueller, P. W. and Herman, H. H. (1981). *J. Biol. Chem.* **256**, 2258–2261.

McEwen, B. S., Lieberburg, I., Chaptal, C. and Krey, L. C. (1977). *Horm. Behav.* **9**, 249–263.

McGeer, P. L. (1967). *Can. J. Biochem.* **45**, 1943–1952.

Meek, J. L. and Neff, N. H. (1973). *J. Neurochem.* **21**, 1–9.

Melchior, C. and Collins, M. A. (1982). *CRC Crit. Rev. Toxicol.* **9**, 313–356.

Melchior, C. L. and Myers, R. D. (1977). *Pharmacol. Biochem. Behav.* **7**, 19–35.

Metcalf, B. W., Wright, C. L., Burkhart, J. P. and Johnston, J. O. (1981). *J. Am. Chem. Soc.* **103**, 3221–3222.

Meyerson, L. R. and Clement-Cormier, Y. C. (1980). *In* "Alcoholism: A perspective." Proceedings Annual Conference on Alcohol 1977–1978. pp. 383–412.

Milby, K., Oke, A. and Adams, R. N. (1982). *Neuroscience Lett.* **28**, 169–174.

Milthers, K. (1962). *Acta Pharmacol. Toxicol.* **19**, 235–240.

Misra, A. L., Mitchell, C. L. and Woods, L. A. (1971). *Nature* **232**, 48–50.

Misra, A. L., Vadlamani, N. L., Pontani, R. B. and Mulé, S. J. (1973). *Biochem. Pharmacol.* **22**, 2129–2139.

Misra, A. L., Vadlamani, N. L., Pontani, R. B. and Mulé, S. J. (1974). *J. Pharm. Pharmacol.* **26**, 990–992.

Mitchard, M. (1971). *Xenobiotica* **1**, 469–481.

Morton, D. J. and Potgieter, B. (1982). *S. Afr. J. Sci.* **78**, 43–45.

Moura, D., Azevedo, I. and Osswald, W. (1977). *J. Pharm. Pharmacol.* **29**, 255–256.

Mukhtar, H., Baars, A. J. and Breimer, D. D. (1981a). *Xenobiotica* **11**, 367–371.

Mukhtar, H., Zoetemelk, C. E. M., Baars, A. J., Wijnen, J. T., Blankenstein-Wijnen, L. M. M., Khan, P. M. and Breimer, D. D. (1981b). *Pharmacology* **22**, 322–329.

Mullis, K. B., Perry, D. C., Finn, A. M., Stafford, B. and Sadée, W. (1979). *J. Pharmacol. Exp. Ther.* **208**, 228–231.

Nabeshima, T., Fontenot, J. and Ho, I. K. (1981). *Biochem. Pharmacol.* **30**, 1142–1145.

Naftolin, F., Ryan, K. J., Davies, I. J., Petro, Z. and Kuhn, M. (1975a). *Adv. Biosci.* **15**, 105–121.

Naftolin, F., Ryan, K. J., Davies, I. J., Reddy, V. V., Flores, F., Petro, Z., White, R. J., Takaoka, Y. and Wolin, L. (1975b). *Rec. Progr. Horm. Res.* **31**, 295–319.

Nagamatsu, K., Kido, Y., Terao, T., Ishida, T. and Toki, S. (1983). *Drug Metab. Disposit.* **11**, 190–194.

Nagatsu, T. (1981). *Trends Pharmacol. Sci.* **2**, 276–279.

Nebert, D. W. and Negishi, M. (1982). *Biochem. Pharmacol.* **31**, 2311–2317.

Nelson, N. A., Kelly, R. C. and Johnson, R. A. (1982). *Chem. Eng. News* **60** (33), 30–44.

Norman, B. J. and Neal, R. A. (1976). *Biochem. Pharmacol.* **25**, 37–45.

Nousiainen, U. and Hänninen, O. (1981). *Acta Pharmacol. Toxicol.* **49**, 77–80.

Nugteren, D. H. and Hazelhof, E. (1973). *Biochem. Biophys. Acta* **326**, 448–461.

O'Brien, P. J. (1978). *Pharmacol. Ther. A* **2**, 517–536.

O'Brien, M. M., Schofield, P. J. and Edwards, M. R. (1983). *Biochem. J.* **211**, 81–90.

O'Donnell, J. P. (1982). *Drug Metab. Rev.* **13**, 123–159.

Oesch, F. (1979). *In* "Progress in Drug Metabolism" (J. W. Bridges and L. F. Chasseaud, eds), Vol. 3, pp. 253–301. Wiley, Chichester, UK.

Oesch, F. (1980). *In* "Enzymatic Basis of Detoxication" (W. B. Jakoby, ed.), Vol. II, pp. 277–290. Academic Press, Orlando, New York and London.

Oftebro, H., Stormer, F. C. and Pedersen, J. I. (1979). *J. Biol. Chem.* **254**, 4331–4334.

Ogino, T. and Suzuki, K. (1981). *J. Neurochem.* **36**, 776–779.

Oguri, K. (1980). *J. Pharm. Soc. Jap.* **100**, 117–125.

Omiecinski, C. J., Namkung, M. J. and Juchau, M. R. (1980). *Molec. Pharmacol.* **17**, 225–232.

Omura, T. and Sato, R. (1962). *J. Biol. Chem.* **237**, 1375–1376.

Omura, T. and Sato, R. (1964). *J. Biol. Chem.* **239**, 2370–2378, 2379–2385.

Oommen, A., George, S. T. and Balasubramanian, A. S. (1980). *Life Sci.* **26**, 2129–2136.

Origitano, T. C. and Collins, M. A. (1980). *Life Sci.* **26**, 2061–2065.

204   M. MESNIL, B. TESTA AND P. JENNER

Osmond, H. and Smythies, J. R. (1952). *J. Ment Sci.* **98**, 309–315.
Patterson, E., Radtke, H. E. and Weber, W. W. (1980). *Molec. Pharmacol.* **17**, 367–373.
Paul, S. M., Axelrod, J. and Diliberto, E. J. (1977). *Endocrinology* **101**, 1604–1610.
Paul, S. M., Hoffman, A. R. and Axelrod, J. (1980). *In* "Frontiers in Neuro-endocrinology" (L. Martini and W. F. Ganong, eds), Vol. 6, pp. 203–217. Raven Press, New York.
Percy, V. A. and Shanley, B. C. (1979). *J. Neurochem.* **33**, 1267–1274.
Perez-Reyes, E. and Mason, R. P. (1981). *J. Biol. Chem.* **256**, 2427–2432.
Perry, T. L., Godin, D. V. and Hansen, S. (1982). *Neuroscience Lett.* **33**, 305–310.
Player, T. J. and Horton, A. A. (1981). *J. Neurochem.* **37**, 422–426.
Powell, G. M. and Roy, A. B. (1980). *In* "Extrahepatic Metabolism of Drugs and Other Foreign Compounds" (T. E. Gram, ed.), pp. 389–423. MTP Press, Lancaster, UK.
Powis, G., Svingen, B. A. and Appel, P. (1981). *Molec. Pharmacol.* **20**, 387–394.
Prohaska, J. R. and Ganther, H. E. (1976). *J. Neurochem.* **27**, 1379–1387.
Rajagopalan, K. V. (1980). *In* "Enzymatic Basis of Detoxication" (W. B. Jakoby, ed.), Vol. I, pp. 295–309. Academic Press, Orlando, New York and London.
Rakonczay, Z., Vincendon, G. and Zanetta, J.-P. (1981). *J. Neurochem.* **37**, 662–669.
Raskin, N. H. and Sokoloff, L. (1970). *J. Neurochem.* **17**, 1677–1687.
Raskin, N. H. and Sokoloff, L. (1974). *J. Neurochem.* **22**, 427–434.
Recknagel, R. O., Glende, E. A. Jr. and Hvuszkewycz, A. M. (1977). *In* "Free Radicals in Biology" (W. A. Pryor, ed.), Vol. 3, pp. 97–132. Academic Press, Orlando, New York and London.
Reichert, D. (1981). *Angew. Chem. Int. Ed.* **20**, 135–142.
Rein, G., Glover, V. and Sandler, M. (1982). *Biochem. Pharmacol.* **31**, 1893–1897.
Reis, D. J. and Molinoff, P. P. (1972). *J. Neurochem.* **19**, 195–204.
Renskers, K. J., Feor, K. D. and Roth, J. A. (1980). *J. Neurochem.* **34**, 1362–1368.
Reyes, E. and Barela, T. D. (1980). *Neurochem. Res.* **5**, 159–169.
Rice, J. M., Joshi, S. R., Shenefelt, R. E. and Wenk, M. L. (1978). *In* "Carcino-genesis" (R. Freudenthal and P. W. Jones, eds), Vol. 3, "Polynuclear Aromatic Hydrocarbons", pp. 413–422. Raven Press, New York.
Rifkind, A. B. and Petschke, T. (1981). *J. Pharmacol. Exp. Ther.* **217**, 572–578.
Rivett, A. J., Smith, I. L. and Tipton, K. F. (1981). *Biochem. J.* **197**, 473–481.
Rosengarten, H. and Friedhoff, A. J. (1976). *Schizophrenia Bull.* **2**, 90–105.
Roth, J. A. (1980). *Biochem. Pharmacol.* **29**, 3119–3122.
Rouet, P., Alexandrov, K., Markovits, P., Frayssinet, C. and Dansette, P. M. (1981). *Carcinogenesis* **2**, 919–926.
Rousseau, A. and Gatt, S. (1979). *J. Biol. Chem.* **245**, 7741–7745.
Rutledge, C. O. and Hoehn, N. M. (1973). *Nature* **244**, 447–450.
Sandler, M., Carter, S. B., Hunter, K. R. and Stern, G. M. (1973). *Nature* **241**, 439–443.
Sasame, H. A., Ames, M. M. and Nelson, S. D. (1977). *Biochem. Biophys. Res. Commun.* **78**, 919–926.
Satoh, T., Fukumori, R., Minegishi, A., Kitagawa, H. and Yanaura, S. (1979). *Res. Commun. Chem. Pathol. Pharmacol.* **23**, 297–311.
Sattin, A. and Rall, T. W. (1970). *Molec. Pharmacol.* **6**, 13–23.
Savolainen, H. (1978). *Res. Commun. Chem. Pathol. Pharmacol.* **21**, 173–176.
Savov, V. M., Eluashvili, I. A., Pisarev, V. A., Prilipko, L. L. and Kagan, V. E. (1980). *Bull. Exp. Biol. Med.-Engl. Transl.* **90**, 555–557.

Sawyer, D. T. and Valentine, J. S. (1981). *Acc. Chem. Res.* **14**, 393–400.
Schaeffer, J. M. and Hsueh, A. J. W. (1980). *Obstet. Gynecol. Surv.* **35**, 162–163.
Schenkman, J. B. and Gibson, G. G. (1981). *Trends Pharmacol. Sci.* **2**, 150–152.
Schoepp, D. and Azzaro, A. J. (1981). *J. Neurochem.* **36**, 2025–2031.
Schurr, A., Ho, B. T. and Schoolar, J. C. (1981). *J. Pharm. Pharmacol.* **33**, 165–170.
Shigezane, J., Oguri, K., Mishima, M. and Yoshimura, H. (1982). *J. Pharmacobio-Dynam.* **5**, S-61.
Siesjö, B. K., Rehncrona, S. and Smith, D. (1980). *Acta Physiol. Scand. Suppl.* **492**, 121–128.
Sietsema, W. K. and DeLuca, H. F. (1982). *J. Biol. Chem.* **257**, 4265–4270.
Sikic, B. I. (1980). *In* "Extrahepatic Metabolism of Drugs and Other Foreign Compounds" (T. E. Gram, ed.), pp. 533–549. MTP Press, Lancaster, UK.
Sinet, P. M., Heikkila, R. E. and Cohen, G. (1980). *J. Neurochem.* **34**, 1421–1428.
Singer, S. S., Federspiel, M. J., Green, J., Lewis, W. G., Martin, V., Witt, K. R. and Tappel, J. (1982). *Biochim. Biophys. Acta* **700**, 110–117.
Sitaramayya, A., Wright, L. S. and Siegel, F. L. (1980). *J. Biol. Chem.* **255**, 8894–8900.
Sivarajah, K., Lasker, J. M., Eling, T. E. and Abou-Donia, M. B. (1982). *Molec. Pharmacol.* **21**, 133–141.
Sligar, S. G., Cinti, D. L., Gibson, G. G. and Schenkman, J. B. (1979). *Biochem. Biophys. Res. Commun.* **90**, 925–932.
Slojkowska, Z., Krasuska, H. J. and Pachecka, J. (1982). *Xenobiotica* **12**, 359–364.
Snipes, C. A. and Shore, L. S. (1982). *Andrologia* **14**, 81–85.
Strittmatter, P. and Dailey, H. A. (1982). *In* "Membranes and Transport" (A. N. Martonosi, ed.), Vol. 1, pp. 71–82. Plenum Publishing Co., New York.
Stubley, C. and Stell, J. G. P. (1980). *J. Pharm. Pharmacol.* **32**, 51P.
Stubley, C., Stell, J. G. P. and Mathieson, D. W. (1979). *Xenobiotica* **9**, 475–484.
Svingen, B. A., Buege, J. A., O'Neal, F. O. and Aust, S. D. (1979). *J. Biol. Chem.* **254**, 5892–5899.
Takeshita, M., Miki, M. and Yubisui, T. (1982). *J. Neurochem.* **39**, 1047–1049.
Tampier, L. (1978). *Pharmacol. Res. Commun.* **10**, 823–829.
Tate, S. S. (1980). *In* "Enzymatic Basis of Detoxication" (W. B. Jakoby, ed.), Vol. II, pp. 95–120. Academic Press, Orlando, New York and London.
Taylor, K. B. (1974). *J. Biol. Chem.* **249**, 454–458.
Testa, B. and Jenner, P. (1976), "Drug Metabolism. Chemical and Biochemical Aspects." Dekker, New York.
Testa, B. and Jenner, P. (1978). *Drug Metab. Rev.* **7**, 325–369.
Testa, B. and Jenner, P. (1981). *Drug Metab. Rev.* **12**, 1–117.
Testa, B., Di Carlo, F. J. and Jenner, P. (1981). *In* "Concepts in Drug Metabolism" (P. Jenner and B. Testa, eds), Part B, pp. 515–535. Dekker, New York.
Thyagarajan, P. (1981a). *Experientia* **37**, 449–451.
Thyagarajan, P. (1981b). *Ind. J. Biochem. Biophys.* **18**, 286–290.
Tiffany-Castiglioni, E., Saneto, R. P., Proctor, P. H. and Perez-Polo, J. R. (1982). *Biochem. Pharmacol.* **31**, 181–188.
Tipton, K. F. (1980). *In* "Enzymatic Basis of Detoxication" (W. B. Jakoby, ed.), Vol. I, pp. 355–370. Academic Press, Orlando, New York and London.
Trager, W. F. (1980). *In* "Concepts in Drug Metabolism" (P. Jenner and B. Testa, eds), Part A, pp. 177–209. Dekker, New York.
Trager, W. F. (1982). *Drug Metab. Rev.* **13**, 51–69.
Trocewicz, J., Oka, K., Nagatsu, T., Nagatsu, I., Iizuka, R. and Narabayashi, H. (1982). *Biochem. Med.* **27**, 317–324.

Tse, D. C. S., McCreery, R. L. and Adams, R. N. (1976). *J. Med. Chem.* **19**, 37–40.

Uemura, T., Shimazu, T., Miura, R. and Yamano, T. (1980). *Biochem. Biophys. Res. Commun.* **93**, 1074–1081.

Ullrich, V. and Haurand, M. (1983). *In* "Advances in Prostaglandin, Thromboxane and Leukotriene" (B. Samuelson, R. Paoletti and P. W. Ramwell, eds), Vol. 11, pp. 105–110. Raven Press, New York.

Usdin, E., Skolnick, P., Tallman, J. F. Jr., Greenblatt, D. and Paul, S. M. (eds) (1982). "Pharmacology of Benzodiazepines." Macmillan Press, London.

Vaccari, A., Caviglia, A., Sparatore, A. and Biassoni, R. (1981). *J. Neurochem.* **37**, 640–648.

Vainio, H. and Hietanen, E. (1980). *In* "Concepts in Drug Metabolism" (P. Jenner and B. Testa, eds), Part A, pp. 251–284. Dekker, New York.

van Bladeren, P. J., Breimer, D. D., Rotteveel-Smijs, G. M. T., de Jong, R. A. W., Buijs, W., van der Gen, A. and Mohn, G. R. (1980). *Biochem. Pharmacol.* **29**, 2975–2982.

van der Schoot, J. B. and Creveling, C. R. (1965). *In* "Advances in Drug Research" (N. J. Harper and A. B. Simmonds, eds), Vol. 2, pp. 47–88. Academic Press, London, Orlando and New York.

Vander Wende, C. and Spoerlein, M. T. (1963). *Life Sci.* **6**, 386–392.

Vanella, A., Geremia, E., D'Urso, G., Tiriolo, P., Di Silvestro, I., Grimaldi, R. and Pinturo, R. (1982). *Gerontology* **28**, 108–113.

Vickers, S., Duncan, C. A. H., Arison, B. H., Ramjit, H. G., Rosegay, A., Nutt, R. F. and Veber, D. F. (1983). *Drug Metab. Disposit.* **11**, 147–151.

Villela, G. G. (1968). *Experientia* **24**, 1101–1102.

Vogel, K., Platt, K.-L., Petrovic, P., Seidel, A. and Oesch, F. (1982). *Arch. Toxicol. Suppl.* **5**, 360–364.

von Wartburg, J.-P. and Wermuth, B. (1980). *In* "Enzymatic Basis of Detoxication" (W. B. Jakoby, ed.), Vol. I, pp. 249–260. Academic Press, Orlando, New York and London.

Walsh, C. (1977). "Enzymatic Reaction Mechanisms." Freeman, San Francisco.

Walsh, C. (1980). *Ann. Rep. Med. Chem.* **15**, 207–216.

Weber, W. W. and Glowinski, I. B. (1980). *In* "Enzymatic Basis of Detoxication" (W. B. Jakoby, ed.), Vol. II, pp. 169–186. Academic Press, Orlando, New York and London.

Weber, W. W., Radtke, H. E. and Tannen, R. H. (1980). *In* "Extrahepatic Metabolism of Drugs and Other Foreign Compounds" (T. E. Gram. ed.), pp. 493–531. MTP Press, Lancaster, UK.

Weidenfeld, J., Siegel, R. A. and Yanai, J. (1983). *J. Steroid Biochem.* **18**, 201–205.

Weiner, N. (1979). *In* "Aromatic Amino Acid Hydroxylases and Mental Disease" (M. B. H. Youdim, ed.), pp. 141–190. Wiley, Chichester, UK.

Weiner, H. (1980). *In* "Enzymatic Basis of Detoxication" (W. B. Jakoby, ed.) Vol. I, pp. 261–280. Academic Press, Orlando, New York and London.

Wendel, A. (1980). *In* "Enzymatic Basis of Detoxication" (W. B. Jakoby, ed.), Vol. I, pp. 333–350. Academic Press, Orlando, New York and London.

Wermuth, B. (1981). *J. Biol. Chem.* **256**, 1206–1213.

Westcott, J. Y., Weiner, H., Shultz, J. and Myers, R. D. (1980). *Biochem. Pharmacol.* **29**, 411–417.

Westkaemper, R. B. and Hanzlik, R. P. (1981). *Arch. Biochem. Biophys.* **208**, 195–204.

Wheldrake, J. F., Marshall, J., Hewitt, S. and Baudinette, R. V. (1981). *Comp. Biochem. Physiol.* Pt B **68**, 491–496.

White, R. E. and Coon, M. J. (1980). *Ann. Rev. Biochem.* **49**, 315–356.
White, H. L. and Glassman, A. T. (1977). *J. Neurochem.* **29**, 987–997.
Wolfe, L. S., Pappius, H. M. and Marion, J. (1976). *Adv. Prostaglandin Thromboxane Res.* **1**, 345–355.
Yang, H. Y. T. and Neff, N. H. (1976). *Molec. Pharmacol.* **12**, 69–72.
Yeh, S. Y. (1982). *Drug Metab. Disposit.* **10**, 319–325.
Yu, P. H. (1978). *Neurochem. Res.* **3**, 755–762.
Yu, P. H. and Boulton, A. A. (1979). *Can. J. Biochem.* **57**, 1204–1209.
Yu, P. H. and Boulton, A. A. (1980). *J. Neurochem.* **35**, 255–257.
Ziegler, D. M. (1980). *In* "Enzymatic Basis of Detoxication". (W. B. Jakoby, ed.), Vol. I, pp. 201–227. Academic Press, Orlando, New York and London.

Central and Peripheral α-Adrenoceptors. Pharmacological Aspects and Clinical Potential

P. A. VAN ZWIETEN and P. B. M. W. M. TIMMERMANS

Division of Pharmacotherapy, University of Amsterdam, Amsterdam, The Netherlands

1 Introduction

The subdivision of the receptors in the adrenergic system into the α- and β-subtypes is now generally accepted. Ever since the formulation of this subdivision by Ahlquist (1948) the emphasis on research and application has been laid upon β-adrenoceptors. This development is quite understandable in view of the widespread therapeutic application of β-adrenoceptor

ADVANCES IN DRUG RESEARCH VOL. 13
0-12-013313-X

blocking agents (β-blockers) in hypertension, angina pectoris and other forms of myocardial ischemia, cardiac arrhythmia, and more recently glaucoma, migraine and certain forms of tremor. Moreover, β-adrenoceptor stimulants are widely applied in the therapy of bronchial asthma and to a more limited extent in cardiology. From a more theoretical point of view, it is attractive for medicinal chemists and pharmacologists that a well-defined relationship between chemical structure and pharmacological activity has been demonstrated for both β-adrenoceptor agonists and antagonists.

In contrast to the thoroughly investigated β-receptor, much less research has been carried out into the α-receptor until approximately a decade ago, when a renaissance of interest began to develop. Until then, a lack of clear structure–activity relationships, the limited therapeutic interest of α-adrenoceptor agonists and antagonists, as well as a meagre understanding of a possible physiological role of α-adrenoceptors, had caused a neglect of this receptor subtype in pharmacology and physiology as well as in clinical medicine.

More recently, however, interest in the α-adrenoceptor has been greatly stimulated as a result of the following developments:

1. The introduction of the concept of pre- and postjunctional receptors, which is mainly based upon research on α-adrenoceptors.
2. The classification of α-adrenoceptors into the α_1- and α_2-subtypes.
3. The discovery that α-adrenoceptors in the brain stem are involved in the antihypertensive activity of centrally acting drugs, like clonidine, guanfacine and α-methyl-DOPA.
4. The development by the pharmaceutical industry of highly selective agonists and antagonists of the α-adrenoceptor subtype which will most probably lead to new and specific therapeutic agents.
5. The introduction of radioligand binding techniques which have particularly facilitated research on α-receptor subtypes.
6. The recognition of structure–activity relationship patterns in certain subgroups of α-adrenoceptor stimulants, like the imidazolidines.

In this view of this development, which is progressing at a rapid pace, it seems of interest to discuss the newer aspects of the research on α-adrenoceptors in the present survey.

2 Classification and nomenclature of α-adrenoceptors

The nomenclature of α-adrenoceptors and their subtypes has been a matter of confusion for a few years, in particular as a result of the subdivision into pre- and postsynaptic as well as into α_1- and α_2-subpopulations. However, more recently a logical though complicated system of classification has been found acceptable to a majority of experts in the field.

The β-adrenoceptors are to be subdivided into the β_1- and β_2-types (Furchgott, 1967; Lands et al., 1967). This has proved a suitable system both from the theoretical as well as from a more therapeutic point of view. The necessity to introduce a comparable subdivision of α-adrenoceptors was felt in particular after the discovery of α-adrenoceptors at prejunctional (presynaptic) sites, that is at the level of the membranes of the varicosities at the noradrenergic nerve endings. Initially it was thought useful to call the postjunctional receptors α_1 and those at presynaptic sites α_2, since it was demonstrated that the receptor demand for pre- and postsynaptic α-adrenoceptors was different in each case (Langer, 1974). However, the discovery of receptors with a preference for agonists and antagonists identical with that of presynaptic α-receptors at postsynaptic sites (postsynaptic α_2-adrenoceptors) led to confusion in the nomenclature and urged a revised classification. In brief, the following system is now generally agreed upon (Berthelsen and Pettinger, 1977; Langer, 1981; Starke, 1981a, Wikberg, 1979; Starke and Langer, 1979; Timmermans and Van Zwieten, 1981, 1982):

1. The terms pre- and postsynaptic indicate only the location of the receptors with respect to the neuron and the synapse; they do not directly refer to the chemical demand of the receptor involved.
2. The terms α_1- and α_2- (like β_1- and β_2-) indicate only the preference of the receptors for agonists and antagonists; they do not primarily refer to localization with respect to the nerve ending and the synapse.

2.1 PRE- AND POSTJUNCTIONAL (PRE- AND POSTSYNAPTIC) RECEPTORS

As shown in Fig. 1, the receptors of the autonomic nervous system are subdivided according to their anatomical localization into pre- and post-junctional subtypes. The nomenclature pre- and postjunctional is probably more accurate than the originally developed terms pre- and postsynaptic, although these are still widely used.

Receptors situated at the target organs innervated by the adrenergic system are located outside the postganglionic neuron and they are called post-junctional or postsynaptic. Their stimulation by an agonist, either an endogenous neurotransmitter (noradrenaline) or a sympathomimetic drug, evokes a physiological or pharmacological effect, like for instance vasoconstriction resulting into a rise in arterial blood pressure when postsynaptic α-receptors in vascular smooth muscle are involved.

The existence of prejunctional (presynaptic) adrenoceptors has been demonstrated convincingly in recent years (reviews by Langer, 1977, 1981;

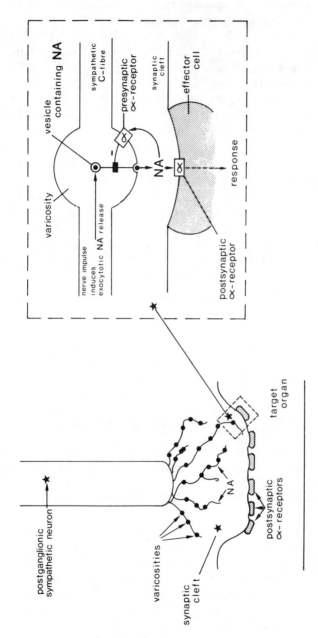

Fig. 1. Adrenergic synapse. Nerve activity releases the endogenous neurotransmitter noradrenaline (NA) and also adrenaline from the varicosities. Noradrenaline and adrenaline reach the post-synaptic α- (or β-) adrenoceptors on the cell membrane of the target organ by diffusion. Upon receptor stimulation, a physiological or pharmacological effect is initiated. Presynaptic α-adrenoceptors on the membrane (see insertion) when activated by endogenous noradrenaline or by exogenous agonists inhibit, and when blocked increase, the amount of transmitter noradrenaline released per nerve impulse.

Starke, 1977, 1981b; Westfall, 1977; Vizi, 1979). They are located at the membranes of the varicosities of the postganglionic sympathetic neurons, as depicted in Fig. 1. The stimulation of the presynaptic α-adrenoceptors at prejunctional sites inhibits the release of the neurotransmitter noradrenaline from the storage sites (vesicles) of the nerve ending per single nerve impulse. Accordingly, noradrenaline inhibits its own release from the nerve ending; presynaptic α-adrenoceptors control a negative feedback of the release of neurotransmitter.

Blockade of the presynaptic α-adrenoceptor by an α-sympatholytic agent (e.g. phentolamine, phenoxybenzamine) facilitates the release of noradrenaline from the nerve ending, thus enhancing the amount of transmitter released per nerve impulse.

2.2 α_1- AND α_2-ADRENOCEPTORS; AGONISTS/ANTAGONISTS

We have already noted that the distinction between α_1- and α_2-adrenoceptors is based solely upon the selectivity and preference of either receptor subtype for agonists and antagonists. At present selective agonists and antagonists for either of the α-adrenoceptor subtypes are available. In Fig. 2 a collection of formulae of agonists and antagonists of α_1- and α_2- is given. For instance, methoxamine and cirazoline are selective α_1-adrenoceptor agonists, whereas α_2-receptors are preferentially stimulated by experimental drugs like B-HT 920 or azepexole (B-HT 933); prazosin and corynanthine are selective antagonists of α_1-adrenoceptors, whereas yohimbine and rauwolscine are recognized as highly selective α_2-adrenoceptor blocking agents.

It should be realized that the endogenous catecholamines noradrenaline and adrenaline are non-selective agonists which stimulate both α_1- and α_2-adrenoceptors about equally well; classical α-adrenoceptor blockers like phentolamine and phenoxybenzamine are also non-selective agents with a comparable affinity for both α_1- and α_2-adrenoceptors.

In Table 1 different α-adrenoceptor agonists and antagonists, together with their preference for both receptor subtypes and their possible therapeutic applications, have been listed.

In this connection the diastereoisomers corynanthine and rauwolscine should be mentioned. Corynanthine is a highly selective α_1-adrenoceptor blocking agent, whereas rauwolscine displays particular selectivity as an antagonist of α_2-adrenoceptors. Since both compounds are diastereoisomers, their physicochemical properties are very similar. For instance their penetration should be expected to be virtually the same because of comparable lipophilicity. For these reasons rauwolscine and corynanthine have become valuable pharmacological tools for the pharmacological differentiation of α_1- and α_2-adrenoceptor mediated processes.

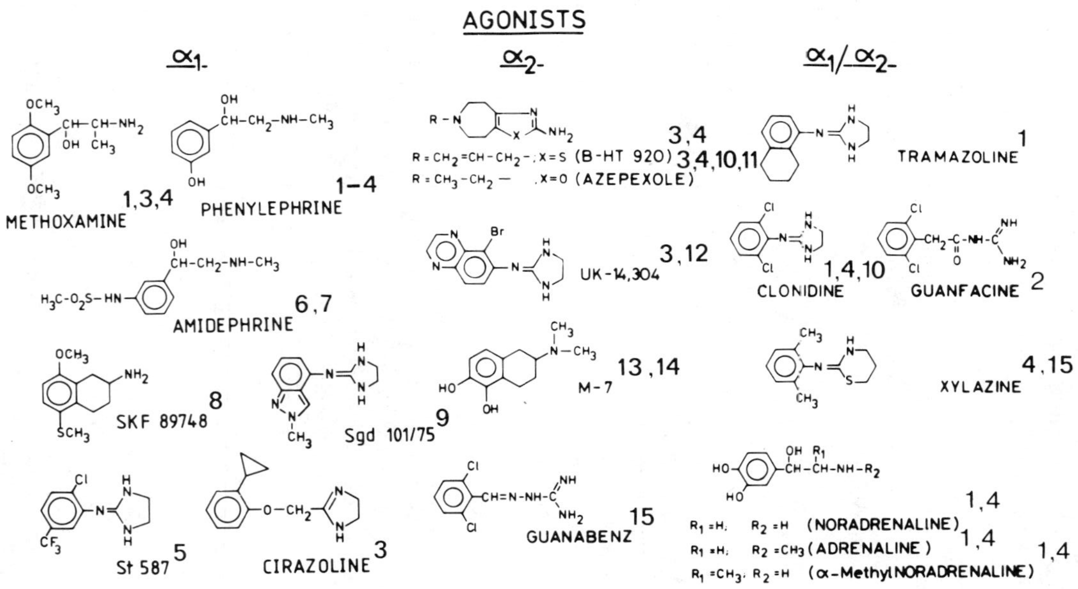

AGONISTS

α_1

METHOXAMINE 1,3,4

PHENYLEPHRINE 1-4

AMIDEPHRINE 6,7

SKF 89748 8

St 587 5

CIRAZOLINE 3

Sgd 101/75 9

α_2

R=CH₂=CH-CH₂-; x=S (B-HT 920) 3,4
R=CH₃-CH₂- ; x=0 (AZEPEXOLE) 3,4,10,11

UK-14,304 3,12

M-7 13,14

GUANABENZ 15

α_1/α_2

TRAMAZOLINE 1

CLONIDINE 1,4,10

GUANFACINE 2

XYLAZINE 4,15

R₁=H, R₂=H (NORADRENALINE) 1,4
R₁=H, R₂=CH₃ (ADRENALINE) 1,4
R₁=CH₃, R₂=H (α-Methyl NORADRENALINE) 1,4

214

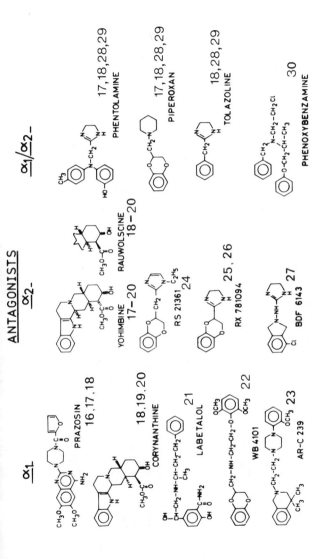

ANTAGONISTS

α₁   α₂   α₁/α₂

PRAZOSIN 16,17,18

CORYNANTHINE 18,19,20

LABETALOL 21

WB 4101 22

AR-C 239 23

YOHIMBINE 17-20

RAUWOLSCINE 18-20

RS 21361 24

RX 781094 25, 26

BDF 6143 27

PHENTOLAMINE 17,18,28,29

PIPEROXAN 17,18,28,29

TOLAZOLINE 18,28,29

PHENOXYBENZAMINE 30

FIG. 2. Collection of formulae of agonists and antagonists of α₁- and α₂-adrenoceptors.

[1]Starke *et al.* (1975); [2]Timmermans *et al.* (1979); [3]Van Meel *et al.* (1981c); [4]Kobinger and Pichler (1981b); [5]De Jonge *et al.* (1981c); [6]Butler and Jenkinson (1978); [7]Flavahan and McGrath (1981); [8]DeMarinis and Hieble (1983); [9]Thoolen *et al.* (1983); [10]Timmermans and Van Zwieten (1980a); [11]Timmermans and Van Zwieten (1980b); [12]Cambridge (1981); [13]Drew (1980); [14]Timmermans *et al.*, (1983b); [15]Docherty and McGrath (1980); [16]Cambridge *et al.* (1977); [17]Doxey *et al.* (1977); [18]Timmermans *et al.* (1980b); [19]Weitzell *et al.* (1979); [20]Shepperson *et al.* (1981); [21]Drew (1978); [22]Kapur and Mottram (1978); [23]Mouillé *et al.* (1980); [24]Michel *et al.* (1981); [25]Dabiré *et al.* (1981); [26]Chapleo *et al.* (1981); [27]Docherty *et al.* (1982); [28]Borowski *et al.* (1977); [29]Starke (1981a); [30]Langer (1973).

215

TABLE 1

α-Adrenoceptor agonists and antagonists. Characterization with respect to their selectivity for α_1- and α_2-adrenoceptors. Possible therapeutic applications

Agents	Receptor stimulated or blocked	Application
Agonists		
Noradrenaline (neurotransmitter)	$\alpha_1 + \alpha_2 + \beta_1$	vasoconstrictor ($\alpha_1 + \alpha_2$)
Adrenaline (neurotransmitter)	$\alpha_1 + \alpha_2 + \beta_1 + \beta_2$	vasoconstrictor ($\alpha_1 + \alpha_2$)
Phenylephrine (Boralin®, Visadron®)	$\alpha_1 > \alpha_2$	vasoconstrictor (α_1), decongestant (α_1)
Clonidine (Catapres®, Catapresan®)	$\alpha_2 > \alpha_1$	antihypertensive (central α_2)
Guanfacine	$\alpha_2 \ll \alpha_1$	antihypertensive (central α_2)
Azepexole (B-HT 933)	α_2	antihypertensive (central α_2)
B-HT 920	α_2	antiglaucomatous (experimental)
UK 14, 304	α_2	tool in experimental pharmacology
Antagonists		
Phentolamine (Regitine®)	$\alpha_1 + \alpha_2$	phaeochromocytoma, preoperative phase ($\alpha_1 + \alpha_2$)
Tolazoline	$\alpha_2 > \alpha_1$	vasodilator ($\alpha_1 + \alpha_2$)
Prazosin (Minipress®)	α_1	antihypertensive (peripheral α_1)
Corynanthine } diastereoisomers	α_1	} tools in experimental pharmacology
Rauwolscine } diastereoisomers	α_2	} tools in experimental pharmacology
Yohimbine	α_2	} tools in experimental pharmacology

2.3 LOCALIZATION OF α_1- AND α_2-ADRENOCEPTORS AT THE CELLULAR LEVEL

Prejunctional α-adrenoceptors are predominantly of the α_2-subtype, as concluded from their preference for selective α_2-adrenoceptor agonists and antagonists, although Kobinger and Pichler (1980a, 1982a) have suggested that a minor proportion of the presynaptic α-adrenoceptor display α_1-characteristics.

At postsynaptic sites, both α_1- and α_2-adrenoceptors are present, probably in proportion not greatly different from 1:1. Particularly in vascular smooth muscle the presence of both α_1- and α_2-adrenoceptors is of great importance, both fundamentally and also as a target for drugs.

Postjunctional α-adrenoceptors in vascular smooth muscle shall be dealt with in a separate paragraph.

More recently, evidence has been produced that postjunctional α_1- and α_2-receptors, respectively, display subtle but relevant differences concerning their anatomical position with respect to the synapse. Postjunctional α_1-adrenoceptors are presumed to be located intrasynaptically and thus to be readily accessible to the endogenous neurotransmitter noradrenaline. However, postjunctional α_2-adrenoceptors are likely to be located extrasynaptically (Langer et al., 1980, 1981a, 1981b; Yamaguchi and Kopin, 1980; Wilffert et al., 1982a, 1982b). Accordingly, they are not very well accessible to intrasynaptically released noradrenaline. In contrast, they will rather react to circulating catecholamines, like adrenaline. In this respect there exists a certain resemblance to the situation of the postjunctional vascular β_2-adrenoceptors, which have been demonstrated to occur mainly extra-synaptically (Glick et al., 1967; Russell and Moran, 1980). Accordingly, it seems justified to state that both postjunctional α_2- and β_2-adrenoceptors are mainly not innervated, in contrast to α_1- and β_1-adrenoceptors at post-junctional, intrasynaptical sites.

3 Distribution of α-adrenoceptors in various tissues

Once the subclassification of α-adrenoceptors with pre/postsynaptic and α_1/α_2-subtypes had been accepted, the necessity was felt to study the distribution of these subtypes in various organs and tissues of the organism. This investigation has been initiated only a few years ago and it is far from being complete. Nevertheless a certain pattern of distribution can be recognized and it should be reported here in spite of its incompleteness.

In view of the particular situation and properties of α-adrenoceptors in the central nervous system, this region will be dealt with in a separate paragraph. For the same reasons the α-adrenoceptors in the eye will be treated separately.

3.1 PREJUNCTIONAL (PRESYNAPTIC) α-ADRENOCEPTORS

We have already mentioned that presynaptic α_2-adrenoceptors have been found at almost all noradrenergic axons where they had been assumed to exist, for example in various types of innervated blood vessels (for reviews see Starke, 1977, 1981b; Doxey and Roach, 1980; Langer, 1981), in the spleen (Langer, 1973), cat autoperfused hindlimb (Steppeler *et al.*, 1978), heart (Starke, 1972; Drew, 1976; Pichler and Kobinger, 1978; Lokhandwala *et al.*, 1977) and vas deferens (Doxey *et al.*, 1977; Drew, 1977).

Presynaptic α_2-adrenoceptors have initially been discovered and thereafter intensively studied in the rabbit pulmonary artery preparation (Starke, 1977, 1981b). The presynaptic α_2-receptors in the other tissues mentioned are probably very similar to those found on the rabbit pulmonary artery.

Receptors with characteristics of α_2-adrenoceptors at prejunctional sites have been identified at cholinergic nerve endings (Drew, 1978; Wikberg, 1979; reviews by Starke, 1977, 1981b), at serotonergic nerve endings (Göthert and Huth, 1980) and at the cell bodies of noradrenergic neurons (Brown and Caulfield, 1979).

3.2 POSTJUNCTIONAL (POSTSYNAPTIC) α-ADRENOCEPTORS

3.2.1 Vascular smooth muscle

This receptor subtype has been studied thoroughly in vascular smooth muscles. The simultaneous existence of postjunctional α_1- and α_2-adrenoceptors has been first demonstrated in various types of vascular smooth muscle (for reviews see Starke, 1981a; McGrath, 1982; Timmermans and and Van Zwieten, 1981, 1982; Langer and Shepperson, 1982). Accordingly, the postsynaptic α-adrenoceptor has been first described in vascular smooth muscle tissue and it was this discovery which led to the view that the nomenclature α_1/α_2 is not necessarily related to pre/postsynaptic location of the receptors. The presence of postsynaptic α_2-adrenoceptors has been made plausible by means of a careful pharmacological analysis, using some of the highly selective agonists and antagonists to either α_1- or α_2-adrenoceptors. *In vivo*, such studies can for instance be carried out in a convenient manner in the pithed rat preparation, where the presynaptic part of the autonomic innervation of the circulatory system has been disrupted. In this model, as well as in other pithed animal preparations, it can be demonstrated that the stimulation of postsynaptic α_1-adrenoceptors by α_1-selective agonists like methoxamine, cirazoline and phenylephrine causes a rise in arterial blood pressure, reflecting the constriction of resistance vessels (Fig. 3). This pressor effect is effectively antagonized by selective α_1-adrenoceptor blocking agents like prazosin or corynanthine (Fig. 3). The parallel shift in the dose–response curves indicates a competitive antagonism. Selective α_2-adrenoceptor blocking agents like yohimbine or rauwolscine are much less active in antagonizing the vasoconstriction induced by α_1-adrenoceptor stimulants (Fig. 3).

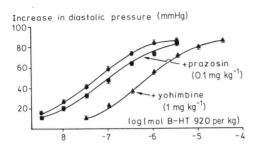

FIG. 3. Influence of α-adrenoceptor blocking drugs on the pressor effect of B-HT 920, a selective α_2-adrenoceptor agonist. Experiments in pithed normotensive rats. The α_2-adrenoceptor antagonist yohimbine causes a parallel shift of the dose–response curve, indicating a competitive antagonism at the level of peripheral postsynaptic vascular α_2-adrenoceptors. The α_1-adrenoceptor prazosin is virtually ineffective. Experiments by the authors. Means $\pm$ S.E.M. ($n = 6$–7).

In the same preparation, selective α_2-adrenoceptor agonists like B-HT 920, UK-14,304 or azepexole (B-HT 933) also cause pressor responses which reflect the constriction of the resistance vessels (Fig. 4). Selective α_2-adrenoceptor blocking agents are effective as antagonists of the α_2-mediated pressor response. The parallel shift of the dose–response curve implicates a competitive antagonism (Fig. 4). Selective α_1-adrenoceptors are but poor antagonists of the α_2-adrenoceptor mediated pressor response.

Similar results have been obtained (Van Meel et al., 1983a) in the isolated perfused hindquarters of rats pretreated with reserpine, as developed by Kobinger and Pichler (1981a).

α_2-Adrenoceptors at postsynaptic sites have been suggested to be present in the dog isolated basilar artery (Timmermans et al., 1982). The receptors involved seem predominantly of the α_2-subtype, as concluded from agonists/antagonists experiments with noradrenaline and clonidine (agonists) versus yohimbine, corynanthine and prazosin.

The α-adrenoceptors present in the rat aorta seem to have a somewhat aberrant receptor demand and it has been virtually impossible so far to force them into the classification of either α_1- or α_2-receptors (Ruffolo et al., 1980, 1981, 1982; Randriantsoa et al., 1981).

By using higher selective α_2-adrenoceptor agonists such as M-7 and UK-14, 304, it is possible to identify postjunctional constitution via α_2-adrenoceptors in the dog saphenous vein *in vitro* (Davey, 1980; Shepperson and Langer, 1981).

The studies carried out in various types of human arteries *in vitro*, obtained postmortem or during surgery, do not allow a firm classification of both subtypes of α_1- and α_2-adrenoceptors (Jauernig *et al.*, 1978; Stevens and Moulds, 1981, 1982). However, preliminary experiments in healthy humans have suggested that in the resistance vessels of the human forearm both α_1- and α_2-adrenoceptors are present. Their stimulation with the appropriate selective agonist causes vasoconstriction, which can be antagonized by the corresponding α_1- or α_2-adrenoceptor antagonists, respectively (Van Brummelen *et al.*, 1982).

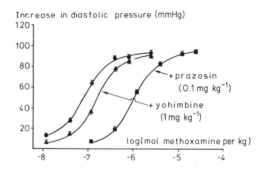

FIG. 4. Influence of α-adrenoceptor blocking drugs on the pressor effect of methoxamine, a selective α_1-adrenoceptor agonist. Experiments in pithed normotensive rats. The α_1-adrenoceptor antagonist prazosin causes a parallel shift of the dose–response curve, indicating a competitive antagonism at the level of peripheral postsynaptic vascular α_1-adrenoceptors. The α_2-adrenoceptor antagonist yohimbine is virtually ineffective. Experiments by the authors. Means $\pm$ S.E.M. ($n = 6$–7).

As a whole, it can be stated that the existence of postsynaptic vasoconstrictor α_1- and α_2-adrenoceptors can easily be demonstrated *in vivo* in the resistance vessels of various types of laboratory animals.

In vitro, the situation appears more complicated. There seems to be no particular difficulty in demonstrating the existence of postsynaptic α_1-adrenoceptors. However, in spite of considerable research investment it has proved rather difficult to demonstrate unequivocally the occurrence of postsynaptic α_2-adrenoceptors *in vitro*. Only in the dog saphenous vein and in the isolated perfused hindquarters of the rat (sensitized by pretreatment of the animal *in vivo* with reserpine) could vasoconstriction be demonstrated unequivocally when induced by highly selective α_2-adrenoceptor stimulants.

Finally, it has been suggested that veins would display a higher density of postsynaptic α_2-adrenoceptors than arteries, but the evidence is obscured by the fact that the α-adrenoceptor blockers investigated display a substantial degree of non-competitive antagonism (De Mey and Vanhoutte, 1981; Vanhoutte, 1982). Accordingly, no firm conclusion can be reached so far.

3.2.2 Platelets

Platelet aggregation can be induced with adrenaline, noradrenaline and α-methylnoradrenaline, but not in a substantial manner with other phenethylamines or imidazoli(di)ne derivatives like clonidine or tramazoline (O'Brien, 1963; Jakobs, 1978; Grant and Scrutton, 1979; Hsu et al., 1978; Lasch and Jacobs, 1979). These experimental findings would suggest the implication of α-adrenoceptors in the aggregation process and therefore put forward the question whether α_1- and/or α_2-adrenoceptors may be involved. In fact, radioligand binding studies using α-adrenoceptor stimulants suggest that the receptors involved are of the α_2-subtype. Moreover, adrenaline-induced aggregation proved counteracted by yohimbine (α_2) and phentolamine ($\alpha_1 + \alpha_2$), whereas prazosin (α_1) remained ineffective (Grant and Scrutton, 1979; Lasch and Jacobs, 1979).

However, the situation is more complex when biological effects, that is platelet aggregation per se, are concerned. Not all α_2-agonists induce platelet aggregation and, as already stated, only adrenaline, noradrenaline and α-methylnoradrenaline are active stimulants of platelet aggregation, whereas a variety of other compounds with an α_2-adrenoceptor stimulant component are virtually ineffective.

For these reasons the significance of α_2-adrenoceptors, in spite of their demonstrability in radioligand binding studies (Hoffmann et al., 1979; Wood et al., 1979; Garcia-Sevilla et al., 1979; Shattil et al., 1981), remains unanswered. This conclusion once more emphasizes the necessity to interpret receptor binding studies with great caution and stresses the necessity to compare the results from such studies with biological data.

3.2.3 Pancreatic islets

In fasted mice, the release of immunoreactive insulin (IRI) from pancreatic β-cells is inhibited by α-adrenergic stimulation, for instance by means of adrenaline, which simultaneously causes hyperglycemia. Both phentolamine ($\alpha_1 + \alpha_2$) and yohimbine (α_2) significantly increases the release of IRI, whereas adrenaline-induced hyperglycemia is inhibited. These findings suggest that the inhibitory receptors involved in the release of IRI are rather of the α_2-subtype with respect to their receptor demand (Smith and Porte, 1976; Nakadate et al., 1980).

3.2.4 Adipocytes

In human and hamster adipocytes lipolysis can be stimulated by theophylline via inhibition of phosphodiesterase and a concomitant rise in cyclic AMP. This effect of theophylline is inhibited by α-adrenoceptor agonists. In this respect clonidine ($\alpha_2 > \alpha_1$) and adrenaline ($\alpha_1 + \alpha_2$) proved more effective agonists than phenylephrine (α_1) and methoxamine (α_1). The inhibitory effect of the α-receptor agonists can be counteracted effectively by yohimbine but much less so by prazosin.

These experimental findings suggest that α_2-adrenoceptors are involved in lipolysis (Schimmel, 1976; Aktories et al., 1980; Lafontan and Berlan, 1980, 1981).

3.2.5 Melanocytes

The melanocyte stimulating hormone (MSH) is known to induce darkening of the skin in lizards and frogs. Melanophores on the skin, which mediate the MSH-action, are assumed to contain α_2-adrenoceptors which are involved in the effect of MSH.

This conclusion has been drawn from a pharmacological analysis with the appropriate selective receptor agonists and antagonists (Berthelsen and Pettinger, 1977; Pettinger, 1977; Carter and Shuster, 1982).

3.3 THE CENTRAL NERVOUS SYSTEM

3.3.1 Central α-adrenoceptors involved in circulatory regulation

The interest in the possibility that α-adrenoceptors might exist in the brain was aroused by the fact that certain drugs exert hypotensive activity via a primary influence on the central nervous system. Prototypes of centrally acting hypotensive drugs are clonidine and a large series of related imidazolidine derivatives, as well as guanfacine, lofexidine and α-methyl-DOPA. The latter in fact is a prodrug, its in vivo conversion into α-methylnoradrenaline being essential for the drug's hypotensive effect. Clonidine and related compounds have been subjected to detailed investigations in the course of the past 15 years. It cannot be doubted that the discovery of clonidine has greatly improved our insight not only into the mode of action of centrally antihypertensive drugs, but also into the central regulation of blood pressure and the functional involvement of central α-adrenoceptors therein.

It was the merit of Schmitt (1971) to propose the functional role of central α-adrenoceptors in the hypotensive effect of clonidine. His theory was based upon the following experimental findings:

1. clonidine is known to activate peripheral α-adrenoceptors, owing to its structural relationship with naphazoline and similar imidazolidine-decongestant drugs;

2. the central hypotensive effect of clonidine is antagonized by yohimbine, piperoxan and other α-adrenoceptor blocking agents, which are sufficiently lipophilic to allow adequate brain penetration. The antagonism is dose-dependent and competitive in nature.

Accordingly, clonidine should be considered an *agonist* of central α-adreno-ceptors, whereas the α-adrenoceptor blocking drugs act as antagonists towards the same receptors. A similar mechanism has been demonstrated to occur for a variety of clonidine-related imidazolidine-derivatives (for review see Timmermans *et al.*, 1980a) and also for guanfacine (see Dollery and Jerie, 1980).

More recently, a new series of highly selective α_2-adrenoceptor agonists like azepexole (B-HT 933) and B-HT 920 (already discussed in preceding paragraphs) have been demonstrated to possess central hypotensive potency mediated via central α-adrenoceptors, although their chemical structure (Fig. 2) is not clearly related to clonidine and its congeners (Kobinger and Pichler, 1977; Van Zwieten and Timmermans, 1980; Pichler and Kobinger, 1981a). Other experimental drugs with α-receptor mediated central hypotensive activity like lofexidine, guanabenz and UK-14,304 (Timmermans *et al.*, 1980a) should be mentioned for the sake of completeness. For chemical structures see Fig. 2.

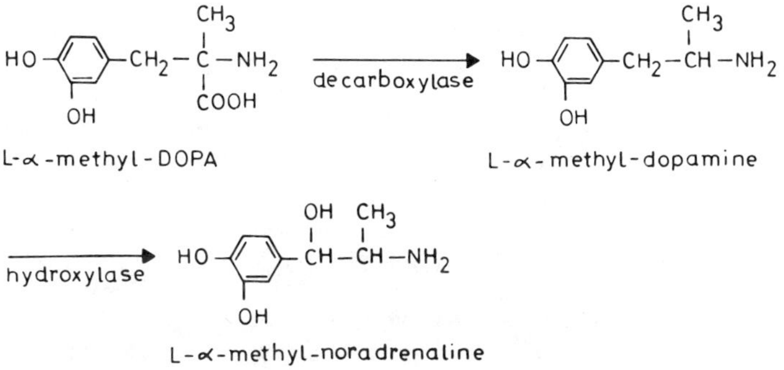

FIG. 5. Biotransformation of L-α-methyl-DOPA in cerebral structures, to yield L-α-methyldopamine and finally L-α-methylnoradrenaline. L-α-methylnoradrenaline is the pharmacologically active compound which stimulates central α_2-adrenoceptors, thus causing a fall in blood pressure.

The concept of the central α-adrenoceptors is also the basis of the explanation of the central hypotensive effect of α-methyl-DOPA (Aldomet®). After oral ingestion and transport via the blood stream the drug penetrates into the brain stem, where it is decarboxylated enzymatically to yield α-methyl-dopamine, which is converted upon enzymatic hydroxylation into α-methyl-noradrenaline (Fig. 5). The latter amine will stimulate the central α-adreno-ceptor in a similar manner as does clonidine and hence cause a hypotensive effect (for review see Henning, 1983). Accordingly, α-methylnoradrenaline appears to be the active compound and α-methyl-DOPA should be classified as a prodrug.

In the organism, the stimulation of central α-adrenoceptors by clonidine and related drugs and also by α-methylnoradrenaline (from α-methyl-DOPA) leads to a reduction in peripheral sympathetic tone. This could be demon-strated experimentally by Schmitt (1971), who established a decreased fre-quency and intensity in discharges of the splanchnic nerve. Simultaneously, plasma catecholamines and plasma renin activity are decreased by clonidine, partly as a result of the reduced peripheral sympathetic activity which is initiated at the level of central α-adrenoceptors.

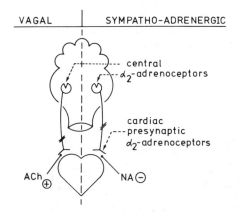

FIG. 6. Schematic representation of the central and peripheral α_2-adrenoceptors involved in the bradycardia caused by clonidine. The stimulation of central α_2-adrenoceptors induces a diminished peripheral sympathetic tone and simultaneously an enhanced vagal activity. In the periphery, the stimulation of cardiac presynaptic α_2-adrenoceptors causes a reduction in the release to endogenous noradrenaline from presynaptic sites. Experiments in pentobarbitone-anesthetized rats by De Jonge et al. (1981a, 1982a). (Modified after Kobinger, 1978.)

The bradycardia, induced by clonidine and related drugs is due to a complex mechanism. It probably consists of at least three different com-ponents, which have been demonstrated in experimental animals. Two of these components are central, the third is peripheral.

As proposed and reviewed by Kobinger (1978) there are at least two central components:

1. the centrally induced reduction of peripheral sympathetic tone which brings about the decrease in blood pressure also diminishes heart rate;
2. clonidine reinforces vagal reflex bradycardia; this mechanism is initiated at the level of the aforementioned central α-adrenoceptors.

The peripheral mechanism involved in the clonidine-induced bradycardia runs as follows: Clonidine (and related imidazolidines) will stimulate the very sensitive presynaptic α_2-adrenoceptors, thus causing a diminished release of noradrenaline from the nerve endings and hence a reduction in peripheral sympathetic tone towards the heart, as reflected by bradycardia. This mechanism has been demonstrated to occur in anesthetized dogs (Cavero and Roach, 1980) as well as in pentobarbitone-anesthetized rats, as studied for a series of imidazolidines including clonidine (De Jonge et al., 1981a, 1982a). The negative chronotropic mechanisms proposed are shown schematically in Fig. 6.

3.3.2 The localization of central α-adrenoceptors

Although the concept of central α-adrenoceptors is more than ten years old, the precise location of these receptors in the central nervous system has not been determined with certainty yet. However, a considerable effort in neuropharmacological research has been invested. There is general agreement that central α-adrenoceptors involved in central blood pressure regulation and in the central hypotensive effect of drugs are mainly located in the brain stem and not in higher centres. A hypothalamic site of attack has been proposed for clonidine, as concluded from stereotactic injections in that particular region, but excessively high doses were required and the involvement of α-adrenoceptors has not been convincingly demonstrated (Struyker Boudier, 1975).

Schmitt (1971) and also Chalmers (1975) have proposed that the α-receptors are located in the nucleus of the solitary tract, since in this region a high density of noradrenergic synapses has been demonstrated to occur and also because of the participation of these structures in the baroreceptor pathway. However, the vasomotor centre and the nucleus of the vagus nerve (NX) may also be involved, as well as the various neuronal interconnections between these nuclei.

Figure 7 visualizes the position of the aforementioned nuclei, their interconnections and their links to the periphery, partly via the spinal cord. It may well be conceived that the α-receptors are not located in one circumscript centre or nucleus but rather by a more or less diffuse pattern over a more extended region in the ponto-medullary area.

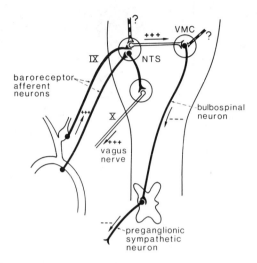

FIG. 7. Schematic representation of the neuronal connections between the medullary centres, baroreceptors (aortic arch and carotid sinus), vagus nerve (NX)-nucleus, and the peripheral sympathetic system. NTS, nucleus of the solitary tract; VMC, vasomotor centre; ═══, facilitating neuron; ▄▄▄, inhibitory neuron; ■ ■ ■, neuron (whether facilitating or inhibitory is not known) connection between the hypothalamic region and NTS/VMC. (From Chalmers, 1975.)

3.3.3 Classification of the central α-adrenoceptors which mediate the central hypotensive activity of drugs

In order to classify the central α-adrenoceptors primarily involved in the hypotensive action of drugs both their location with respect to the synaps and subtype (α_1 or α_2) should be determined. These questions are more difficult to answer than for peripheral organs because of the extremely complex structure of the central nervous system.

The existence of presynaptic α_2-adrenoceptors in the brain involved in a negative feedback circuit and sensitive to the appropriate agonists and antagonists has indeed been demonstrated (review by Starke, 1977; Langer, 1981; Timmermans and Van Zwieten, 1982). Accordingly, a subdivision of central α-adrenoceptors appears necessary.

In case of a postsynaptic mechanism underlying the central hypotensive effect of clonidine, the excitation of the postsynaptic α-receptor will enhance the activity of the inhibitory bulbospinal neuron and hence depress peripheral sympathetic activity, as shown in Fig. 8.

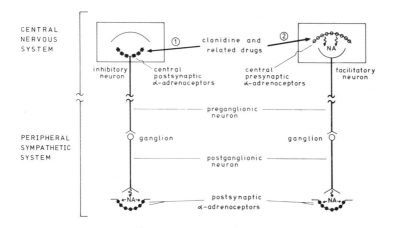

FIG. 8. Schematic representation of the interaction of clonidine (and related drugs) with postsynaptic and presynaptic α-adrenoceptors in the brainstem, as a basis for the central hypotensive effect. Two possibilities exist: (1) *Left*. Clonidine stimulates central postsynaptic α-adrenoceptors; accordingly, an inhibitory neuron is activated and the peripheral sympathetic activity is diminished, thus causing a hypotensive effect. (2) *Right*. Clonidine stimulates presynaptic α-adrenoceptors; accordingly, central noradrenaline release is diminished, the facilitatory neuron is less activated, and peripheral sympathetic activity is diminished, thus causing a hypotensive effect. The first possibility (left) is likely to be the correct one.

If, however, a presynaptic mechanism would be predominant, the stimulation of presynaptic α-adrenoceptors would implicate the impairment of noradrenaline release at the level of central (nor)adrenergic nerve endings, thus depressing the activity of a facilitatory neuron. Finally, a depression of peripheral sympathetic tone and a concomitant fall in blood pressure will result.

The complexity of the central nervous system as well as methodological problems and limitations have impaired the final answer to the question, whether the α-receptors involved are of the pre- or postsynaptic subtype. Various authors have demonstrated that the pharmacological destruction of the central presynaptic neurons and receptors by means of 6-hydroxydopamine or reserpine does not abolish the central hypotensive effect of clonidine and related drugs (reviews by Kobinger, 1978; Häusler, 1982; Van Zwieten and Timmermans, 1979; Timmermans and Van Zwieten, 1982). These results, which should be interpreted cautiously, would indicate that a postsynaptic rather than a presynaptic mechanism is involved in the hypotensive effect of clonidine and related drugs.

From an intellectual point of view a presynaptic mechanism would seem more attractive and easier to accept than a postsynaptic process, which implies that an α-adrenoceptor agonist lowers blood pressure, an unusual event in classical pharmacology. Nevertheless the experimental findings mentioned above rather favour the cerebral postsynaptic α-adrenoceptors as primary target of the central hypotensive action of clonidine and related drugs.

The availability of specific agonists and antagonists towards either α_1- or α_2-adrenoceptors has greatly facilitated the answer to the question whether central α_1- or α_2-adrenoceptors are involved. This matter has been settled satisfactorily by means of the diastereoisomers yohimbine, rauwolscine and corynanthine. Yohimbine and rauwolscine are selective α_2-adrenoceptor antagonists, whereas corynanthine is a selective α_1-adrenoceptor antagonist. Being diastereoisomers these compounds will differ little with respect to physical chemical properties and brain penetration.

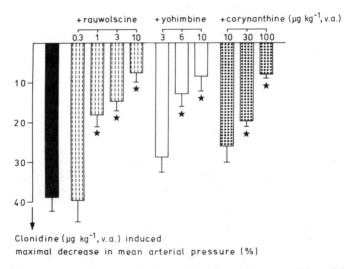

FIG. 9. The antagonism by rauwolscine, yohimbine and corynanthine of the central hypotensive action of clonidine in cats. Drugs were injected into the left vertebral artery (v.a.). Black column: maximal depressor effect of clonidine (1 μg kg^{-1}) without pretreatment. Striped columns: rauwolscine (μg kg^{-1}, v.a.). White columns: yohimbine (μg kg^{-1}, v.a.). Stippled columns: corynanthine (μg kg^{-1}, v.a.). The doses of the three α-sympatholytic drugs are listed at the top. Means ± S.E.M. (n = 5–9). (From Timmermans et al., 1981a.)

In a careful analysis, it could be demonstrated that the central hypotensive effect of clonidine obtained after its injection into the cat's left vertebral artery is effectively antagonized by the α_2-adrenoceptor blocking agents yohimbine and rauwolscine injected via the same route prior to clonidine (see Fig. 9). However, the α_1-adrenoceptor antagonist corynanthine had less influence on the central hypotensive effect of clonidine (Timmermans et al., 1981a).

Recent correlation studies also stress the participation of central α_2-, but not of α_1-adrenoceptors in the acute blood pressure lowering effect of α-adrenoceptor agonists (Kobinger and Pichler, 1980b; De Jonge et al., 1981b, 1982b; Timmermans et al., 1981b).

In conclusion, it can be stated that the α-adrenoceptors in the brain stem which mediate the central hypotensive action of clonidine are probably located postsynaptically and are of the α_2-subtype with respect to their receptor demands. Central and presumably peripheral presynaptic cardiac α_2-adrenoceptors are involved in the bradycardic action of clonidine.

α_1-Adrenoceptors are present in the brain, as concluded from radio-ligand binding studies (Greenberg et al., 1976; U'Prichard et al., 1977; Greengrass and Bremner, 1979; Hornung et al., 1979; Lyon and Randall, 1980; Miach et al., 1980). However, their functional role with respect to circulatory events and drug action remains unclear.

It has been suggested that central α_1-adrenoceptors inhibit the vagally mediated bradycardia in anesthetized β-adrenoceptor-blocked dogs (Huchet et al., 1981). Furthermore, the selective α_1-adrenoceptor blocking agent prazosin selectively antagonizes neuronal responses mediated by α_1-adrenoceptors in the brain (Menkes et al., 1981). However, prazosin does not display any central hypotensive activity whatsoever, in spite of its lipophilic character which allows a substantial degree of brain penetration.

Furthermore, the selective α_1-adrenoceptor agonist St 587 (for structure see Fig. 2), a lipophilic α_1-adrenoceptor agonist which can be assumed to achieve sufficiently high brain concentrations, does not display any central hypotensive or hypertensive activity (De Jonge et al., 1981c).

In conclusion, no evidence at all has been provided in favour of a mediatory role of α_1-adrenoceptors in the initiation of a central hypotensive effect of drugs. Conversely, firm evidence has been put forward which identifies the α-adrenoceptors mediating the central hypotensive activity of drugs as being postsynaptic and of the α_2-subtype.

3.3.4 Structure–activity relationships of α-adrenoceptor agonists which display central hypotensive activity

This question has only been studied thoroughly for clonidine and related imidazolidines. α-Methyl-DOPA, the other prototype of centrally acting hypotensive drugs interfering with α-adrenoceptors (through α-methylnoradrenaline), is unique in that no congener of this drug is known so far which displays substantial central hypotensive activity.

The quantitative structure–activity relationships within a series of imidazolidines comprising clonidine and several of its congeners has been studied in full detail. The results have been dealt with in a monography on this subject (Timmermans *et al.*, 1980a). We shall limit ourselves to a brief discussion of the most important conclusions achieved in this monography.

As shown in Fig. 10 the clonidine molecule contains at least three fundamental structural units which can be subject to chemical manipulation for the investigation of possible structure–activity relationships in a series of imidazolidines. In spite of several attempts to synthesize more potent drugs, clonidine is still one of the most active compounds in the present series. Chemical alterations in the structure of the heterocyclic nucleus or in the substitution pattern of the phenyl moiety invariably lead to agents which are less potent than clonidine or in a few cases equipotent, but usually not more active.

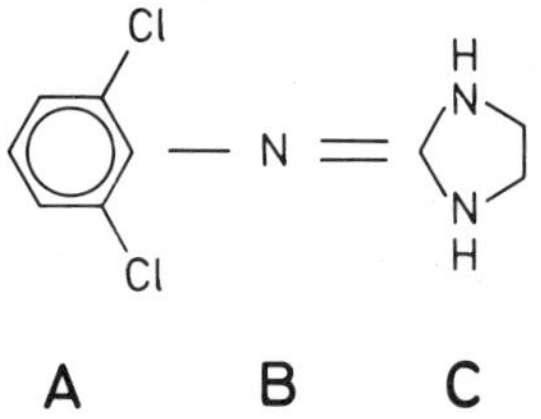

A   B   C

Fig. 10. Subdivision of clonidine into three fundamental structural units.

Quantitative structure–activity relationship (QSAR) studies have demonstrated that particular and well-defined steric and electronic requirements of the molecule are involved. Rather stringent demands are made upon the steric occupation at the phenyl ring of the imidazolidines. Lipophilicity also plays an important role, in particular since it largely determines the degree of brain penetration and therefore the concentration of the drug at the level of the central α-adrenoceptor.

Correlation studies on a series of related imidazolidines have been translated into a hypothetical working model which may provide insight into the mechanism of interaction between clonidine-like drugs and the central α_2-adrenoceptor, as shown in Fig. 11. The following sites of interaction are presumed to be relevant to the hypotensive potency of the drugs involved:

1. the aromatic phenyl ring of the imidazolidine possibly interacts by means of electron donation with an electron-deficient area of the receptor;
2. a positively charged nitrogen of the imidazolidine nucleus interacts with a negatively charged site at the receptor;

3. a third type of interaction is based upon the formation of a hydrogen bond with the bridge nitrogen, although this type of interaction is probably less imporatnt quantitatively.

From the steric point of view it seems likely that probably one side of the substituted phenyl nucleus determines the fitting with the receptor. This side appears to be the one which bears an *ortho*-substituent with a steric bulk close to that of chlorine. The orientation of the imidazolidine ring is partly determined by the other *ortho*-substituent of the phenyl nucleus, when present.

For full details the reader should consult the monograph by Timmermans *et al.* (1980a).

Recently, 2,6- and 2,3-substitutions have been combined in one molecule. The resulting 2,3,6-trisubstituted analogues showed pronounced (central) hypotensive activity, the 2,3,6-trichlorosubstituted derivative being more potent than clonidine itself (Timmermans *et al.*, 1982; De Jonge *et al.*, 1983). This outcome is in agreement with the proposed mode of interaction between clonidine-like imidazolidines and central (hypotensive) α_2-adrenoceptors outlined above.

3.3.5 α-Adrenoceptors involved in the bradycardia induced by clonidine and related imidazolidines

Clonidine and related imidazolidines are known to cause bradycardia. As already discussed in a preceding paragraph, the mechanisms underlying this phenomenon are complex and involve at least three different components. The two central components result from the stimulation of central α_2-adrenoceptors, causing both a reduction in peripheral sympathetic tone and a reinforcement of vagally induced reflex bradycardia. The involvement of peripheral cardiac presynaptic α_2-adrenoceptors was already mentioned (De Jonge *et al.*, 1981a, 1982a).

3.3.6 α-Adrenoceptors involved in the sedation and the dry mouth induced by centrally acting antihypertensive drugs

Sedation is a general feature of various centrally acting drugs, including the centrally acting hypotensive agents. Since in animal experiments sedation by clonidine can be counteracted by yohimbine and piperoxan, Schmitt (1971) has proposed that central α-adrenoceptors may be involved, possibly located in cerebral structures. More recently, various authors (Cavero and Roach, 1978; Drew *et al.*, 1979; Timmermans *et al.*, 1981a), using selective agonists and antagonists, have concluded that the α-adrenoceptors involved are rather of the α_2-subtype. The pharmacological methods available at present do not allow a definite decision as to whether these α_2-adrenoceptors are located pre- or postjunctionally. However, after depletion of catecholamine stores or destruction of noradrenergic nerve endings, clonidine causes excitation rather than sedation (Strömbom, 1975; Zebrowska-Lupina et al., 1977; Pichler and Kobinger, 1981b). A preferential agonist of α_2-adrenoceptors, like B-HT 920, is then without effect (Pichler and Kobinger, 1981b). These data are indicative of a presynaptic mechanism involved in α_2-adrenoceptor-mediated sedation.

Since both the central hypotensive effect and the side-effect of sedation are mediated by central α-adrenoceptors of the α_2-subtype, it would seem very difficult if not impossible to develop molecules which are effective central hypotensives devoid of sedative activity. Although both types of central α_2-adrenoceptors are located in different brain regions, this differentiation probably does not offer a possibility to separate antihypertensive and sedative properties. It can hardly be expected that both receptor populations greatly differ with respect to their accessibility to drugs which have penetrated into the central nervous system.

The dry mouth frequently observed as a side-effect of clonidine is due to the reduced secretion of saliva. A more detailed pharmacological analysis (Green et al., 1979) has revealed that clonidine reduces peripheral parasympathetically and electrically evoked submaxillary salivation via the activation of presynaptic α-adrenoceptors which inhibit cholinergic transmission. In view of the receptor demand of clonidine and related compounds the receptors involved are probably of the α_2-subtype.

3.3.7 The eye

So far the distribution of α- and β-adrenoceptors over various ocular tissues has been a matter of confusion. In recent experiments, however, we could demonstrate a net difference between the functional role of ocular α_1- and α_2-adrenoceptors, respectively. In conscious rabbits the topical application of selective α_2-adrenoceptor agonist as azepexole (B-HT 933) and B-HT 920 caused a marked and dose-dependent ocular hypotensive response (Innemee et al., 1981). The decrease in ocular pressure induced by these drugs was antagonized by the selective α_2-adrenoceptor blocking agent yohimbine. However, selective stimulation of ocular α_1-adrenoceptors with appropriate, topically applied agonists, induced an elevation in intraocular pressure accompanied by mydriasis. These results suggest that the selective stimulation of α_2-adrenoceptors in the eye will induce ocular hypotension. It cannot be decided yet whether the α_2-adrenoceptors are located at pre- or postjunctional sites. α_2-Adrenoceptor agonists induced neither macroscopic ocular side-effects nor any substantial effect on the pupil size. As such they might offer a new possibility to treat glaucomatous disease with drugs. This possibility, however, so far remains limited to animal experiments and it will require clinical substantiation.

4 A comparison between central and peripheral α-adrenoceptors

Ever since the concept of central α-adrenoceptors mediating the hypotensive effect of clonidine and related drugs had been submitted by Schmitt (1971) the question has been asked whether central and peripheral α-adrenoceptors would be different or not. Schmitt (1971) originally expressed the opinion that both receptor subtypes are rather different, as concluded from a pharmacological analysis using the agonists and antagonists available at that time. The availability of more selective agonists and antagonists as tools and also the possibility of performing correlation studies by means of computer techniques have somewhat modified the conclusion reached by Schmitt (1971).

We have already reported that the central nervous system contains α_1-adrenoceptors as concluded from radioligand binding studies. In view of their affinity for selective agonists and antagonists these central α_1-adrenoceptors are very similar to α_1-adrenoceptors at postjunctional sites in peripheral vascular structures (Timmermans et al., 1981c; Hieble et al., 1982). However, it should be emphasized as already discussed in a preceding paragraph that central α_1-adrenoceptors do not play a relevant role, in any case not in the mediation of the central hypotensive and bradycardic effects of clonidine and similar drugs.

Both radioligand binding experiments (see e.g. U'Prichard et al., 1977; Rouot et al., 1979; Perry et al., 1981) and the various functional studies (outlined previously in this paper) suggest the presence of α_2-adrenoceptors in the brain and their involvement in the central hypotensive effect of clonidine and related drugs.

Various correlation studies have compared the central hypotensive potency of clonidine and related drugs (including azepine derivatives like azepexole and B-HT 920) and their peripheral effects on α_2-adrenoceptors (Hammer et al., 1980; Kobinger and Pichler, 1980b; Timmermans et al., 1981b; De Jonge et al., 1981b, 1982b). All these studies suggest a close similarity between the α-adrenoceptors in the peripheral blood vessels and those present in the brain and involved in the central hypotensive action of clonidine and related drugs.

The QSAR study on imidazolidine agonists (Timmermans et al., 1980a) which activate central α_2-adrenoceptors and hence decrease arterial blood pressure has led to the hypothetical α_2-receptor model depicted in Fig. 11.

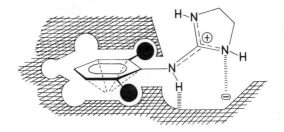

FIG. 11. Schematic working model of the mode of interaction between clonidine-like imidazolidines and the central alpha receptor. Note the steric requirements and position of the (black) substituents at the phenyl ring, the hydrogen bonding between the bridge nitrogen and the receptor, and the charge transfer between the imidazolidine moiety and the receptor. The receptor is represented by the hatched area. (From Timmermans *et al.*, 1980a).

The central receptor described hypothetically by this model is assumed to be very similar to peripheral α_2-adrenoceptors in vascular smooth muscle. Indeed, the classical model for peripheral (nor)adrenergic receptors proposed by Belleau does not exclude a similarity between central and peripheral α-adrenoceptors, as concluded from correlation studies, from the selectivity of agonists and antagonists, and from other indirect arguments as presented in the present paragraph.

5 Mechanisms at a cellular level

5.1 PRESYNAPTIC α_2-ADRENOCEPTORS

Presynaptic α_2-adrenoceptors appear to be involved in the regulation of noradrenaline release from noradrenergic nerve endings. However, little is known about the intricate mechanisms involved at a cellular level.

A variety of plausible mechanisms have been proposed, all of which require more experimental evidence.

1. The presynaptic α_2-adrenoceptor could modify the release of noradrenaline by regulating the influx of extracellular calcium ions. Accordingly, the activation of presynaptic α_2-adrenoceptors will inhibit the transmembrane calcium influx via potential sensitive permeability channels (Göthert, 1977, 1979; Göthert *et al.*, 1979; De Langen and Mulder, 1980). However, the relevance of this mechanism is questioned by the observation that calcium entry blockers like nifedipine do not substantially influence the process triggered by the activation of presynaptic α_2-adrenoceptors (Timmermans *et al.*, 1983a).

2. As proposed by Stjärne (1978, 1979) the presynaptic inhibition of noradrenaline release is achieved by hyperpolarization of the axons, thus inducing an impairment of impulse propagation and of the recruitment of varicosities.

3. An association has been proposed between the release of noradrenaline from nerve endings, as mediated via presynaptic α_2-adrenoceptors on the one hand, and the activity of Na^+/K^+-ATP-ase on the other hand (Vizi, 1977, 1979). Accordingly, the stimulation of α_2-adrenoceptors at the membrane would increase Na^+/K^+-ATP-ase activity and thus reduce the release of the endogenous neurotransmitter (noradrenaline) by increasing the efflux of calcium ions from the nerve endings (Vizi, 1977, 1979). However, the validity of this hypothesis remains to be demonstrated (Powis, 1981).

4. Cyclic nucleotides, like cyclic AMP or cyclic GMP, have been implicated in the process of noradrenaline release, as regulated by presynaptic α_2-adrenoceptors, although the evidence available is limited and sometimes conflicting (see e.g. Langer, 1981). An intracellular decrease in cyclic AMP concentration can be induced by α_2-adrenergic inhibition of adenylate cyclase (Fain and Garcia-Sainz, 1980; Schultz et al., 1980; Jakobs and Schultz, 1982).

5.2 POSTSYNAPTIC α_1- AND α_2-ADRENOCEPTORS

The stimulation of non-neuronal postsynaptic α_2-adrenoceptors located at the membranes of platelets, pancreatic islets, adipocytes and neuroblastoma x glioma hybrid cells has been shown to respond with an inhibition of the accumulation of cyclic AMP independent from the presence of calcium ions (see Atlas and Sabol, 1981). In vivo, considerable differences have been demonstrated between the events which follow the stimulation of post synaptic α_1- and α_2-adrenoceptors, respectively. This difference has become particularly obvious with respect to ionic movements following the excitation of vascular α_1- and α_2-adrenoceptors, respectively, by their selective agonists.

In general, it seems likely that calcium movements in particular play a part in the development of the stimulus generated by the formation of the agonist–receptor complex. The older work of Bohr (1963), who demonstrated that only part of the vasoconstriction induced by noradrenaline is dependent upon the presence of extracellular calcium ions, prompted us to study the role of calcium fluxes involved in the vasoconstriction induced by the selective stimulation of α_1- and α_2-adrenoceptors, respectively. In these investigations calcium entry blockers were appreciated as useful pharmacological tools. The experiments were carried out in pithed normotensive rats and in a later stage also in similar preparations of various other animal species.

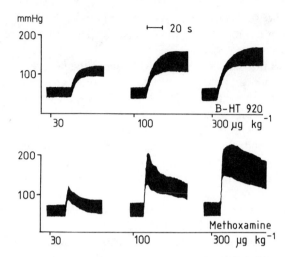

FIG. 12. The onset of the pressor response induced by B-HT 920 (α_2) and methoxamine (α_1) in the pithed rat. Note a slower increase in arterial blood pressure for B-HT 920 in comparison with a rapid rise in pressure caused by methoxamine. (Unpublished data from the authors.)

Firstly, the vasoconstriction process due to selective stimulation of α_1- and α_2-adrenoceptors was investigated as such. As clearly shown in Fig. 12, the rise in blood pressure reflecting constriction of the precapillary arterioles (resistance vessels) occurred more rapidly upon selective stimulation of postsynaptic α_1-adrenoceptors (e.g. by methoxamine) and the pressor effect induced by selective stimulation of postsynaptic α_2-adrenoceptors (e.g. by B-HT 920). Not only the rate of the rise in pressure, but also the course of the dose–response characteristics, were rather different in both cases: as a rule, the dose–response curve reflecting the pressor effect due to α_1-stimulation is steeper and achieves a higher maximum than representing the pressor response to α_2-adrenoceptor excitation (compare Figs 3 and 4). These obvious differences in the contractile process following selective stimulation of either α-adrenoceptor subtype strongly suggests that the generation of the stimuli, following the formation of the agonist–receptor complex, is greatly different in both cases. These obvious differences were further accentuated when the influence of calcium entry blockade was investigated. In brief, it appeared that the response to α_2-receptor activation was sensitive to impairment of calcium entry, whereas the α_1- response was virtually not (Van Meel *et al.*, 1981a, 1981b, 1982a).

Figure 13 illustrates this principle. In pithed rats the pressor response to methoxamine, a selective α_1-adrenoceptor agonist, is not significantly influenced by pretreatment with nisoldipine, a potent derivative of the well-known calcium antagonist nifedipine. In contrast, a very marked and dose-dependent shift and flattening of the dose–response curve of B-HT 920, a highly selective α-adrenoceptor stimulant, was observed as a result of the pretreatment with nisoldipine. This finding not only holds for nisoldipine and B-HT 920, but could be demonstrated for several calcium channel blockers on the one hand and some other α_2-adrenoceptor agonists as well. Moreover, it could also be demonstrated in other animal species like the rabbit and cat (Van Meel *et al.*, 1982b; Timmermans *et al.*, 1983a). A series of other examples, confirming the aforementioned principle, is depicted in Fig. 14.

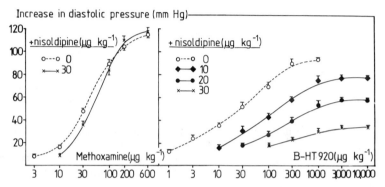

FIG. 13. Log dose–pressor response curves to intravenous methoxamine (left) and B-HT 920 (right) in pithed normotensive rats after intraarterial pretreatment with the calcium entry blocker nisoldipine. Note the pronounced depression of the slope and maximum of the dose-response curve to B-HT 920 by very low doses of nisoldipine and the negligible effect of this calcium antagonist on the hypotensive action of methoxamine. (From Van Zwieten *et al.*, 1982b.)

Apart from blockade of the calcium influx by representatives of various classes of calcium antagonists, Na_2-EDTA, a compound known to inactivate ionized calcium, depresses the effect of α_2-receptor stimulation much more than the α_1-induced pressor response. More recently, the differential effect of calcium entry blockade on pressor responses mediated by α_1- and α_2-adrenoceptor stimulation could also be demonstrated in an *in vitro* model involving isolated perfused hindlimbs of reserpine-treated rats, as introduced by Kobinger and Pichler (1981a). Again, the vasoconstrictor responses (reductions in flow) due to selective α_1-adrenoceptor stimulation remained virtually uninfluenced by calcium antagonism, whereas those to α_2-adrenoceptor activation were effectively impaired by the prior administration of a calcium entry blocker. The interference of nisoldipine with the reduction in flow in isolated perfused hindquarters of rats pretreated with reserpine is demonstrated in Fig. 15 (Van Meel *et al.*, 1983a).

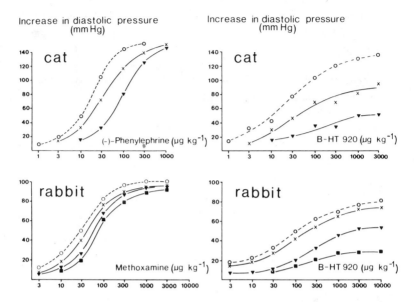

FIG. 14. Influence of nifedipine on the pressor responses caused by phenylephrine (α_1), methoxamine (α_1) and B-HT 920 (α_2) in pithed cats and ganglion-blocked, vagotomized and atropine-treated rabbits, respectively. The results are similar to those obtained in rats (see Fig. 13). (From Van Zwieten et al., 1982b.)

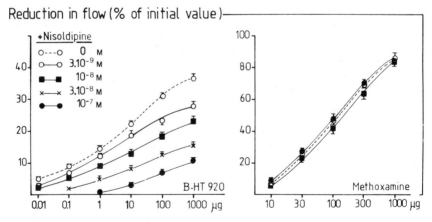

FIG. 15. Influence of nisoldipine on the vasoconstrictor response induced in the perfused hindquarters of the rat by B-HT 920 (α_2) and methoxamine (α_1), respectively. The degree of vasoconstriction is expressed by the reduction in flow. Similarly, as in the in vivo model of the pithed rat, nisoldipine reduces the vasoconstriction mediated by α_2-receptor stimulation in a dose-dependent and noncompetitive manner. The vasoconstriction induced via α_1-receptor stimulation remains unaffected by the calcium entry blocker. (From Van Meel et al., 1983a.)

The differential influence of calcium channel blockers and Na_2-EDTA on pressor effects mediated by α_1- and α_2-adrenoceptors, respectively, has shed some new light upon the role of calcium movements in the generation of the stimulus initiated by the stimulation of vascular α-adrenoceptors.

Before discussing this hypothesis two other points should be clarified. Firstly, it should be considered that the calcium slow channel blockers possess α_2-adrenoceptor blocking activity, thus impairing the formation of the α_2-agonist–receptor complex. However, this possibility could be ruled out by means of radioligand binding studies. In such studies we could not establish substantial affinity for α_1- or α_2-adrenoceptors (Van Meel et al., 1981b). In other words, the calcium antagonists at issue are not α_2-adrenoceptor antagonists. Secondly, the impairment of the vasoconstriction due to α_2-adrenoceptor stimulation is not necessarily caused by inhibition of the calcium influx but might theoretically also be the result of some other mechanism. This possibility was investigated by comparing, in a quantitative manner, the inhibitory potency of a series of calcium slow channel blockers with respect to the depressant effect on α_2-adrenoceptor mediated vasoconstriction in vivo on the one hand and a parameter reflecting calcium entry blockade in vitro on the other hand (Van Meel et al., 1983b). The in vitro parameter was established as follows: increasing the potassium concentration in the extracellular fluid induces the contraction of rabbit isolated aorta strips, owing to the influx of extracellular calcium ions. The inhibition of the calcium inward flux by the so-called calcium entry blockers is selective and competitive in nature. Accordingly, the quantitative evaluation of the inhibition of the K^+-induced vasoconstriction is a satisfactory and reproducible measure for the degree of calcium entry blockade exerted by one particular compound.

A close and highly significant correlation was established between the following two parameters (Van Meel et al., 1983b):

1. Calcium entry blockade in vitro, derived from the inhibition by K^+-induced vasoconstriction, pD_2' (in vitro);
2. The depressant effect on α_2-adrenoceptor mediated pressor responses in vivo, pD_2' (in vivo).

The correlation, established for a series of 10 rather divergent calcium slow channel blockers, is shown in Fig. 16. From this obvious and close correlation it may be concluded that the depressant influence of the calcium antagonists on the α_2-adrenoceptor mediated vasoconstriction should indeed be attributed to the impairment of the transmembrane influx of calcium ions.

With respect to the role of calcium movements in the vasoconstriction mediated by the stimulation of vascular postsynaptic α_2-adrenoceptors the following hypothesis is submitted:

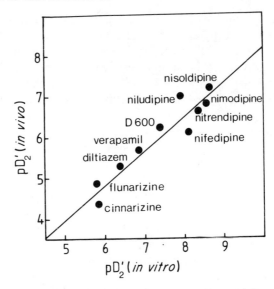

FIG. 16. Relationship between the activities of various calcium antagonists to attenuate the B-HT 920-induced, α_2-adrenoceptor mediated vasoconstriction in pithed normotensive rats, pD_2' (*in vivo*) (see also Fig. 13) and K^+-induced contraction of rabbit thoracic aorta strips, pD_2' (*in vitro*). (From Van Meel *et al.*, 1983b.)

1. The formation of the α_2-agonist–receptor complex generates a stimulus initiated by the influx of extracellular calcium ions. This stimulus contributes to the activation of intracellular contractile proteins, thus causing vascular smooth muscle contraction. The calcium inward flux is sensitive to blockade by proper drugs (calcium entry blockers) which impair vasoconstriction by reducing the number of Ca^{2+}-ions entering the cell. However, the calcium antagonists do not interfere with the formation of the α_2-agonist–receptor complex, which occurs normally. Na_2-EDTA also impairs the α_2-adrenoceptor induced vasoconstriction although via a different mechanism: this compound complexates with extracellular Ca^{2+}-ions, thus preventing their inward flux across the cell membrane.

2. For the α_1-adrenoceptor the stimulation is rather different. The formation of the α_1-agonist–receptor complex does not trigger directly the influx of extracellular calcium ions, but rather induces membrane depolarization. This process initiates the release of ionized activator calcium from various intracellular storage sites, for instance from the sarcoplasmatic reticulum or from the inner side of the sarcolemma. Probably no substantial calcium influx across the membrane occurs, thus explaining why α_1-adrenoceptor mediated vasoconstriction is insensitive to calcium channel blockers.

A schematic representation of this hypothesis is depicted in Fig. 17.

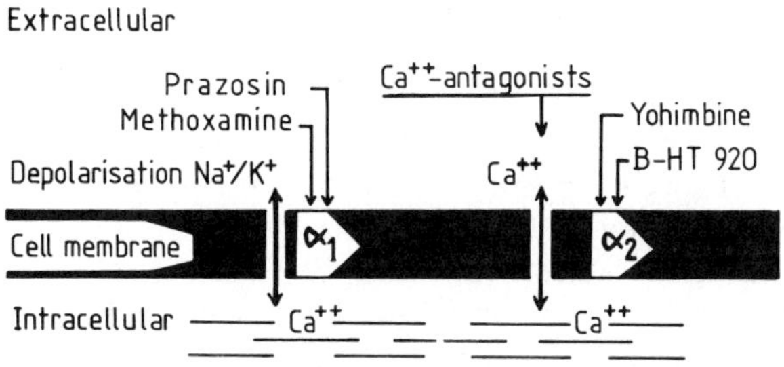

FIG. 17. Schematic representation of a vascular smooth muscle cell membrane. Note the (hypothesized) differences between the consequences of the stimulation of α_1- or α_2-adrenoceptors, respectively. Stimulation of an α_1-adrenoceptor induces membrane depolarization, based upon Na^+ and K^+ fluxes; this process is not sensitive to calcium entry blockers. However, the stimulation of the α_2-adrenoceptor with an appropriate agonist is accompanied by the influx of Ca^{2+}-ions, which will induce the activation of the intracellular contractile proteins. Blockade of this calcium influx with a calcium entry blocker prevents vasoconstriction, in spite of the unhampered formation of the agonist/α_2-receptor complex.

This concept is supported by Godfraind's experiments on isolated aorta preparations, using $^{45}Ca^{2+}$ as a tracer for the determination of calcium fluxes (Godfraind et al., 1982). From these experiments the authors have concluded that α_2-receptor stimulation will open up calcium channels, whereas the stimulation of α_1-adrenoceptors will induce depolarization and subsequently the release of calcium ions from intracellular stores.

The aforementioned hypothesis conflicts with the findings by Vanhoutte and his group who, using various types of isolated vessels, concluded from their experiments that rather α_1-adrenoceptor stimulation is accompanied by a calcium influx which is sensitive to blockade by calcium antagonists (Vanhoutte, 1982; Vanhoutte and Rimele, 1982).

The discrepancy between our results and hypothesis and those described by Vanhoutte can only be attributed to fundamental differences in the experimental models employed. The vascular beds studied are significantly different, and the difference between in vivo and in vitro conditions obviously also plays an important part. Apart from the hypothesis submitted for the role of calcium movements involved in the α_2-adrenoceptor mediated vasoconstriction, the present findings may also be interpreted as a basis for the explanation of vasodilator effects of the calcium entry blockers. The endogenous circulating catecholamines noradrenaline and adrenaline are nonselective agonists which will stimulate both α_1- and α_2-adrenoceptors at postsynaptic sites. It should be assumed, therefore, that vascular tone is maintained by the stimulation of both receptor subtypes. In the presence of a calcium slow channel blocker, however, the constrictor effect due to α_2-adrenoceptor stimulation is diminished according to the hypothesis previously described in detail. The concomitant reduction in vascular tone may explain the arteriolar dilatation and reduction in peripheral vascular resistance which may be the basis of the vasodilator activity observed for all calcium antagonists. In this connection, it should be added that in our experimental model not only the constrictor effects of the selective α_2-agonists, but also the α_2-component of the noradrenaline effect, were diminished by calcium entry blockers, whereas the α_1-component remained intact (Van Meel *et al.*, 1982a).

The proposed mode of action of the calcium antagonists, causing a decrease in vascular tone, would represent a rather subtle mechanism which could satisfactorily explain the vasodilator activity of this class of drugs. The vasodilator effect, which most certainly involves the relaxation of the resistance vessels, is the obvious basis of the now well-established antihypertensive potency of calcium entry blockers.

6 Drugs which interact with α_1- and α_2-adrenoceptors

We have already discussed the various selective or non-selective agonists and antagonists of α_1- and α_2-adrenoceptors. It thus appears that we now have at our disposal a large variety of drugs and experimental compounds able to interact with either α_1- or α_2-adrenoceptors, or with both (Fig. 2, Table 1). In this connection both agonists and antagonists are available, with either selective or non-selective properties.

At presynaptic sites the α_2-adrenoceptors are targets for circulating catecholamines (noradrenaline, adrenaline), which are known to be non-selective stimulants of both α_1- and α_2-adrenoceptors. As such, the presynaptic α_2-adrenoceptors may be regarded as inhibitory autoreceptors for the release of the endogenous neurotransmitter from the sympathetic nerve endings. This feedback mechanism may be of physiological relevance under *in vivo* circumstances (Graham and Pettinger, 1979; Graham *et al.*, 1980; Majewski *et al.*, 1982), although this concept is subject to debate (Dollery *et al.*, 1979; Hamilton *et al.*, 1982). At present there is insufficient experimental evidence to decide upon a definite acceptance or rejection of the hypothesis. Presynaptic α_2-adrenoceptors can also be stimulated by exogenous compounds which reach the presynaptic sites via the blood stream. We have already discussed the possible important role of presynaptic α_2-adrenoceptors in the generation of bradycardia induced by clonidine.

The blockade of presynaptic α_2-adrenoceptors by classical, non-selective α-adrenoceptor antagonists like phentolamine and phenoxybenzamine satisfactorily explains the older observation that these α-blocking drugs cause an enhanced release of noradrenaline from the nerve endings.

At postsynaptic sites, both α_1- and α_2-adrenoceptors are present and as such are targets of endogenous, circulating catecholamines as well as of exogenous drugs. It seems very likely that postsynaptic α_1-adrenoceptors contribute to the maintenance of total peripheral resistance in humans. Preliminary evidence (Van Brummelen et al., 1982) suggests that vascular postsynaptic α_2-adrenoceptors also contribute to the generation of total peripheral resistance.

As discussed in detail in a preceding paragraph, vascular postsynaptic α_2-adrenoceptors may be involved in a complex manner in the vasodilation induced by calcium entry blockers. The recent observation that vasoconstriction via postsynaptic α_2-adrenoceptors is influenced by the presence of endogenous angiotensin II (De Jonge et al., 1981d, 1982c) and also by circulating adrenaline and by corticosteroids (Van Meel et al., 1983c) is in agreement with the presumption that postsynaptic α_2-adrenoceptors are hormone receptors. As such they are not under direct noradrenergic control, so that a modulation of their response by blood-borne substances is conceivable.

In view of the structural demand of α_2-adrenoceptors at pre- and postsynaptic sites it should be expected that all α_2-adrenoceptor agonists display a comparable activity at pre- and postsynaptic sites, respectively. However, it must be realized that the accessibility of pre- and post-synaptic α_2-adrenoceptors to drugs is probably somewhat different. Postsynaptic α_2-adrenoceptors are located at extrasynaptic sites and hence particularly sensitive to circulating hormones (adrenaline) and to drugs administered via the blood stream, but less so to endogenous neurotransmitters released from the nerve endings, since these tend to remain located to the synapse as such. In this connection, it is of interest to draw the reader's attention to a new development: the experimental compound B-HT 958 (Pichler et al., 1982; for structure see Fig. 18) is a partial agonist of vascular postjunctional α_2-adrenoceptors in the rat, with predominant stimulatory activity on presynaptic cardiac α_2-adrenoceptors. Postsynaptically the antagonistic effect of B-HT 958 dominates and this explains the apparent high pre/post-activity ratio. Moreover, within a series of 2,5-disubstituted clonidine analogues, some derivatives appear able to discriminate between cardiac pre- and vascular postsynaptic α_2-adrenoceptors (De Jonge et al., 1981d). In addition, the α-adrenoceptor antagonist BE 2254 (see Fig. 18) has been reported to differ in potency at pre- and postsynaptic α_2-adrenoceptors (Hicks, 1981). It thus appears possible to develop drugs with differential activities towards pre- and postsynaptic α_2-adrenoceptors.

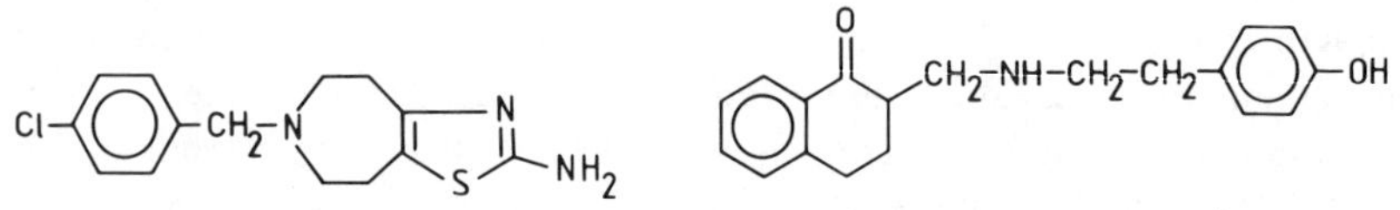

FIG. 18. Structural formulae of B-HT 958 and BE 2254.

7 Clinical potential of drugs interacting with α-adrenoceptors

The clinical applicability of classical α-adrenoceptor agonists and antagonists is briefly mentioned in Table 1 and does not require a detailed discussion here. In brief, α-adrenoceptor agonists may be of use in certain forms of circulatory shock, in particular when extreme vasodilation occurs, as is the case in anaphylactic shock; another indication is as nasal and conjunctival decongestants and as vasoconstrictor agents administered together with local anesthetic agents. α-Adrenoceptor blocking agents, like phentolamine or phenoxybenzamine, are mainly used temporarily in the treatment of phaeochromocytoma, prior and during surgical intervention in this condition. The treatment of hypertension and of disturbances of peripheral circulation (claudicatio intermittens, etc.) with non-selective α-adrenoceptor blockers has proved disappointing and should no more be attempted. Some beneficial effect has been observed, however, in vasospastic conditions, like Raynaud's syndrome, although various other vasodilators may be of use as well; the effect of the α-blocking drug is by no means specific. Phentolamine is studied as an unloading drug in congestive heart failure (Georgopoulos et al., 1978; Gould et al., 1980). The beneficial effect is due to vasodilatation and is not particularly specific. The cautious use of α-blockers in conditions of circulatory shock has been studied, with the aim to block the vasoconstrictor effects of excessive quantities of endogenous catecholamines released by reflex mechanisms.

A new development in the field of α-adrenoceptor blocking drugs was the introduction of prazosin and related agents (trimazosin, doxazosin), which are selective antagonists of postsynaptic α_1-adrenoceptors. Prazosin is a useful antihypertensive drug and it can also be applied as an unloading drug in the treatment of congestive heart failure. It causes dilatation of both arteriolar and venous vessels, thus reducing both cardiac afterload and pre-load. The reduction in total peripheral resistance fully explains its antihypertensive effect. The lowering of blood pressure by prazosin is accompanied by a reflex tachycardia which remains much more modest than observed in the treatment with non-selective α-blockers like phentolamine. This modest degree of reflex tachycardia is attributed to the absence of presynaptic α_2-receptor blockade, although this explanation is not fully satisfactory.

The possibility to develop compounds with differential effects on pre- and postsynaptic α_2-adrenoceptors, as discussed in the preceding paragraph, may lead to potentially interesting new drugs in the treatment of hypertension, angina and congestive heart failure.

The central hypotensive action of clonidine, guanfacine and α-methyl-DOPA (mediated by α-methylnoradrenaline) has already been discussed in full detail. It seems unlikely that highly selective new antihypertensive drugs based upon an interaction with central α_2-adrenoceptors can be anticipated. The similarity of the α_2-adrenoceptors involved in either the therapeutic effect or the adverse reactions (sedation, dry mouth) would seem to prohibit the separation of both desired and unwanted effects.

Clonidine has been demonstrated to suppress certain symptoms of the opiate withdrawal syndrome, both in laboratory animals and in human addicts (Gold et al., 1978; Aghajanian, 1978; references quoted). This action, which may be of certain interest in the pretreatment of opiate addiction, is possibly due to a stimulation of central presynaptic α_2-adrenoceptors which inhibit the firing of the locus coeruleus. In this connection we must mention the role of central α_2-adrenoceptors involved in the withdrawal syndrome following cessation of long-term antihypertensive treatment with clonidine (Hoobler and Kashima, 1977; Chrysand and Whitsett, 1978; Weber, 1980). A recently developed animal model (Thoolen et al., 1981a-e, 1982) has allowed us to study this phenomenon on a reproducible and quantitative basis. The drug is infused continuously over 2 weeks by means of ALZET osmotic minipumps implanted into conscious unrestrained spontaneously hypertensive rats. Extirpation of the minipump interrupts the treatment and hence triggers the withdrawal phenomenon, which is characterized by tachycardia, blood pressure upswings and behavioural changes (Figs 19–21). There is no overshoot in blood pressure (Fig. 20). The role of central and peripheral α_2-adrenoceptors in the generation of the withdrawal phenomenon may be based upon the development of clonidine-induced subsensitivity of the receptors involved. However, in spite of this desensitization of α_2-adrenoceptors as suggested, there occurs no increased tolerance against the antihypertensive effect of clonidine.

An unexpected potential therapeutic application of α_2-adrenoceptor stimulants is the lowering of intraocular pressure in glaucoma simplex. In animal experiments it has been demonstrated (Innemee et al., 1981), that the selective α_2-adrenoceptor agonist B-HT 920 induces a substantial decrease in intraocular pressure. Experiments with appropriate antagonists have shown that the lowering of the intraocular pressure is mediated by α_2-adrenoceptors

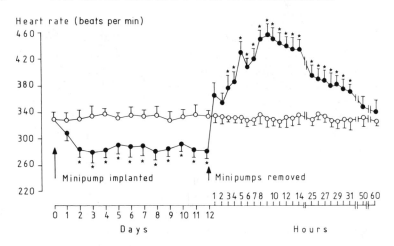

FIG. 19. Heart rate of conscious unrestrained spontaneously hypertensive rats during continuous subcutaneous infusion of clonidine (500 μg kg⁻¹ day⁻¹, ●) or saline (○). The drug or saline was infused by subcutaneously implanted mini-osmopumps, which allow a continuous infusion. After day 12 the infusions were abruptly stopped from surgical extirpation of the mini-pumps. Note the pronounced degree of tachycardia which develops after a few hours and wears off after approximately 30 hours. Asterisks indicate values significantly different from control ($p < 0.05$). Symbols represent means $\pm$ S.E.M. ($n = 5$–10). (From Thoolen *et al.*, 1982.)

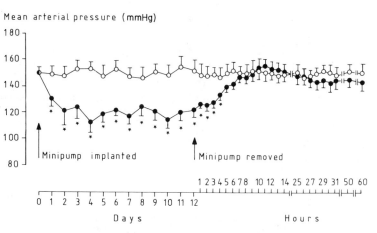

FIG. 20. Mean arterial pressure of conscious unrestrained spontaneously hypertensive rats during continuous subcutaneous infusion of clonidine (500 μg kg⁻¹ day⁻¹, ●) or saline (○) and after withdrawal of treatment. Same experiments and details as in Fig. 19. Note the hypotensive effect during infusion and the lack of overshoot hypertension after the interruption of the clonidine administration. (From Thoolen *et al.*, 1982.)

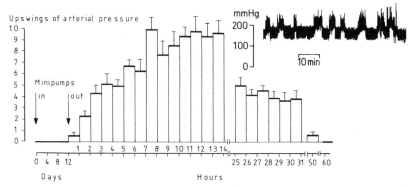

FIG. 21. Upswings of blood pressure after sudden cessation of a continuous subcutaneous infusion of clonidine (500 μg kg⁻¹ day⁻¹). Same experiments as in Fig. 20. *Insertion:* blood pressure upswings, occurring spontaneously. *Columns:* number of blood pressure upswings after withdrawal of clonidine (means ± S.E.M., $n = 8$–10). (From Thoolen *et al.*, 1982.)

in the eye but it is so far unknown whether these receptors are pre- or postsynaptic. Neither do we know in which anatomical structures of the eye the α₂-adrenoceptors are located. In this context, it may be of relevance that the potent ocular hypotensive effect of B-HT 920 is not accompanied by any effects on pupil size or on the eye lids. Macroscopic ocular side-effects and the influence on pupil size are probably mediated by α₂-adrenoceptors. As such, this type of drug would offer the possibility to develop a new series of antiglaucomatous drugs. However, studies in glaucomatous patients have not yet been carried out on any substantial scale.

Finally, we speculate that α₂-adrenoceptor antagonists might have a beneficial effect in depressive illness, since they facilitate neurotransmission also in the central nervous system. It has been submitted that depression may be causally related to impaired noradrenergic transmission in the central nervous system. At present, some selective antagonists of α₂-adrenoceptors are tested clinically as potential therapeutics in mood disorders.

8 Conclusions

The renaissance of interest in α-adrenoceptors which has developed during the past decade has proved most rewarding, both from a fundamental, molecular pharmacological point of view as well as for physiological and therapeutic reasons. The subdivision of the α-adrenoceptors into α₁/α₂ and pre/postjunctional subtypes, respectively, has led to a logical although complex classification. After a period of confusion in the nomenclature this is a most welcome development. The introduction of highly selective agonists and antagonists towards α_1/α_2-adrenoceptors as well as sophisticated radioligand binding studies have substantiated the concept of the existence of two types of α-adrenoceptors with rather different structural demands. Furthermore, considerable differences have been demonstrated to exist between α_1- and α_2-adrenoceptor stimulation, respectively. Apart from a certain fundamental interest, this differential behaviour of α_1- and α_2-adrenoceptor subtypes is probably of capital importance in the explanation of the vasodilator action of calcium entry blockers, vascular postsynaptic α-adrenoceptors probably playing a major role.

More recently, particular attention has been paid to the precise location of the postsynaptic α_2-adrenoceptor with respect to the synapse. All evidence available at present points towards a hormonal character of the postsynaptic α_2-adrenoceptor.

A few years ago several investigators have initiated studies on the distribution of α_1/α_2-adrenoceptors over the various organs and tissues in the organism. These studies have not been completed yet, although a global pattern of distribution has emerged. A functional role of α_1/α_2-adrenoceptors is particularly obvious in vascular smooth muscle and in the central nervous system, although the presence of these receptors can be demonstrated in various other organs or subcellular structures.

The central α-adrenoceptors have been recognized as the targets of centrally acting clonidine, guanfacine and α-methyl-DOPA. It has been well documented that they are of the α_2-subtype, whereas their location seems likely to be postjunctional. The central α_2-adrenoceptors are probably very similar to α_2-adrenoceptors in the periphery.

More recently, the existence of α_2-adrenoceptors in the eye has been postulated. Their stimulation by selective agonists induces a substantial reduction of intraocular pressure, without causing any other macroscopic ocular changes with respect to pupil size, eye lids etc. As such, these drugs may offer a new possibility to treat glaucoma simplex.

In the history of drug design it has always been observed that a more precise localization and subdivision of receptors leads to the development of selective agonists and antagonists, some of which lead to therapeutic applications. Well-known examples of such a development are the subdivision of cholinergic receptors (nicotinic, muscarinic), β-adrenoceptors (β_1/β_2), histamine receptors (H_1/H_2), serotonine receptors (S_1/S_2) and possibly also dopaminergic receptors (various subtypes). Clinically useful drugs have emerged from the development of selective agonists and antagonists. Little imagination is required to predict a similar development in the field of α-adrenoceptors in the course of the next few years.

References

Aghajanian, G. K. (1978). *Nature* **276**, 186–188.
Ahlquist, R. P. (1948). *Am. J. Physiol.* **153**, 586–599.
Aktories, K., Schultz, G. and Jakobs, K. H. (1980). *Naunyn-Schmiedeberg's Arch. Pharmacol.* **312**, 167–173.
Atlas, D. and Sabol, L. (1981). *Eur. J. Biochem.* **113**, 521–529.
Berthelsen, S. and Pettinger, W. A. (1977). *Life Sci.* **21**, 595–606.
Bohr, D. F. (1963). *Science* **139**, 579–599.
Borowski, E., Starke, K., Ehrl, H. and Endo, T. (1977). *Neuroscience* **2**, 285–296.
Brown, D. A. and Caulfield, M. P. (1979). *Br. J. Pharmacol.* **65**, 435–445.
Butler, M. and Jenkinson, D. H. (1978). *Eur. J. Pharmacol.* **52**, 303–311.
Cambridge, D., Davey, M. J. and Massingham, R. (1977). *Br. J. Pharmacol.* **59**, 514 P.
Cambridge, D. (1981). *Eur. J. Pharmacol.* **72**, 413–415.
Carter, R. J. and Shuster, S. (1982). *Br. J. Pharmacol.* **75**, 169–175.
Cavero, I. and Roach, A. G. (1978). *Br. J. Pharmacol.* **62**, 468P–469P.
Cavero, I. and Roach, A. G. (1980). *Br. J. Pharmacol.* **70**, 269–276.
Chalmers, J. P. (1975). *Circ. Res.* **36**, 469–480.
Chapleo, C. B., Doxey, J. C., Meyers, P. L. and Roach, A. G. (1981). *Br. J. Pharmacol.* **74**, 824P.
Chrysand, S. G. and Whitsett, T. L. (1978). *JAMA* **239**, 2241.
Dabiré, H., Mouillé, P., Andréjak, M., Fournier, B. and Schmitt, H. (1981). *Arch. int. Pharmacodyn.* **254**, 252–270.
Davey, M. J. (1980) *J. Cardiovasc. Pharmacol.* **2**, S287–S301.
De Jonge, A., Timmermans, P. B. M. W. M. and Van Zwieten, P. A. (1981a). *Naunyn-Schmiedeberg's Arch. Pharmacol.* **317**, 8–12.
De Jonge, A., Slothorst-Grisdijk, F. P., Timmermans, P. B. M. W. M. and Van Zwieten, P. A. (1981b). *Eur. J. Pharmacol.* **71**, 411–420.
De Jonge, A., Van Meel, J. C. A., Timmermans, P. B. M. W. M. and Van Zwieten, P. A. (1981c). *Life Sci.* **28**, 2009–2016.
De Jonge, A., Wilffert, B., Kalkman, H. O., Van Meel, J. C. A., Thoolen, M. J. M. C., Timmermans, P. B. M. W. M. and Van Zwieten, P. A. (1981d). *Eur. J. Pharmacol.* **74**, 385–386.
De Jonge, A., Santing, P. N., Timmermans, P. B. M. W. M. and Van Zwieten, P. A. (1981e). *J. Auton. Pharmacol.* **1**, 377–383.
De Jonge, A., Santing, P. N., Timmermans, P. B. M. W. M. and Van Zwieten (1982a). *J. Auton. Pharmacol.* **2**, 87–96.
De Jonge, A., Timmermans, P. B. M. W. M. and Van Zwieten, P. A. (1982b). *J. Pharmacol. Exp. Ther.* **222**, 705–711.
De Jonge, A., Knape, J. Th. A., Van Meel, J. C. A., Kalkman, H. O., Wilffert, B., Thoolen, M. J. M. C., Timmermans, P. B. M. W. M. and Van Zwieten, P. A. (1982c). *Naunyn-Schmiedeberg's Arch. Pharmacol.* **321**, 309–313.
De Jonge, A., Timmermans, P. B. M. W. M. and Van Zwieten, P. A. (1983). *Brit. J. Pharmacol.* In press.
De Langen, C. D. J. and Mulder, A. H. (1980). *Brain Res.* **185**, 399–408.
DeMarinis, R. M. and Hieble, J. P. (1983). *J. Med. Chem.* In press.
De Mey, J. G. and Vanhoutte, P. M. (1981). *Circ. Res.* **48**, 875–884.
Docherty, J. R. and McGrath, J. C. (1980). *Naunyn-Schmiedeb. Arch. Pharmacol.* **312**, 107–116.

250   P. A. VAN ZWIETEN AND P. B. M. W. M. TIMMERMANS

Docherty, J. R., Göthert, M., Dieckhöfer, C. and Starke, K. (1982). *Arzneim.- Forsch.* (*Drug Res.*) **32**, 1534–1539.
Dollery, C. T. and Jerie, P. (1980). *Br. J. Clin. Pharmacol.* **10** (Supplement 1).
Dollery, C. T., Fitzgerald, G. A. and Watkins, J. (1979). *Br. J. Clin. Pharmacol.* **8**, 396P.
Doxey, J. C. and Roach, A. G. (1980). *J. Auton. Pharmacol.* **1**, 73–99.
Doxey, J. C., Smith, C. F. C. and Walker, J. M. (1977). *Brit. J. Pharmacol.* **60**, 91–96.
Drew, G. M. (1976). *Eur. J. Pharmacol.* **36**, 313–320.
Drew, G. M. (1977). *Eur. J. Pharmacol.* **42**, 123–130.
Drew, G. M. (1978). *Br. J. Pharmacol.* **64**, 293–300.
Drew, G. M. (1980). *Eur. J. Pharmacol.* **65**, 85–87.
Drew, G. M., Gower, A. J. and Mariott, A. S. (1979). *Br. J. Pharmacol.* **67**, 133–138.
Fain, J. N. and Garcia-Sainz, J. A. (1980). *Life Sci.* **26**, 1183–1194.
Flavahan, N. A. and McGrath, J. C. (1981). *Br. J. Pharmacol.* **72**, 585P.
Furchgott, R. F. (1967). *Ann. N.Y. Acad. Sci.* **139**, 553–570.
Garcia-Sevilla, J. A., Hollingswort, P. J. and Smith, C. B. (1981). *Eur. J. Pharmacol.* **74**, 329–341.
Georgopoulos, A. J., Valasidis, A. and Siourthas, D. (1978). *Eur. J. Clin. Pharmacol.* **13**, 325–329.
Glick, G., Epstein, S. E., Wechsler, A. S. and Braunwald, E. (1967). *Circ. Res.* **21**, 217–227.
Godfraind, T., Miller, R. C. and Socrates Lima, J. (1982). *Br. J. Pharmacol.* **77**, 597–604.
Gold, M. S., Redmond, D. E. and Kleber, H. D. (1978). *The Lancet* **I**, 599–602.
Göthert, M. (1977). *Naunyn-Schmiedeb. Arch. Pharmacol.* **300**, 267–272.
Göthert, M. (1979). *Naunyn-Schmiedeb. Arch. Pharmacol.* **307**, 29–37.
Göthert, M., Pohl, I. M. and Wehking, E. (1979). *Naunyn-Schmiedeb. Arch. Pharmacol.* **307**, 21–27.
Göthert, M. and Huth, H. (1980). *Naunyn-Schmiedeb. Arch. Pharmacol.* **313**, 21–26.
Gould, L., Becker, W. H. and Macklin, E. E. (1980). *Angiology* **31**, 120–125.
Graham, R. M. and Pettinger, W. A. (1979). *J. Cardiovasc. Pharmacol.* **1**, 497–502.
Graham, R. M., Stephenson, W. H. and Pettinger, W. A. (1980). *Naunyn-Schmiedeb. Arch. Pharmacol.* **311**, 129–138.
Grant, J. A. and Scrutton, M. C. (1979). *Nature* **277**, 659–661.
Grant, J. A. and Scrutton, M. C. (1980). *Br. J. Pharmacol.* **71**, 121–134.
Green, G. J., Wilson, H. and Yates, M. S. (1979). *Eur. J. Pharmacol.* **56**, 331–336.
Greenberg, D. A., U'Prichard, D. C. and Snyder, S. H. (1976). *Life Sci.* **19**, 69–76.
Greengrass, P. and Bremner, R. (1979). *Eur. J. Pharmacol.* **55**, 323–326.
Hamilton, C. A., Reid, J. L. and Zamboulis, C. (1982). *Br. J. Pharmacol.* **75**, 417–424.
Hammer, R., Kobinger, W. and Pichler, L. (1980). *Eur. J. Pharmacol.* **62**, 277–285.
Häusler, G. (1982). *J. Cardiovasc. Pharmacol.* **4**, S72–S76.
Henning, M. (1983). *In* "Handbook of Hypertension" (W. H. Birkenhäger and J. L. Reid, eds). *In* "The Pharmacology of Antihypertensive Drugs" (P. A. van Zwieten, ed.), pp. 154–193. Elsevier, Amsterdam.
Hicks, P. E. (1981). *J. Auton. Pharmacol.* **1**, 391–397.
Hieble, J. P., Sarau, H. M., Foley, J. J., DeMarinis, R. M. and Pendleton, R. G. (1982). *Naunyn-Schmiedeb. Arch. Pharmacol.* **318**, 267–273.
Hoffman, B. B., De Lean, A., Wood, C. L., Schocken, D. D. and Lefkowitz, R. J. (1979). *Life Sci.* **24**, 1739–1746.

Hoobler, S. W. and Kashima, T. (1977). *Mayo Clin. Proc.* **52**, 395–398.
Hornung, R., Presell, P. and Glossmann, H. (1979). *Naunyn-Schmiedeb. Arch. Pharmacol.* **308**, 223–230.
Hsu, C. Y., Knapp, D. R. and Halusha, P. V. (1979). *J. Pharmacol. Exp. Ther.* **208**, 366–370.
Huchet, A. M., Chelby, J. and Schmitt, H. (1981). *Eur. J. Pharmacol.* **71**, 455–461.
Innemee, H. C., De Jonge, A., Van Meel, J. C. A., Timmermans, P. B. M. W. M. and Van Zwieten, P. A. (1981). *Naunyn-Schmiedeberg's Arch. Pharmacol.* **316**, 294–298.
Jakobs, K. H. (1978). *Nature* **274**, 819–820.
Jakobs, K. H. and Schultz, G. (1982). *J. Cardiovasc. Pharmacol.* **4**, S63–S67.
Jauernig, R. A., Moulds, R. F. W. and Shaw, J. (1978). *Arch. Int. Pharmacodyn.* **231**, 81–89.
Kobinger, W. (1978). *Rev. Physiol. Biochem. Pharmacol.* **81**, 39–100.
Kobinger, W. and Pichler, L. (1977). *Naunyn-Schmiedeberg's Arch. Pharmacol.* **300**, 39–46.
Kobinger, W. and Pichler, L. (1980a). *Eur. J. Pharmacol.* **65**, 393–402.
Kobinger, W. and Pichler, L. (1980b). *Naunyn-Schmiedeberg's Arch. Pharmacol.* **315**, 21–27.
Kobinger, W. and Pichler, L. (1981a). *Eur. J. Pharmacol.* **76**, 101–105.
Kobinger, W. and Pichler, L. (1981b). *Eur. J. Pharmacol.* **73**, 313–321.
Kobinger, W. and Pichler, L. (1982a). *Eur. J. Pharmacol.* **82**, 203–206.
Kapur, H. and Mottram, D. R. (1978). *Biochem. Pharmacol.* **27**, 1879–1880.
Lafontan, M. and Berlan, M. (1980). *Eur. J. Pharmacol.* **66**, 87–93.
Lafontan, M. and Berlan, M. (1981). *TIPS* **2**, 126–129.
Lands, A. M., Arnold, A., McAuliff, J. P., Luduena, F. P. and Brown, T. G. (1967). *Nature*, **214**, 597–598.
Langer, S. Z. (1973). *In* "Frontiers in Catecholamine Research" (E. Usdin, S. H. Snyder, eds), pp. 543–549. Pergamon Press, New York.
Langer, S. Z. (1974). *Biochem. Pharmacol.* **23**, 1793–1800.
Langer, S. Z. (1977). *Br. J. Pharmacol.* **60**, 481–497.
Langer, S. Z. (1981). *Pharmacol. Rev.* **32**, 337–360.
Langer, S. Z. and Shepperson, N. B. (1982). *Trends Pharmacol. Sci.* **3**, 440–444.
Langer, S. Z., Massingham, R. and Shepperson, N. B. (1980). *Clin. Sci.* **59**, 225s–228s.
Langer, S. Z., Massingham, R. and Shepperson, N. B. (1981a). *Br. J. Pharmacol.* **72**, 123P.
Langer, S. Z., Shepperson, N. B. and Massingham, R. (1981b). *Hypertension* **3**, (Suppl I), I-112—I-118.
Lasch, P. and Jacobs, K. H. (1979). *Naunyn-Schmiedeberg's Arch. Pharmacol.* **306**, 119–125.
Lokhandwala, M. F., Coats, J. T. and Buckley, J. P. (1977). *Eur. J. Pharmacol.* **42**, 257–265.
Lyon, T. F. and Randall, W. C. (1980). *Life Sci.* **26**, 1121–1129.
Majewski, H., Hedler, L. and Starke, K. (1982). *Naunyn-Schmiedeberg's Arch. Pharmacol.* **321**, 20–27.
McGrath, J. C. (1982). *Biochem. Pharmacol.* **31**, 467–484.
Menkes, D. B., Baraksan, J. M. and Aghajanian, G. K. (1981). *Naunyn-Schmiedeberg's Arch. Pharmacol.* **317**, 273–275.
Miach, P. J., Dausse, J. P., Cardot, A. and Meyer, P. (1980). *Naunyn-Schmiedeberg's Arch. Pharmacol.* **312**, 23–26.

Michel, A. D., Nahorski, S. R. and Whiting, R. L. (1981) *Br. J. Pharmacol.* **74**, 845P–846P.

Mouillé, P., Huchet, A. M., Chelly, J., Lucet, B., Doursout, M. F. and Schmitt, H. (1980). *J. Cardiovasc. Pharmacol.* **2**, 175–183.

Nakadate, T., Nakaki, T., Muraki, T. and Kato, R. (1980). *Eur. J. Pharmacol.* **65**, 421–424.

O'Brien, J. R. (1963). *Nature* **200**, 763–764.

Pettinger, W. A. (1977). *J. Pharmacol. Exp. Ther.* **210**, 622–626.

Perry, B. D. and U'Prichard, D. C. (1981). *Eur. J. Pharmacol.* **76**, 461–464.

Pichler, L. and Kobinger, W. (1978). *Eur. J. Pharmacol.* **52**, 287–295.

Pichler, L. and Kobinger, W. (1981a). *J. Cardiovasc. Pharmacol.* **3**, 269–277.

Pichler, L. and Kobinger, W. (1981b). *Naunyn Schmiedeberg's Arch. Pharmacol.* **317**, 180–182.

Pichler, L., Hörtnagl, H. and Kobinger, W. (1982). *Naunyn Schmiedeberg's Arch. Pharmacol.* **320**, 110–114.

Powis, D. A. (1981). *Biochem. Pharmacol.* **30**, 2389–2397.

Randriantsoa, A., Heitz, C. and Stoclet, J. C. (1981). *Eur. J. Pharmacol.* **75**, 57–60.

Rouot, B. M. and Snyder, S. H. (1979). *Life Sci.* **25**, 769–774.

Ruffolo, R. R., Yaden, E. L. and Waddell, J. E. (1980). *J. Pharmacol. Exp. Ther.* **213**, 557–561.

Ruffolo, R. R., Waddell, J. E. and Yaden, E. L. (1981). *J. Pharmacol. Exp. Ther.* **217**, 235–240.

Ruffolo, R. R., Waddell, J. E. and Yaden, E. L. (1982). *J. Pharmacol. Exp. Ther.* **221**, 309–314.

Russell, M. P. and Moran, N. C. (1980). *Circ. Res.* **46**, 344–352.

Schimmel, R. J. (1976). *Biochim. Biophys. Acta* **428**, 379–387.

Schmitt, H. (1971). *Actual. Pharmacol.* **24**, 93–131.

Schultz, G., Jakobs, K. H. and Hofman, F. (1980). *Arzneim.-Forsch.* **30**, 1981–1986.

Shattil, S. J., McDonough, M., Turnbull, J. and Insel, P. A. (1981). *Molec. Pharmacol.* **19**, 179–182.

Shepperson, N. B. and Langer, S. Z. (1981). *Naunyn-Schmiedeberg's Arch. Pharmacol.* **318**, 10–13.

Shepperson, N. B., Duval, N., Massingham, R. and Langer, S. Z. (1981), *J. Pharmacol., Exp. Ther.* **219**, 540–546.

Smith, P. H. and Porte, D. (1976). *Ann. Rev. Pharmacol. Toxicol.* **16**, 269–284.

Starke, K. (1972). *Naunyn-Schmiedeberg's Arch. Pharmacol.* **274**, 18–45.

Starke, K. (1977). *Rev. Physiol. Biochem. Pharmacol.* **77**, 1–124.

Starke, K. (1981a). *Rev. Physiol. Biochem. Pharmacol.* **88**, 199–236.

Starke, K. (1981b). *Ann. Rev. Pharmacol. Toxicol.* **21**, 7–30.

Starke, K. and Langer, S. Z. (1979). *In* "Presynaptic Receptors, Advances in the Biosciences" S. Z. Langer, K. Starke and M. L. Dubocovich, eds), Vol. 18, pp. 1–3. Pergamon Press, Oxford.

Starke, K., Endo, T. and Taube, H. D. (1975). *Naunyn-Schmiedeberg's Arch. Pharmacol.* **291**, 55–78.

Steppeler, A., Tanaka, T. and Starke, K. (1978). *Naunyn-Schmiedeberg's Arch. Pharmacol.* **304**, 223–230.

Stevens, M. J. and Moulds, R. F. W. (1981). *Arch. int. Pharmacodyn.* **254**, 43–57.

Stevens, M. J. and Moulds, R. F. W. (1982). *J. Cardiovasc. Pharmacol.* **4**, S129–S133.

Stjärne, L. (1978). *Neuroscience* **3**, 1147–1155.

Stjärne, L. (1979). *In* "Catecholamines; Basic and Clinical Frontiers" (E. Usdin, I. J. Kopin and J. Barchas, eds), pp. 240–243. Pergamon Press, New York.

Strömbom, U. (1975). *J. Neural. Transm.* **37**, 229–235.
Struyker Boudier, H. A. J. (1975). Catecholamine Receptors in Nervous Tissue. Ph.D. Thesis, University of Nijmegen, The Netherlands.
Thoolen, M. J. M. C., Timmermans, P. B. M. W. M. and van Zwieten, P. A. (1981a). *Life Sci.* **28**, 2103–2109.
Thoolen, M. J. M. C., Timmermans, P. B. M. W. M. and van Zwieten, P. A. (1981b). *J. Pharm. Pharmacol.* **33**, 232–235.
Thoolen, M. J. M. C., Timmermans, P. B. M. W. M. and van Zwieten, P. A. (1981c). *Gen. Pharmacol.* **12**, 303–308.
Thoolen, M. J. M. C., Timmermans, P. B. M. W. M. and van Zwieten, P. A. (1982). *Naunyn-Schmiedeberg's Arch. Pharmacol.* **319**, 82–86.
Thoolen, M. J. M. C., Mathy, M. J., Timmermans, P. B. M. W. M. and van Zwieten, P. A. (1983). *Br. J. Clin. Pharmacol.* **15**, 491S–505S.
Timmermans, P. B. M. W. M., Kwa, H. Y. and van Zwieten, P. A. (1979). *Naunyn-Schmiedeberg's Arch. Pharmacol.* **310**, 189–193.
Timmermans, P. B. M. W. M. and van Zwieten, P. A. (1980a). *Eur. J. Pharmacol.* **63**, 199–202.
Timmermans, P. B. M. W. M. and van Zwieten, P. A. (1980b). *Naunyn-Schmiedeberg's Arch. Pharmacol.* **313**, 17–20.
Timmermans, P. B. M. W. M., Hoefke, W., Stähle, H. and van Zwieten, P. A. (1980a). *Prog. Pharmacol.* **3**, 1–104.
Timmermans, P. B. M. W. M., van Meel, J. C. A. and van Zwieten, P. A. (1980b). *J. Auton. Pharmacol.* **1**, 53–60.
Timmermans, P. B. M. W. M. and van Zwieten, P. A. (1981). *J. Auton. Pharmacol.* **1**, 171–183.
Timmermans, P. B. M. W. M., Schoop, A. M. C., Kwa, H. Y. and van Zwieten, P. A. (1981a). *Eur. J. Pharmacol.* **70**, 7–15.
Timmermans, P. B. M. W. M., De Jonge, A., van Meel, J. C. A., Slothorst-Grisdijk, F. P., Lam, E. and van Zwieten, P. A. (1981b). *J. Med. Chem.* **24**, 502–507.
Timmermans, P. B. M. W. M., Karamat Ali, F., Kwa, H. Y., Schoop, A. M. C., Slothorst-Grisdijk, F. P. and van Zwieten, P. A. (1981c). *Molec. Pharmacol.* **20**, 295–301.
Timmermans, P. B. M. W. M. and van Zwieten, P. A. (1982). *J. Med. Chem.* **25**, 1389–1401.
Timmermans, P. B. M. W. M., De Jonge, A., van Zwieten, P. A., de Boer, J. J. J. and Speckamp, W. N. (1982). *J. Med. Chem.* **25**, 1122–1124.
Timmermans, P. B. M. W. M., De Jonge, A., van Meel, J. C. A., Mathy, M. J. and van Zwieten, P. A. (1983a). *J. Cardiovasc. Pharmacol.* **5**, 1–11.
Timmermans, P. B. M. W. M., Wilffert, B., Davidesko, D., Mathy, M. J., Dijkstra, D., Horn, A. S. and van Zwieten, P. A. (1983b). *J. Pharmacol. Exp. Ther.* **225**, 407–409.
U'Prichard, D. C., Greenberg, D. A. and Snyder, S. H. (1977). *Molec. Pharmacol.* **13**, 454–473.
Van Brummelen, P., Vermey, P., Timmermans, P. B. M. W. M. and Van Zwieten, P. A. (1982). *Br. J. Clin. Pharmacol.* **15**, 134P–135P.
Vanhoutte, P. M. (1982). *J. Cardiovasc. Pharmacol.* **4**, S91–S96.
Vanhoutte, P. M. and Rimele, T. J. (1982). *J. Cardiovasc. Pharmacol.* **4**, S280–S286.
Van Meel, J. C. A., De Jonge, A., Wilffert, B., Kalkman, H. O., Timmermans, P. B. M. W. M. and Van Zwieten, P. A. (1981a). *Eur. J. Pharmacol.* **69**, 205–208.

Van Meel, J. C. A., De Jonge, A., Wilffert, B., Kalkman, H. O., Timmermans, P. B. M. W. M. and Van Zwieten, P. A. (1981b). *Naunyn-Schmiedeberg's Arch. Pharmacol.* **316**, 288–293.

Van Meel, J. C. A., De Jonge, A., Timmermans, P. B. M. W. M. and Van Zwieten, P. A. (1981c). *J. Pharmacol. Exp. Ther.* **219**, 760–767.

Van Meel, J. C. A., Wilffert, B., De Zoeten, K., Timmermans, P. B. M. W. M. and Van Zwieten, P. A. (1982a). *Arch Int. Pharmacodyn.* **260**, 206–217.

Van Meel, J. C. A., De Zoeten, K., Timmermans, P. B. M. W. M. and Van Zwieten, P. A. (1982b). *J. Auton. Pharmacol.* **2**, 13–20.

Van Meel, J. C. A., Timmermans, P. B. M. W. M. and Van Zwieten, P. A. (1983a). *J. Cardiovasc. Pharmacol.* **5**, 580–585.

Van Meel, J. C. A., Towart, R., Kazda, S., Timmermans, P. B. M. W. M. and Van Zwieten, P. A. (1983b). *Naunyn-Schmiedeberg's Arch. Pharmacol.* **322**, 34–37.

Van Meel, J. C. A., Qian Jiaqing, Wilffert, B., De Jonge, A., Timmermans, P. B. M. W. M. and Van Zwieten, P. A. (1983c). *Eur. J. Pharmacol.* **92**, 27–34.

Van Zwieten, P. A. and Timmermans, P. B. M. W. M. (1979). *TIPS* **1**, 39–41.

Van Zwieten, P. A. and Timmermans, P. B. M. W. M. (1980). *Pharmacology* **21**, 327–332.

Van Zwieten, P. A., van Meel, J. C. A. and Timmermans, P. B. M. W. M. (1982a). *J. Cardiovasc. Pharmacol.* **4**, S273–S279.

Van Zwieten, P. A., Van Meel, J. C. A., De Jonge, A., Wilffert, B. and Timmermans, P. B. M. W. M. (1982b). *J. Cardiovasc. Pharmacol.* **4**, S19–S24.

Vizi, E. S. (1977). *J. Physiol.* **267**, 261–280.

Vizi, E. S. (1979). *Prog. Neurobiol.* **12**, 181–290.

Weber, M. A. (1980). *J. Cardiovasc. Pharmacol.* **2**, (Suppl. 1), S73–S89.

Weitzell, R., Tanaka, T. and Starke, K. (1979). *Naunyn-Schmiedeberg's Arch. Pharmacol.* **308**, 127–136.

Westfall, T. C. (1977). *Physiol. Rev.* **57**, 659–728.

Wilffert, B., Timmermans, P. B. M. W. M. and van Zwieten, P. A. (1982a). *J. Pharmacol. Exp. Ther.* **221**, 762–768.

Wilffert, B., Gouw, M. A. M., De Jonge, A., Timmermans, P. B. M. W. M. and van Zwieten, P. A. (1982b). *J. Pharmacol. Exp. Ther.* **223**, 219–223.

Wikberg, J. E. S. (1979). *Acta Physiol. Scand.* **468** (Suppl), 1–89.

Wood, C. L., Arnett, C. D., Clarke, W. R., Tsai, B. S. and Lefkowitz, R. J. (1979). *Biochem. Pharmacol.* **28**, 1277–1282.

Yamaguchi, I. and Kopin, I. J. (1980). *J. Pharmacol. Exp. Ther.* **214**, 275–281.

Zebrowska-Lupina, I., Przegalinski, E., Sloniec, M. and Kleinrock, Z. (1977). *Naunyn-Schmiedeberg's Arch. Pharmacol.* **297**, 227–231.

Novel Approaches to the Design of Safer Drugs: Soft Drugs and Site-Specific Chemical Delivery Systems

NICHOLAS BODOR

*Department of Medicinal Chemistry, College of Pharmacy, J. Hillis Miller
Health Center, University of Florida, Gainesville, Florida, USA*

1 Introduction

1.1 GENERAL CONSIDERATIONS

The rational design of new drugs is still considered by most practitioners to mean maximization of the desired drug activity within certain structural limits. That is, the main objective is to modify the structure of the lead compound in such a way as to enhance the specific pharmacological activity which is desired. Medicinal chemists are using for this purpose a variety of empirical and semi-empirical structure–activity relationships which more or

ADVANCES IN DRUG RESEARCH VOL. 13
0-12-013313-X

less help to predict the chemical structure of the compound which will have the maximal desired activity within a logical structural class of analogs. Most of these structure–activity relationships, particularly the ones based on simple empirical or semi-empirical substituent effects, are essentially hindsight and of limited use.

Sometimes the design process goes further. Drugs usually have multiple pharmacological effects, and, recognizing this, the drug designer tries to improve selectivity as well—in other words, to optimize and not only to maximize the activity. In this process, one is trying not only to design a better drug structure by altering its measurably active moiety but also to provide better affinity or binding properties to the target receptors. In this case, however, the main problem is that we know even less about the structure of the receptors than about the structure–activity relationship of the drugs. Despite all these attempts to introduce rational and logical drug design processes in drug discovery, the success ratio is alarmingly low. Still, very few compounds having maximal or even optimal activity will become clinically useful drugs, the main and most frequent reason being the *toxicity of the compounds*—toxicity which is often said to be "unexpected" or "unpredicted". Compounds which show very high activity in various *in vitro* tests or *in vivo* models may prove later to be highly toxic. Actually this happens so frequently that drug designers became accustomed to it. Everybody has his own story about a newly discovered highly active drug which had ultimately to be discarded because of its unexpected high toxicity. But since this happens so often, we have to recognize that there must be something basically missing in the general drug design process. In many cases, this deficiency is clearly related to a *lack of prediction of toxicities* beyond the known pharmacological selectivity. Thus, we have to conclude that *the main objective* of drug design should not be the activity of the drug but its *therapeutic index*.

The therapeutic index (TI) is the most important characteristic of a drug. It reflects its selectivity and margin of safety by expressing the ratio between activity and toxicity, and it is often defined as the ratio between the median toxic dose and the median effective dose (TD_{50}/ED_{50}) in which the effective dose refers to its characteristic and most desired therapeutic effect. This apparently simple definition is, however, much more complex than it would appear since the concept of toxicity is even more intricate than that of activity. Toxicity results from a combination of many processes and factors including not only all other pharmacological effects of the drug itself, but also the various effects of its metabolites, reactive intermediates, and various compounds resulting from direct or indirect interactions with cell components. In order to introduce into drug design logical steps based on toxicity considerations, we have to analyze in some detail the variety of processes a drug undergoes after its administration, as summarized in Scheme 1.

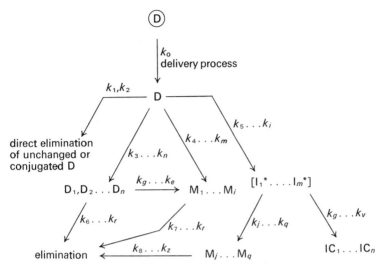

SCHEME 1

This rather simple scheme shows that the drug after its administration can undergo a variety of processes including (a) direct elimination in unchanged or conjugated form, and (b) transformation into structurally close analogs represented by $D_1 \ldots D_n$ (active metabolites having similar type and extent of activity as the drug itself but with altered pharmacokinetic properties), into metabolites $M_1 \ldots M_i$ (having activities different from that of the drug), and also the reactive intermediates represented by $I_1^* \ldots I_m^*$ which can further metabolize ($M_j \ldots M_g$) or form toxic species like $IC_1 \ldots IC_n$ by reacting with cellular components. The overall toxicity of the drug $T(D)$ can now be described as a combination of the toxicity due to the drug itself which is essentially its lack of selectivity or *intrinsic toxicity* (T_i) and the *toxicity due to the various metabolic products*. This obviously includes the different selectivities of the active metabolites $D_1 \ldots D_n$ as well as the different types of activities of the metabolites $M_1 \ldots M_i$ and the toxicity such as carcinogenicity and mutagenicity of the reactive intermediates $I_1^* \ldots I_m^*$. Thus, we can write the toxicity as

$$T(D) = T_i + T(D_1 \ldots D_n) + T(M_1 \ldots M_i) + T(I_1^* \ldots I_n^*).$$

The T_i is a molecular property, and it is in most cases optimized by the structure–activity studies used. Since this includes primarily the selectivity aspect of the compound, it can further be manipulated and affected by site-specific delivery manipulations, among which the simplest is the obvious alteration of the route of administration or formulation. Simple prodrug approaches could be included here which might alter toxicity and selectivity by changing the pharmacodynamic aspects of the drug delivery. Ideally, a prodrug (PD) is inactive, and it is transformed *in vivo* into the active drug without substantial direct elimination or unwanted metabolism (Scheme 2):

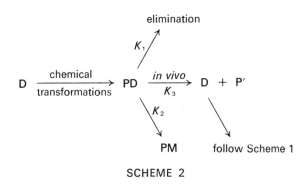

SCHEME 2

Essentially, the prodrugs are designed in such a way that their major or preferably single metabolic pathway is the one leading to the active drug ($K_3 \gg K_1 + K_2$). The simple prodrug approach, however, even in the best cases, can only optimize the delivery and elimination processes and indirectly affect some toxic effects which are due to specific rate dependent processes, e.g. saturation of enzymatic conjugation reactions. Prodrugs might effectively reduce some toxicities by protecting the drug from unwanted degradations, particularly those occurring in the gastrointestinal tract prior and during absorption or possibly during the first passage through the liver. Several recent reviews on prodrugs discuss these aspects (Sinkula and Yalkowsky, 1975; Bodor, 1981a, 1981b, 1982c). It is clear, however, that prodrug manipulations will not substantially influence the formation of active or highly reactive species. Simple prodrug manipulations cannot, in most cases, affect site specificity of the drugs. In contrast, the site-specific delivery via chemical delivery systems has great potential to improve the therapeutic index of drugs. This novel aspect of drug design will be discussed later.

   Metabolic studies indicate that many drugs, like other xenobiotics, are not always metabolized by transformation into more hydrophilic, less toxic substances, but may also be transformed in part to *highly reactive chemical species* which then can react with various macromolecules causing tissue damage or eliciting antigen production. In most cases, the damage will take place locally in specific tissues, e.g. the liver, where activation did take place, although some reactive intermediates may be transferred to other organs. Most studies indicate that formation of highly reactive intermediates results from a tendency of the body to eliminate invading chemicals by transforming them into compounds which are more hydrophilic or more easily conjugated. These processes are generally oxidative in nature. Transfer of the active oxygen by the cytochrome P-450 monooxygenase system (Gillette, 1963) may result, however, in highly reactive carcinogenic epoxides and radicals. Based on the toxicity of these reactive species, it must be recognized that formation of relatively small amounts can cause significant toxic effects. Although there are certain mechanisms in the body to capture these active intermediates, e.g. the glutathione route, some highly reactive species may escape these defences and cause short- or long-term damage. Since very low concentrations of the reactive intermediates can cause significant harmful effects, more potent drugs used in lower doses can do at least as much harm as the less effective ones. This is partly due to the fact that the rates of mono-oxygenase reactions are at least two orders of magnitude lower (Mannering, 1981) than the slowest enzymatic reactions transforming endobiotics. The reason for this is that in these reactions it is not the substrate (drug) con-centration, but the concentration of the ferricytochrome P-450 substrate complex which determines the rate. Another important point is that inhibition of, or competition for, the hepatic monooxygenase system can affect the extrahepatic metabolism and thus increase the incidence of extrahepatic tumors, e.g. tumors induced by N-nitrosamines activated locally (Bartsch *et al.*, 1977).

1.2 SOFT DRUGS/HARD DRUGS

Examples of the metabolic activation of drugs to reactive intermediates which then cause toxic side effects are constantly growing in number and cover a variety of pharmacological activities. Reactive intermediates are implicated in the toxicity of phenacetin, isoniazid and paracetamol (Gillette *et al.*, 1974), estrogens (Nelson *et al.*, 1976), β-blockers such as practolol (Orton and Lowery, 1977), as well as a wide variety of other drugs. However, the main objective of this introduction is not to discuss the various metabolic activation routes of drugs or to explain failures of active compounds to be-come pharmacologically useful drugs due to their metabolic toxication. Rather, all the data accumulated on the metabolic activation–toxication of drugs clearly indicate a *necessity of including metabolism considerations in the general drug design processes*.

As a consequence, we now have to combine two basic properties of the drug—its *activity and toxicity*—in order to accomplish the main objective, namely *designing the therapeutic index*. The desired activity is relatively simple to maximize as compared to a rational design in minimizing toxicity. There are, fortunately, a number of new strategies available to achieve this goal.

It must be recognized that predicting metabolism is not only possible, but it can be done on a more rational basis developing *structure–metabolism relationships*. An important generalization was made by Ariëns by identifying "vulnerable moieties" as the parts of the drug molecules which are responsible for bioinactivation or metabolism and elimination of drugs, but these were not used for the rational design of the metabolic disposition of the drugs. The importance of the drug metabolism–disposition considerations was recognized by Ariëns (Ariëns, 1977), but interestingly he suggested a "zero structure–metabolism relationship" as a means of designing drugs of reduced toxicity. In other words, it was suggested to design *non-metabolizable drugs* (Ariëns and Simonis, 1977, 1982; Ariëns, 1981) which we call "hard drugs" to contrast with the soft drug approach. The idea of hard drug design seems quite attractive at first sight, since not only would it solve the problem of toxicity due to reactive intermediates or active metabolites, but the drug pharmacokinetics would be much simplified since it would be controlled primarily by renal extraction. It is very unlikely, however, that this could be a general principle leading to a variety of ideal hard, non-metabolizable drugs. Indeed, it is known that the various xenobiotic-metabolizing enzymes, and particularly cytochrome P-450, can attack and alter even highly stable compounds; and even if this transformation affects only a very small percentage of the administered drug, it can cause toxicity. It appears to be a general rule that the more difficult the metabolism of a chemical, the more likely it is to form highly reactive intermediates. However, the main problem is that theoretically, *non-metabolizable properties can be achieved only when going to pharmacokinetic extremes*. By pharmacokinetic extremes we mean either highly lipophilic structures in which the metabolically sensitive parts are blocked by "steric packing" or by substitution of hydrogen atoms with halogens or, at the other end of the scale, highly water-soluble compounds which lack substrate properties to the metabolizing enzymes. These are called pharmacokinetic extremes because the elimination half-life, in the first case, is extremely prolonged while in the second case it is very much shortened. But in the case of highly lipid-soluble non-metabolizable forms, a good portion of these compounds will deposit and accumulate in adipose tissues and organelles, producing long-term biochemical and physical lesions. On the other hand, in the case of the highly water-soluble compounds, the biological half-life will often be very short, and only very potent compounds (for example, cromoglycic acid) would have a chance to be useful drugs.

The suggestion of Ariëns (Ariëns and Simonis, 1977) to use additional alkyl chains incorporated in the active structure as safe oxidizable handles has more potential. It would direct metabolism and elimination towards a more predictable route by stepwise oxidation of the alkyl chain and elimination with or without prior conjugation. The deliberate *use of the oxygenase systems* for a predictable metabolism and elimination of the drugs, however, *is not recommended* due to some properties of these systems, namely slow rates of reaction, high sensitivity to competition, inhibition, and saturation.

The other major approach to design safe and better drugs, an approach which is much more general and applicable to a variety of drug classes, is to *control and direct metabolism* by drug design and not by avoiding it. This is the concept of "soft drugs" (Bodor, 1981a, 1982a, 1982b) which are defined as biologically active, therapeutically useful chemical compounds (drugs) characterized by a predictable and controllable *in vivo* destruction (metabolism) to non-toxic moieties, after they achieve their therapeutic role.

From the earlier discussions it is clear that one of the main concepts in soft drug design is to *avoid oxidative metabolism as much as possible*. The cytochrome P-450 monooxygenases have a vital role in numerous basic biochemical processes such as steroid synthesis. These enzymes are saturable, and they are subject to competitive inhibition and deactivation as well as to induction and activation. The inherent competition among various drugs administered simultaneously or with endogenous substrates can and always do lead to a rather complex and hardly controllable situation. This problem is most frequently identified by the basically misleading term of "drug interactions". Drug interactions of this kind are essentially competition among the various substrates for the oxidative enzymes. In order to avoid the oxidative metabolism, the soft drug concept advocates the use of hydrolytic enzymes (for example, the various esterases) to achieve *predictable, controllable and directed drug metabolism*. This, however, requires some essential changes in our thinking related to drug structures. It is very important to note that non-specific esterases have no clearcut role in basic biochemical processes, except perhaps such hydrolytic enzymes as lipases. Apparently, the main role of these hydrolytic enzymes should be precisely to get rid of a variety of invading foreign substrates. So why do we not use these enzymes in our rational design of safer, soft drugs? However, it is remarkable to note how little is known about these rather common enzyme systems. In many cases during the design processes using the soft drug approach, it was found that relatively small structural changes can cause rather dramatic differences in the substrate character of various esters and amides.

Therefore, the main objective of the medicinal chemist involved in soft drug design should not be to explain and quantify the various possible metabolic processes depicted in Scheme 1, but rather to simplify them. As shown in Scheme 3, *the soft drug* (SD) which is now replacing D simply eliminates the majority of the unwanted processes and *deliberately simplifies the disposition of the drug*. Ideally, the soft drug is inactivated in one metabolic step. It is possible for the inactive M_1 metabolite to be further metabolized or conjugated again to other inactive products, all of which are eliminated.

Thus, the formation of active metabolites and reactive intermediates is avoided altogether.

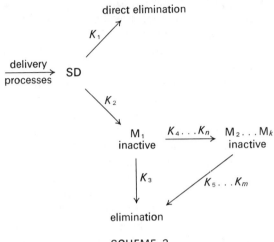

SCHEME 3

At this point, it appears necessary to clarify one recent confusion (Ariëns and Simonis, 1982) between the terms of *prodrug* and *soft drug*. Even such experts as Albert talk about "soft prodrugs" (Albert, 1982) when clearly referring to a soft drug. This confusion is rather unexplainable since, theoretically, the prodrugs and soft drugs are exactly opposite to each other: *A prodrug is inactive and is activated predictably* in vivo *to the active drug while the soft drug is the active species, then to be predictably inactivated* in vivo. A soft drug, as actually any other drug, can be subject to prodrug design or even to the more complex design of chemical delivery systems. Thus, according to the current definitions, there could be (as it will be shown later) a "pro-soft drug" but *not* a "soft-prodrug."

The soft drug design *combines structure–activity* relationships with *structure–metabolism* relationships to ultimately design the therapeutic index. The main advantages that can theoretically be achieved by the soft drug approach can be summarized as follows: improvement of the therapeutic index by *eliminating formation of reactive toxic intermediates*; avoidance of the formation of *active species* (no active metabolites or secondary active species); elimination of many so-called "*drug interactions*" by not competing for saturable highly used enzyme systems; and *simplification of numerous pharmacokinetic problems* caused by multicomponent systems.

It is important to note that since the main objective is an optimal thera-peutic index, the new soft drug of choice does not necessarily have to be the most potent agent in a given series. The "less drug, less toxicity" theorem of Ariëns (Ariëns, 1981) is certainly not the one followed by the soft drug design. This assumption means that as compared to a less active drug, a more potent one necessitating lower doses would be less toxic in proportion. The statement is unsubstantiated for any kind of drugs, and, when the therapeutic index is the objective, a higher dose of a less potent but much less toxic soft compound will be the choice.

There are a number of potential ways by which the rational soft drug design can be approached. In the years to come, it is possible that more general or specific novel strategies will be discovered, but, based on our current knowledge, *soft drugs can be classified* in five different groups: *soft analogs, activated soft compounds, natural soft drugs, soft drugs based on the active metabolite approach*, and *those based on the inactive metabolite approach*. Examples for these classes will be given in section 2. Before that, however, a different but equally successful and promising approach for designing safer drugs will be introduced: chemical delivery systems for site-specific drug delivery.

1.3 CHEMICAL DELIVERY SYSTEMS

In order to define the "chemical delivery system" (CDS), a comparison with the prodrugs has to be made again. As mentioned before, it is evident that simple prodrug approaches cannot solve the variety of transport–delivery problems (Bodor, 1981b), the main value in the prodrugs being to overcome problems of general distribution, pharmacokinetics, premature metabolism, absorption, etc. As compared with prodrugs, chemical delivery systems actually represent a more advanced step forward in which the drug is transformed by several synthetic steps into an inactive derivative which will undergo several predictable enzymatic transformations ultimately resulting in the delivery of the drug at the site of action. The emphasis is on the *several, successive steps* which will result in the *optimization* not only of the *drug delivery* at a certain site of action or organ, but also of the *therapeutic index* by effectively separating the site of action from the rest of the body. This can be achieved by a physical or affinity-based separation, or by using chemical delivery systems in which the intermediate delivery forms are inactive. One single delivery form such as a prodrug cannot effectively achieve site specificity unless a given enzyme is concentrated in certain areas or organs, thus causing specific activation. The chemical delivery system can be illustrated as shown in Scheme 4 where $CS_1 \ldots CS_n$ represent given chemical carriers or transient derivatizing groups which are successively hooked to the drug D. The resulting chemical delivery system will then via a succession of enzymatic reactions eventually release the drug at a given desired site (S)

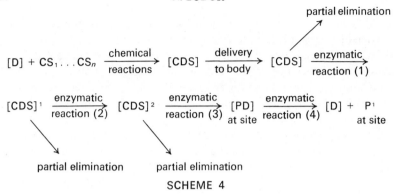

SCHEME 4

while the intermediate transient derivatives (of which the last one could be considered a prodrug) are *all inactive* and will effectively result in the ultimate *separation of activity and toxicity*. This concept was successfully applied to local delivery of steroids or other drugs in specific areas in the eye and most recently, to the brain and to the testes. Specific examples which will be given in section 2.5 should contribute to a better understanding of this general approach.

2 Soft drug approaches

2.1 SOFT ANALOGS

Compounds in this class are close *structural analogs of known active drugs* or bioactive compounds which, however, have a *specific metabolically* (preferably hydrolytic) *sensitive spot* built into their structure which provides their one-step, controllable detoxication. These sensitive structural parts are not oxidizable alkyl chains or functional groups subject to conjugation. The designed detoxication will take place as soon as possible after the desired activity is achieved, not allowing other types of metabolic routes to take place. The basic principles of soft analog design are:

1. the new soft compounds are *close structural analogs*, isosteric and/or isoelectronic with the lead compounds;
2. a metabolically, *preferentially hydrolytic sensitive part* is built in the molecule;
3. the metabolically weak spot is located in such a part of the molecule that *little or no effect on the transport, affinity and activity* of the drug will take place—that is, the overall physical, physicochemical, steric and complementarity properties of the soft analog are very close to those of the lead compound;
4. the built-in metabolism is the *major or preferentially the only metabolic* route for deactivation of the drug;

5. the *rate* of the predictable metabolism can be *controlled by structural modifications*;

6. the *products* resulting from the metabolism are *nontoxic* and have no significant biological activity;

7. the predicted metabolism does *not* require enzymatic processes leading to *highly reactive intermediates.*

The type of *designed metabolism* should produce a *profound structural change* in the molecule leading to complete loss of binding and affinity properties and to a breakdown of the active sites of the molecule. This is how one can avoid formation of the usual active metabolites resulting in multi-component active systems. The requirement for the facile deactivation is very important, meaning that the rate of the designed metabolism should be relatively high, not allowing, on the one hand, other metabolic routes, and, on the other hand, making it much easier to control penetration, elimination, and consequently concentration, pharmacokinetic and pharmacodynamic factors.

The search towards soft analogs started after the discovery of the "soft quaternary salts" (Bodor, 1977a) generally described as structure **2** and characterized by a chemical or enzymatic hydrolytic cleavage leading to the simultaneous destruction of both the ester and the quaternary ammonium head. Structure **2** can be designed to contain the three basic structural components: an acid, an aldehyde and a tertiary amine, and synthesized accordingly. Hydrolysis of **2** effectively cuts the compounds into the original components, as shown in Scheme 5:

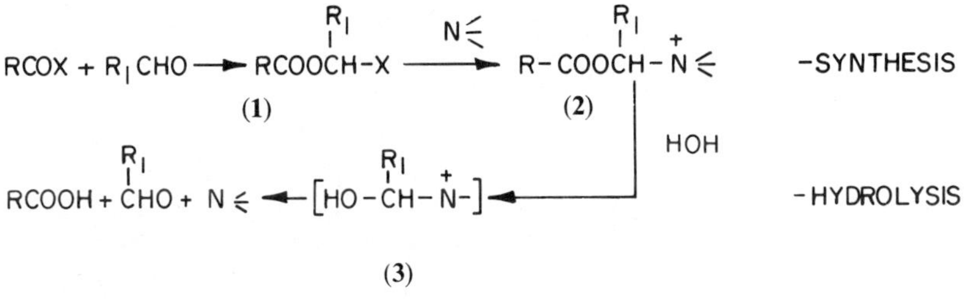

$$RCOX + R_1CHO \longrightarrow R\text{-}COOCH\text{-}X \longrightarrow R\text{-}COOCH\text{-}N\overset{R_1}{\underset{|}{\overset{+}{<}}} \quad \text{–SYNTHESIS}$$

$$(1) \qquad\qquad (2)$$

$$\Big\downarrow HOH$$

$$RCOOH + \overset{R_1}{\underset{|}{CHO}} + N\overset{<}{} \longleftarrow \Big[HO\text{-}\overset{R_1}{\underset{|}{CH}}\text{-}\overset{+}{N}\text{-}\Big] \longleftarrow \quad \text{–HYDROLYSIS}$$

$$(3)$$

SCHEME 5

Kinetic evidence as well as direct measurements indicate that the intermediate (**3**) cleaves instantaneously to the amine and aldehyde. Structure **2** was first used for the improved delivery of tertiary amine-type drugs such as pilocarpine (Bodor, 1977b) and erythromycin (Bodor and Freiberg, 1981). The term 'soft' in connection with these quaternary salts was given to

TABLE 1

Structure of source "soft antimicrobial" agents[a]

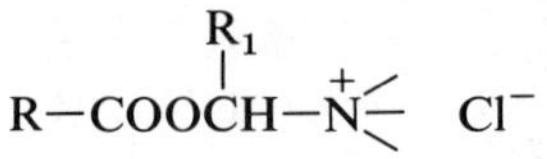

$$R-COOCH-\overset{+}{\underset{|}{N}}\!\!\stackrel{<}{}\quad Cl^-$$
with R_1 on the CH position

Compound	R	R_1	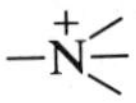 $-\overset{+}{N}\!\!\stackrel{<}{}$
5a	$CH_3(CH_2)_6$	H	1-Pyridinium
5b	$CH_3(CH_2)_{10}$	H	1-Pyridinium
5c	$CH_3(CH_2)_{12}$	H	1-Pyridinium
5d	$CH_3(CH_2)_{14}$	H	1-Pyridinium
5e	$CH_3(CH_2)_{10}$	H	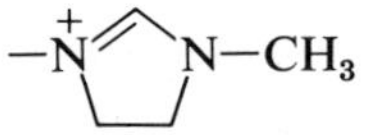 $-\overset{+}{N}\!\!=\!\!\diagdown\,N-CH_3$ (imidazolinium)
5f	$CH_3(CH_2)_{12}$	H	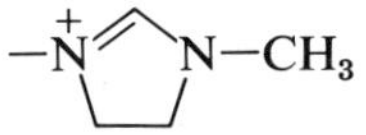 $-\overset{+}{N}\!\!=\!\!\diagdown\,N-CH_3$ (imidazolinium)
5g	$CH_3(CH_2)_{14}$	H	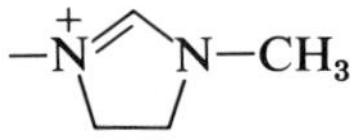 $-\overset{+}{N}\!\!=\!\!\diagdown\,N-CH_3$ (imidazolinium)
5h	$CH_3(CH_2)_{10}$	CH_3	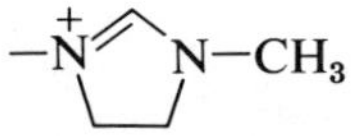 $-\overset{+}{N}\!\!=\!\!\diagdown\,N-CH_3$ (imidazolinium)
5i	$CH_3(CH_2)_{14}$	CH_3	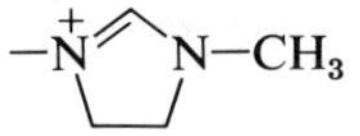 $-\overset{+}{N}\!\!=\!\!\diagdown\,N-CH_3$ (imidazolinium)
5j	$CH_3(CH_2)_{10}$	H	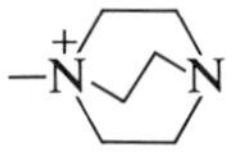 $-\overset{+}{N}\diagdown\!\!\diagup N$ (diazabicyclo)
5k	$CH_3(CH_2)_{10}$	H	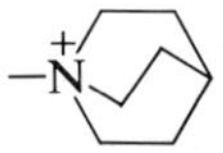 $-\overset{+}{N}$ (bicyclic azonium)
5l	$CH_3(CH_2)_{10}$	H	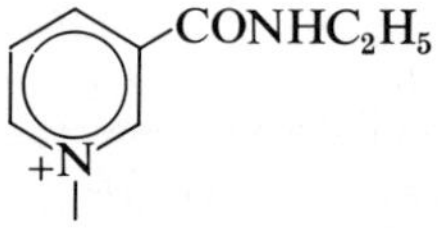 3-($CONHC_2H_5$)-1-pyridinium

[a]Bodor *et al.* (1980a).

reflect their *easy biodegradable properties* as compared to conventional "hard" quaternary salts, which generally require multiple oxidative steps to be metabolized. A direct usefulness of structure **2** in designing active soft drugs was also proposed (Bodor, 1977a).

The simplest example for a useful soft analog is provided by the isosteric analog (**5c**) of cetylpyridinium chloride (**4**) (Bodor *et al.*, 1980a) which is a known "hard" quaternary antimicrobial agent.

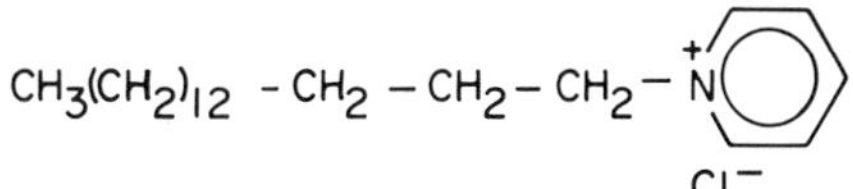

$$CH_3(CH_2)_{12} - CH_2 - CH_2 - CH_2 - \overset{+}{N} \bigcirc$$
$$Cl^-$$

(4)

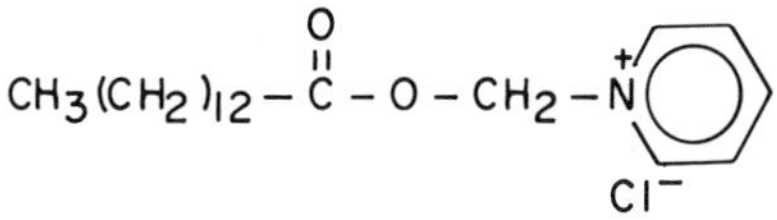

$$CH_3(CH_2)_{12} - \overset{\overset{O}{\|}}{C} - O - CH_2 - \overset{+}{N} \bigcirc$$
$$Cl^-$$

(5c)

Evidently, the side chains, both in **4** and **5c**, are essentially of 16 atom length providing analogous physical properties such as critical micelle concentration. It was found that the soft derivative **5c** as well as a number of its homologs and analogs (obtained by replacing pyridine with other tertiary amines) possess a good antimicrobial activity comparable to that of their hard analogs. The structures of some of these synthesized and studied soft antimicrobial agents are listed in Table 1.

As predicted, these structures undergo facile hydrolytic cleavage and deactivation, as exemplified by the hydrolysis kinetics of the analog **5b** given in Table 2.

Note that the observed rates for the disappearance of the quaternary salt (**5b**) and appearance of pyridine are the same supporting the earlier statement that the intermediate (**3**) is instantaneously cleaving to the amine and aldehyde. Compounds **5** hydrolyse much faster enzymatically than non-enzymatically, and it was found that they are good substrates for cholinesterase. The half-life of most of these compounds in human plasma is around 8–10 minutes. Limited studies of the antimicrobial activity of these compounds are listed in Tables 3 and 4.

Table 3 gives the minimal inhibitory concentrations (MIC) of compounds **5** against five selected bacteria as compared to the structural analogs **4** and **6**. These activities can be considered as an equilibrium thermodynamic activity. The kinetic effect, that is, the time required for bacteriostatic action, was determined by the contact germicidal efficiency (CGE) as given in Table 4.

TABLE 2

Hydrolysis kinetics for $CH_3(CH_2)_{10}COOCH_2Py^+Cl^-$ (**5b**)

Conditions[a]	K_{obsd} (min^{-1})	$t_{\frac{1}{2}}$ (min)
pH 9·3, $\mu = 0·5$, $25 \pm 0·1°C$		
$-(d[\mathbf{5b}]/dt)$	$4·3 \times 10^{-2}$	16
$+(d[Py]/dt)$	$4·3 \times 10^{-2}$	16
pH 7·0, $25 \pm 0·1°C$		
$\mu = 0·0$	$1·5 \times 10^{-3}$	450
$\mu = 0·05$	$1·5 \times 10^{-3}$	450
$\mu = 0·10$	$1·5 \times 10^{-3}$	450
pH 7·0, $\mu = 0·1$		
$40 \pm 0·1°C$	$4·2 \times 10^{-3}$	166
$45 \pm 0·1°C$	$5·6 \times 10^{-3}$	124
$50 \pm 0·1°C$	$1·1 \times 10^{-2}$	64
pH 4·6, $\mu = 0·5$		
$50 \pm 0·1°C$	$5·2 \times 10^{-4}$	1325

[a]High-pressure LC analysis was performed on a Partisil SAX column (Whatman, Inc.). Mobile phase: 0.01 M $NH_4H_2PO_4$, 10% methanol.

TABLE 3

Minimal inhibitory concentrations[a] of selected soft quaternary salts[b]

Compound	S. aureus	B. subtilis	S. typhimurium	P. aeruginosa	S pyogenes
4	<2·0	<2·0	8·0	16·0	<2·0
5a	529·1	529·1	1058·2	1058·2	529·1
5b	8·9	143·1	35·8	511·5	71·5
5c	8·1	8·3	133·0	>1063·9	4·2
5d	16·7	1071·1	1071·1	1071·1	267·5
5e	4·1	16·3	65·3	261·2	<2·0
5f	<2·2	4·4	69·7	>1115·1	<2·2
5g	1·3	>42·4[c]	>42·4[c]	>42·4[c]	>42·4[c]
5i	130·4	32·6	521·7	1043·3	32·6
5j	65·5	32·8	524·2	1048·4	32·8
5k	16·4	32·8	262·1	1048·5	4·1
6[d]	<2·0	2·0	64·3	128·5	<2·0

[a]Minimal inhibitory concentration determined in 0.1 M NaH_2PO_4 adjusted to pH 6.0 expressed in ppm. The decimal points indicate the concentrations of the actual solutions and are not to be interpreted as the accuracy of the MIC.

[b]For compound structures (see Table 1).

[c]Approximately the saturated solubility.

[d]**6** = $CH_3(CH_2)_{14}CH_2N^+(CH_3)_3Br^-$.

TABLE 4

Contact germicidal efficiency (CGE) of selected soft quaternary salts[a]

Compound	Concentration (ppm)[b]	Sterilization time (min)[c]		
		S. aureus	*P. aeruginosa*	*S. pyogenes*
4	1038·7	0·5	0·5	0·5
	936·0	0·5	0·5	0·5
5a	1035·9	> 30	> 30	> 30
5b	1010·9	0·5	0·5	0·5
	896·0	0·5	0·5	0·5
	896·0	0·5	0·5	0·5
5c	1042·1	1	1	0·5
5e	902	0·5	0·5	0·5
	1068	0·5	0·5	0·5
5f	1012·2	0·5	0·5	0·5
5i	1116·0	0·5	3	0·5
5j	1026	0·5	3	0·5
5k	1027	0·5	0·5	0·5
6[d]	1031	0·5	0·5	0·5

[a]In 0.1 M NaH_2PO_4 adjusted to pH 7.0.
[b]The decimal points indicate the concentrations of the actual solutions and are not to be interpreted as the accuracy of the measurements. Amounts were weighed to obtain approximately 1000-ppm solutions; the deviations are due to difference in weighing.
[c]Time intervals screened: 0.5, 1, 2, 3, 4, 5, 6, 7, 8, 9, 10, 15, and 30 min.
[d]**6** = $CH_3(CH_2)_{15}N^+(CH_3)_3Br^-$.

The shortest time interval for which growth of the microorganism is not observed is the sterilization time. It can be seen that a relatively low concentration of about 0.1 % of all compounds except the short side chain (**5a**) are quite effective. The failure of **5a** to be active is expected as it is not surface-active. As shown in Table 5, significant bactericidal activity of a selected compound (**5e**) can be seen at concentrations near to its MIC levels.

The main test was to verify the assumption as to the soft nature of the compounds studied, implying low toxicity due to their facile systemic metabolism. Table 6 compares the relative toxicities of **5e** and **4** indicating that the soft analog is up to 50 times less toxic than its hard counterpart which more than compensates for the somewhat lower activity.

The activity of **5e** is about 10 times less than that of the widely used **4**, but it is still highly effective at the relatively low 0.1 % concentration which actually is less than the concentration of **4** generally used. In conclusion, it is clear that active isosteric soft analogs of the hard antimicrobial quaternary salts can be developed.

TABLE 5

Contact germicidal efficiency as a function of concentration[a]

Compound	Concentration (ppm)	Sterilization time (min)[b]		
		S. aureus	P. aeruginosa	S. pyogenes
5e	1068	0·5	0·5	0·5
	507	1	0·5	0·5
	258	2	0·5	0·5
	125	5	0·5	3
	63	$10 < t \leqslant 15$	1	6
	32	> 30	> 30	> 30

[a]Contact germicidal efficiency determined in 0.1 M NaH_2PO_4, pH 7.0.
[b]Time intervals screened: 0.5, 1, 2, 3, 4, 5, 6, 7, 8, 9, 10, 15, and 30 min.

TABLE 6

Relative toxicity of $CH_3(CH_2)_{10}COOCH_2Im^+Cl^-$ (5e)
versus $CH_3(CH_2)_{15}Py^+Cl^-$ (4)

Mode of administration	LD_{50} (mg kg^{-1}) (white Swiss male mice)	
	5e	4[a]
iv	75–100	
ip	155 (140–160)[b]	10
po	4110 (2800–6000)[b]	108

[a]Toxic Substances List, ACS Edition, American Chemical Society, Washington, D.C., 1974.
[b]Confidence interval.

Another example for the application of the design of soft analogs based on soft quaternary salts was provided by the development of *soft anticholinergic agents* (Bodor *et al.*, 1980b). These soft analogs were designed to have *high local but practically no systemic activity*. It is well known that antimuscarinic compounds have several clinical useful effects among which the local antisecretory activity was long thought (Killmer-McMillan *et al.*, 1965) to be beneficial for inhibiting eccrine sweating. It was confirmed that a wide range of anticholinergic agents are effective as local antiperspirants, but it was concluded that none of them is really safe to use because of the well-known systemic effects of these drugs such as dry mouth and mydriasis. The known CNS effects could be prevented by the use of quaternary ammonium derivatives, but the other peripheral side effects still persisted. Interestingly, it was found that quaternary ammonium antimuscarinics such as oxyphenonium (7), scopolamine methylbromide (8) and others have very good local antisecretory activity, implying good topical absorptivity despite their positively charged structure. Actually, some of these quaternary ammonium salts such as structure 9 are more potent topically than the corresponding tertiary amine.

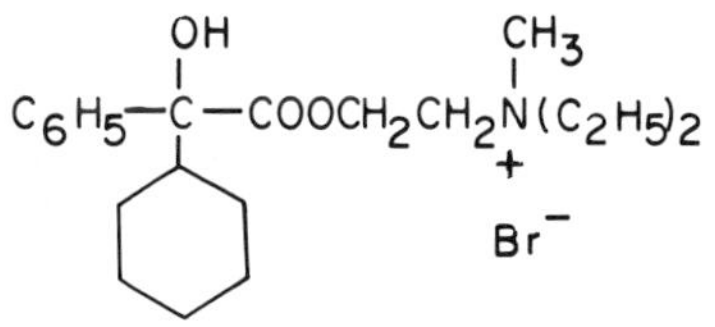

(7) 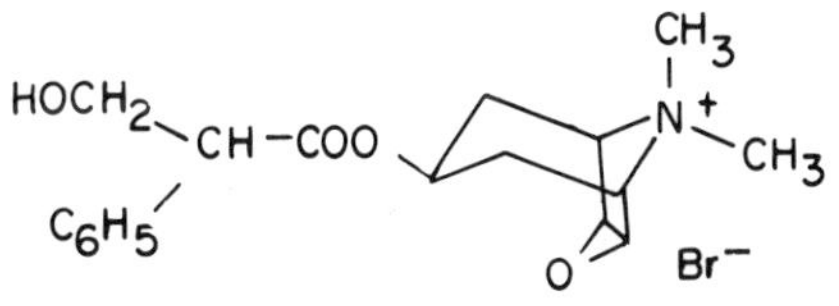   (8)

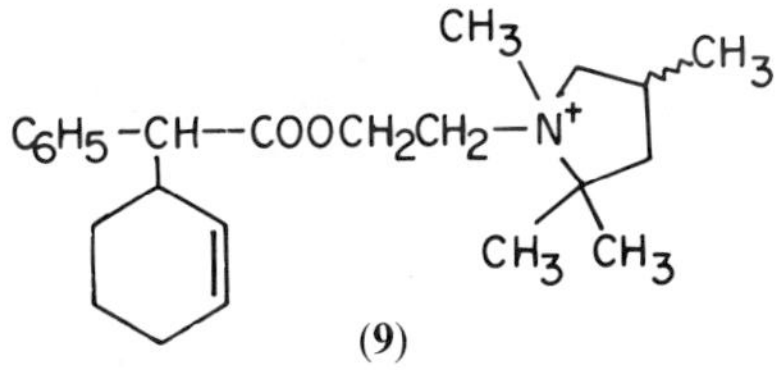

(9)

Based on the general structure of a soft quaternary salt (2), it is clear that anticholinergic agents based on amino alcohol esters could be good candidates for the soft analog type of design. The main difference would be, however, that while in the usual amino alcohol esters (formulae 10 and 11) the oxygen bridge and the quaternary nitrogen are separated by at least two carbon atoms, in a corresponding soft analog (12) there will be just one carbon atom separating these two heteroatoms.

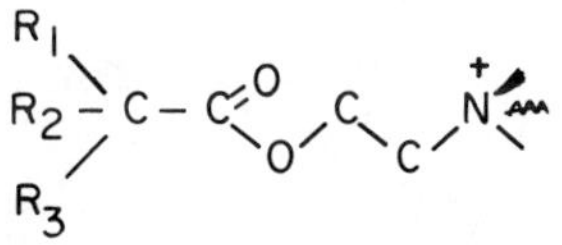

(10) 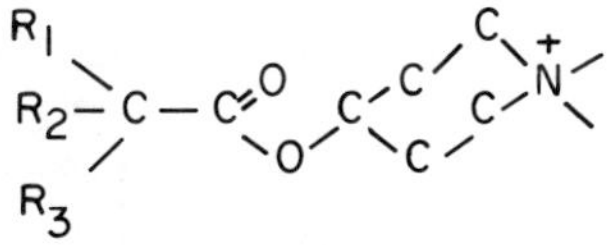   (11)

TABLE 7

Acetylcholine and histamine antagonist potency of some "soft analogs"

Compound	R_1	Structure R_2	R_3	$-\overset{+}{\underset{\diagdown}{N}}\diagup$	Anti-cholinergic[a] pA_2	Anti-histaminic[b] pA_2	Cholinergic[c] potency
12a	C_6H_5	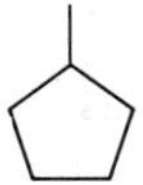 (cyclopentyl)	H	$-\overset{+}{N}(CH_2CH_3)_3$	8·1	No	—
12b	C_6H_5	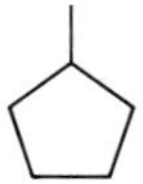 (cyclopentyl)	H	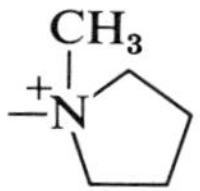 (pyrrolidinium, CH_3)	8·4	No	—
12c	C_6H_5	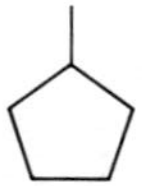 (cyclopentyl)	H	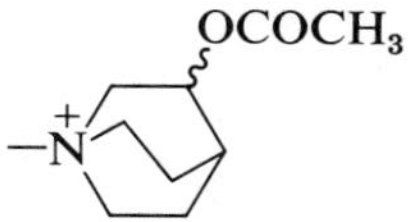 (quinuclidine, $OCOCH_3$)	8·6	5·7	—
12d	C_6H_5	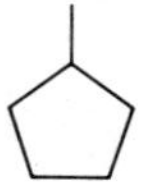 (cyclopentyl)	H	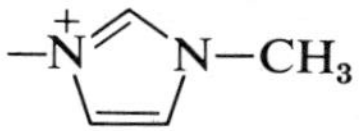 (imidazolium, $N-CH_3$)	7·8	6·3	—
12e	C_6H_5	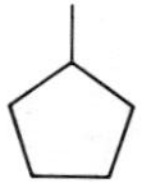 (cyclopentyl)	H	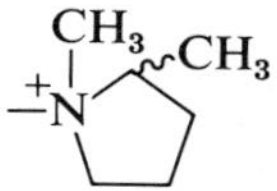 (pyrrolidinium, CH_3, CH_3)	9·3	7·9	—
12f	C_6H_5	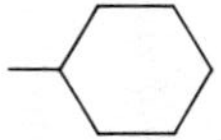 (cyclohexyl)	H	$-\overset{+}{N}(CH_2CH_3)_3$	8·6	5·7	—

272

	R_1	R_2	R_3			
12g	C_6H_5	$-CH_2CH_3$	H	$-\overset{+}{N}(CH_2CH_3)_3$	6·6	6·5	—
12h	C_6H_5	CH_2CH_3	H	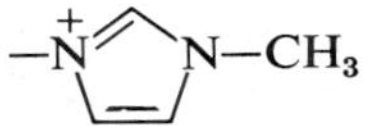 ![imidazolium N–CH₃]	5·9	5·9	—
12i	C_6H_5	C_6H_5	CH_3	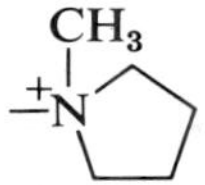 ![pyrrolidinium CH₃]	8·4	—	—
12j	CH_3CH_2	CH_3	H	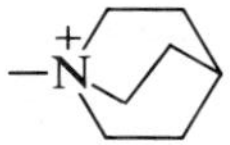 ![bicyclic quaternary N⁺]	—	—	1 : 5 B1 : hexamethonium
12k	CH_3CH_2	CH_3	H	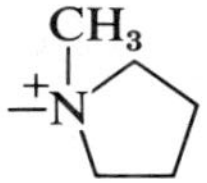 ![pyrrolidinium CH₃]	—	5·6	—
12l	CH_3CH_2	CH_3	H	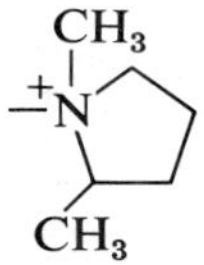 ![pyrrolidinium CH₃ CH₃]	4·9	—	—
12m	H	H	H	$-\overset{+}{N}(CH_2CH_3)_3$	—	—	1 : 10^4 B1 : atropine not hexamethonium

(continued)

273

TABLE 7 (continued)

Compound	R$_1$	Structure R$_2$	R$_3$	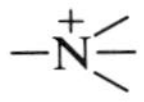	Anti-cholinergic[a] pA$_2$	Anti-histaminic[b] pA$_2$	Cholinergic[c] potency
12n	—	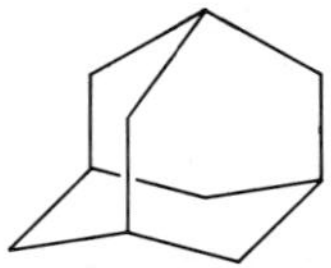 (adamantyl)	—	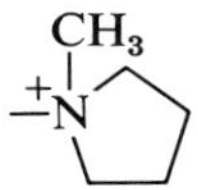 $-\overset{+}{N}$ CH$_3$ (pyrrolidine)	6·9	—	—
12o	—	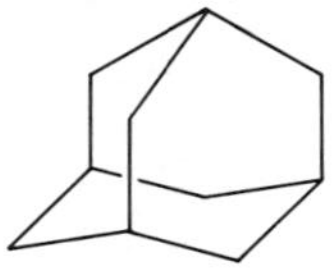 (adamantyl)	—	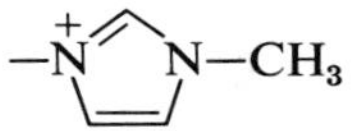 $-\overset{+}{N}$ N$-$CH$_3$ (imidazole)	5·7	5·3	—
12p	C$_6$H$_5$	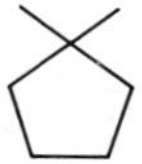 (cyclopentyl)	—	$-\overset{+}{N}(CH_2CH_3)_3$	7·1	—	—

274

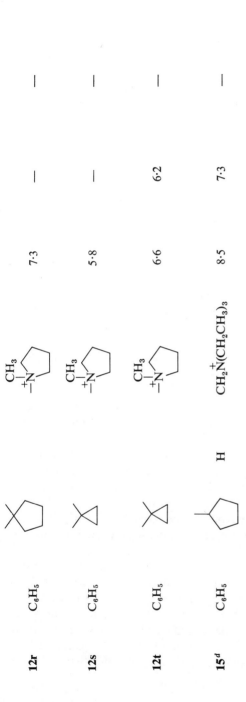

12r	C_6H_5		$\overset{+}{N}$–CH_3 (pyrrolidine)	7·3	—
12s	C_6H_5		$\overset{+}{N}$–CH_3 (pyrrolidine)	5·8	—
12t	C_6H_5		$\overset{+}{N}$–CH_3 (pyrrolidine)	6·6	6·2
15[d]	C_6H_5	H	$CH_2\overset{+}{N}(CH_2CH_3)_3$	8·5	7·3

[a]Anticholinergic activity was assessed using the guinea-pig ileum test: strips of whole ileum were used in McEwen's solution at 37°C. 1 g tension was applied and cumulative concentration response curves were recorded to acetylcholine, then in the presence of antagonists at different concentrations. pA_2 values were then calculated from the dose-ratio obtained. pA_2 for atropine: 8.5.

[b]As a, using histamine instead of acetylcholine.

[c]Cholinergic potency compared to that of acetylcholine. It was checked whether activity could be blocked by hexamethonium or by atropine.

[d]The "hard quaternary" choline analog of **12a**.

275

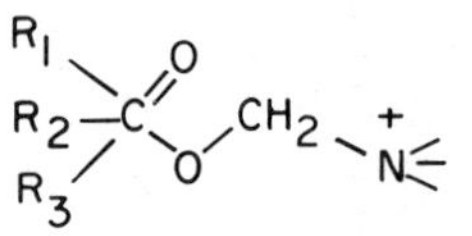

$$R_1, R_2, R_3 - C \overset{O}{\underset{O}{\diagdown}} CH_2 - \overset{+}{N} \diagdown$$

(12)

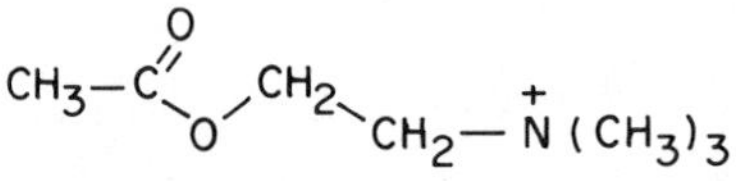

$$CH_3 - C \overset{O}{\underset{O}{\diagdown}} CH_2 - CH_2 - \overset{+}{N} (CH_3)_3$$

(13)

$$CH_3 - C \overset{O}{\underset{O}{\diagdown}} CH_2 - \overset{+}{N}(CH_3)_3$$

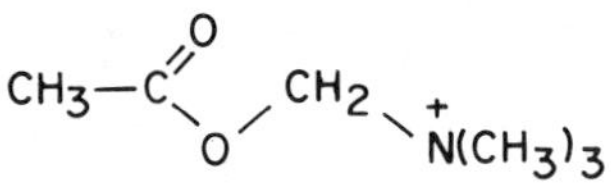

(14)

The corresponding structure 12 would have the main advantage of being deactivated by hydrolytic cleavage, actually falling apart in the three components destroying simultaneously not only the ester but the quaternary head as well (see Scheme 5). The main question was, however, if this kind of structure will have antimuscarinic activity. It is generally believed that the muscarinic receptors require a distance corresponding to at least two carbon atoms separating the quaternary head and the ester oxygen in order to have significant binding and activity. Thus, it was found (Geiger and Alpers, 1964) that acetylcholine (13) is 5000 times more active than acetylnorcholine (14), and it is clear that 14 is basically the typical soft analog of acetylcholine. The second aspect of the soft analog design, that is the fast deactivation upon absorption, does prevent any systemic effects.

The first question was quickly answered by a detailed study of the structure–activity relationships of a series of soft analogs as shown in Table 7, clearly indicating that many of the one-carbon bridge containing compounds are very potent in antagonizing acetylcholine (some of them even more potent than atropine), and the activity depends very much on the steric hindrance of the acyl moiety as well as on the quaternary ammonium portion. Note that the soft analog 12a and its hard counterpart 15 have the same anticholinergic potency. It is interesting to note that compounds derived from small branched fatty acids such as 12j are pretty active as cholinergics, actually much more potent than acetylnorcholine 14.

The next main question was whether these compounds are indeed "soft". To examine this point, their *in vivo* activity to antagonize acetylcholine was determined using anesthetized cats. The test compound was injected and at various intervals acetylcholine was given to check the characteristic vasopressor activity. The duration and extent of the antagonism was followed as the measure for the soft nature. The results are given in Table 8, and they clearly indicate that the highly potent soft anticholinergics have a short duration of action.

TABLE 8

Acetylcholine antagonist effect of selected soft quaternary salts on cat blood pressure

Compound	Concentration (mol kg⁻¹)	Activity										
12a	5.7×10^{-8}	time (min)	1	3	5	7	9					
		% response[a]	0	18	55	82	100					
	5.7×10^{-7}	time (min)	1	3	6	12	15	18	22	27	31	37
		% response[a]	0	0	0	18	36	55	65	73	95	100
12b	5.4×10^{-9}	time (min)	1	2	4	7						
		% response[a]	0	0	67	100						
	5.4×10^{-8}	time (min)	1	2	5	9	13	18	23	28	33	38	44
		% response[a]	0	0	0	0	31	63	63	69	81	88	88
12f	5.4×10^{-8}	time (min)	1	2	4	6	8	10				
		% response[a]	0	0	50	67	83	100				
	5.4×10^{-7}	time (min)	1	3	6	9	12	15	18	21	24	
		% response[a]	0	0	0	0	43	60	78	93	100	

[a]Percentage of the decrease in blood pressure after a dose of acetylcholine in the presence of antagonist, compared to the decrease after the same dose of acetylcholine in the absence of antagonist (100 %).

Thus, the activity of **12a** disappears completely after 9 minutes at a 5.7×10^{-8} mol kg^{-1} dose, and over 50% of the acetylcholine response is back after 18 minutes at a 10 times higher dose level. At the lower dose, atropine will completely inhibit response to acetylcholine for several hours. On the other hand, the slow infusion at a low-dose level of **12a** for an hour did not result in measurable acetylcholine antagonist activity indicating that a sustained low level of input will not lead to buildup of the antagonist due to its facile deactivation.

All these data indicate that the new type of anticholinergics are *highly active* while *"soft"* in nature; consequently, they are promising as local agents. Indeed, preliminary studies indicate that selected compounds from this class are very effective in controlling eccrine sweating in man both in the forearm and the underarm tests, without causing any detectable peripheral anti-secretory activity.

A recent application of the soft quaternary types of analogs involves some *cholinesterase* (*ChE*) *inhibitors* (Bodor and Oshiro, 1983) originally designed to reduce blood cholesterol and specifically low density lipoproteins (LDL). The idea was based on a recent observation of Kutty *et al.* (1975) who found that accidental poisoning with ChE inhibitors, such as organophosphates, resulted in dramatic decrease of serum cholesterol and specifically of the LDL. Subsequent animal studies using other known ChE inhibitors, such as neostigmine bromide (Kutty *et al.*, 1977), have confirmed this finding. The mechanism by which these inhibitors affect LDL is unknown, but is was suggested that cholinesterase is somehow involved in the formation of LDL from pre-LDL; transformation of the latter is inhibited by blocking ChE while the formation of HDL will not be affected (Scheme 6):

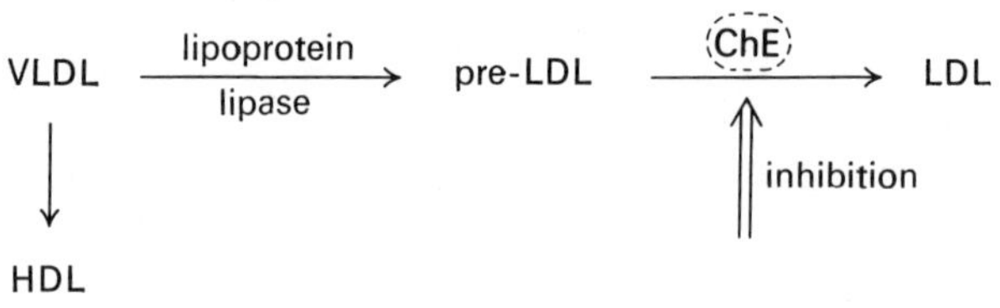

SCHEME 6

Due to their high toxicity, it is, however, inconceivable to use the known potent ChE inhibitors for reducing LDL. Rather, it would be desirable to have inhibitors with much lower toxicity. Soft analogs of pyridostigmine (**16**) were designed and synthetized from the precursor **17**; they are exemplified by structures **18a-e**.

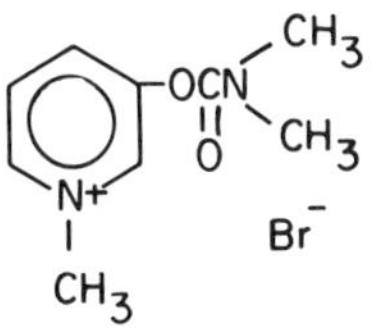

(16)

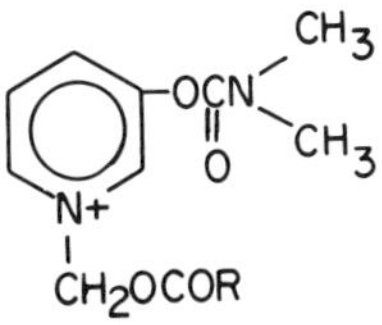

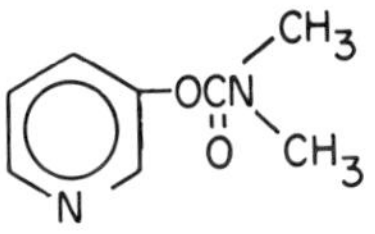

	R
18a	— C_6H_5
b	— $C(CH_3)_3$
c	— CH_2CH_3
d	— CH_2⟨⟩
e	— CH_2⟨⊙⟩

(17)

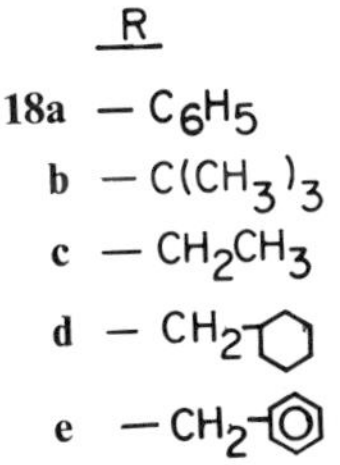

Preliminary studies were done on the analogs **18a** and **b** which were tested in hypercholesterolemic rats together with neostigmine and the hydrolysis product **17**. Thus, it was found that **18b** has a statistically significant lowering effect of about 40% on the total cholesterol and LDL without affecting HDL and phospholipids, while **18a** and **17** were found to be inactive, as shown in Table 9.

TABLE 9

The effect of some soft cholinesterase inhibitor analogs on the plasma lipids of hypercholesterolemic rats[a,b]

Compound	Total cholesterol (mg%)	LDL-cholesterol (mg%)	HDL-cholesterol (mg%)	Phospholipids (mg%)
Saline	125·2 ± 9·3	76·4 ± 12·4	28·0 ± 1·8	139·2 ± 6·3
Neostigmine	131·2 ± 11·8	76·6 ± 10·7	33·4 ± 1·5	134·7 ± 7·2
18a	146·1 ± 27	56·3 ± 15·9	31·7 ± 2·4	165·5 ± 12·8
18b	77·6 ± 6·7[c]	49·1 ± 12·6	27·5 ± 1·6	144·4 ± 12·1
17	127·9 ± 14·3	65·7 ± 12·5	39·4 ± 0·4	148·0 ± 7·9

[a]Each value (mean ± S.E.) is the average of 5 rats. The test compounds were administered intraperitoneally three times at 2-hour intervals and plasma lipids were measured 6 hours after first administration.
[b]Dose of **18a**, **18b**, and **17** was 2 mg kg^{-1}, for neostigmine was 0.2 mg kg^{-1} due to toxicity.
[c]$p < 0.01$.

TABLE 10

Hydrolysis of some soft cholinesterase inhibitors

Compound	Buffer pH 7·40[a]		Human plasma[b]		
	$k_1 \pm$ S.E. (min^{-1})	$t_{\frac{1}{2}}$ (min)	$k_2 \pm$ S.E. (min^{-1})	$t_{\frac{1}{2}}$ (min)	C_0 (M)
18a	$2{\cdot}39 \pm 0{\cdot}02 \times 10^{-3}$	290	$3{\cdot}76 \pm 0{\cdot}05$	0·18	1×10^{-3}
18b	$1{\cdot}07 \pm 0{\cdot}05 \times 10^{-3}$	647	$3{\cdot}22 \pm 0{\cdot}12 \times 10^{-3}$	215	6×10^{-4}

[a] 0.01 M phosphate buffer at $37 \pm 0.2°C$, $\mu = 0.1$ M (NaCl), average of six measurements $\pm$ standard error.
[b] Fresh human plasma at $37 \pm 0.1°C$, $C_0 =$ initial concentration.
Remarks: HPLC method was used to follow the disappearance of the quaternary salts. In both cases, the hydrolysis product was identified as **17**.

On the other hand, neostigmine, **18a** and **18b** were found to be *equipotent in vitro* inhibitors of cholinesterase while **17** was inactive. The *in vivo* toxicities were again very different. While all the animals died after being injected with 0.5 mg kg^{-1} neostigmine, **18a** and **18b** at 2 mg kg^{-1} dose did not cause any visible toxicity. The substantial difference between the *in vivo* activities of the two soft analogs **18a** and **b** can possibly be explained by their unexpectedly different plasma hydrolytic rates. As shown in Table 10, while both compounds are fairly stable in a pH 7.4 buffer ($t_\frac{1}{2} \simeq 5$–10 h), in human plasma the active **18b** has a $t_\frac{1}{2} = 215$ minutes while **18a** cleaves extremely rapidly ($t_\frac{1}{2} = 0.2$ min).

In both cases the inactive **17** is liberated. Thus, it appears that **18b** was successful in separating the desired activity from the unwanted toxicity. Based on earlier observations (Bodor *et al.*, 1980b) on the enzymatic hydrolysis of soft quaternary salts being catalyzed by cholinesterases, it appears that the activity of **18b** is due to its ability to *temporarily* block ChE, while it is also a substrate for this enzyme. The overall result will be a temporary, reversible inhibition of the cholinesterase. It appears that this is enough to interfere with the formation of LDL.

The above three examples clearly illustrate the soft analog design technique. It is a rather general method, obviously not restricted to quaternary salts only. Some of its basic principles of isosteric and/or isoelectronic design are subsequently applied in other soft drug design techniques such as the active metabolite or the inactive metabolite approaches (see Sections 2.3 and 2.6).

2.2 ACTIVATED SOFT COMPOUNDS

Compounds belonging to this class *are not analogs of known drugs*. Their design process starts with a known or designed *nontoxic, inactive compound which is then activated* to perform a certain pharmacological function by introducing in the structure a pharmacophoric group. *The activated* form will lose the activating group and *revert to the original non-toxic compound* and/or will undergo further metabolism to nontoxic moieties while performing its role.

In general, there are much less structural restraints on these kinds of compounds, as it is not expected that the whole molecule will perform as a receptor oriented drug. The actual process of releasing the activating group is the one which is responsible for the desired activity.

During the search for locally active antimicrobial agents of low toxicity, *N*-chloramines based on amino acids, amino alcohol esters and related compounds were developed. These compounds represent a stable source for positive chlorine (Cl$^+$) which will be released before or after penetrating the microbial cell walls, regenerating in this process the original amine (Scheme 7):

$$\text{\textbackslash}N-Cl + H_2O \xrightleftharpoons{K_{cp}} \text{\textbackslash}N-H + HOCl; HOCl \rightleftharpoons Cl^+ + OH^-$$

SCHEME 7

The antimicrobial activity of chloramines was known for quite some time, but most of them could not be used because of their chemical instability. Only the N-chloro derivatives of some amides and imides were of interest. After establishing the mechanism of their decomposition (Kaminski *et al.*, 1976a), it was found that if the α-carbon atoms lack hydrogen, stable N-chloramines can be obtained which, however, have much lower "chlorine potential" and are much less corrosive (Kaminski *et al.*, 1976a, 1976b, 1976c; Kosugi *et al.*, 1976). The types of these low chlorine potential chloramines are represented by structures 19, 20 and 21.

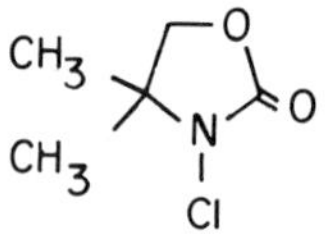

X = Cl
Y = H or Cl

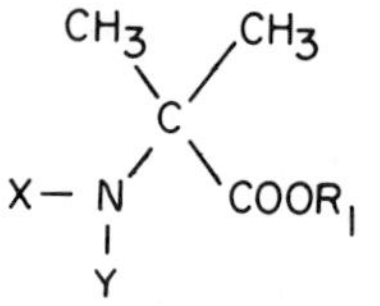

R = alkyl, etc.,

(20)

(19)

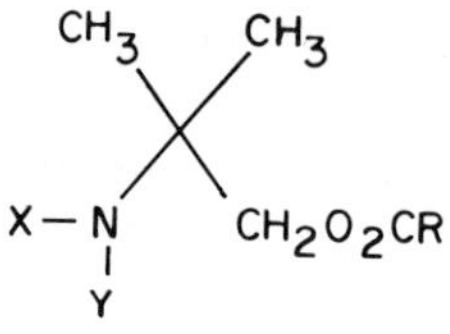

(21)

21a: X = Cl, Y = Cl, R = CH_3

21b: X = H, Y = H, R = $(CH_2)_2CH_3 \cdot HCl$

21c: X = H, Y = Cl, R = $(CH_2)_2CH_3$

21d: X = Cl, Y = Cl, R = $(CH_2)_2CH_3$

21e: X = H, Y = Cl, R = $C(CH_3)_3$

21f: X = Cl, Y = Cl, R = $C(CH_3)_3$

21g: X = H, Y = H, R = $(CH_2)_4CH_3 \cdot HCl$

21h: X = Cl, Y = Cl, R = $(CH_2)_4CH_3$

21i: X = Cl, Y = Cl, R = $(CH_2)_4CH_3$

21j: X = H, Y = H, R = $(CH_2)_6CH_3 \cdot HCl$

21k: X = H, Y = Cl, R = $(CH_2)_6CH_3$

21l: X = Cl, Y = Cl, R = $(CH_2)_6CH_3$

TABLE 11

Contact germicidal efficiency (CGE) of 2-amino-2-methyl-1-propyl carboxylates

Compound	Concentration[a]		Sterilization time[b] (min)				
	ppm	ppm, Cl⁺	S. aureus	S. pyogenes	E. coli	S. typhimurium	B. subtilis
21a	1292	458	5	2·5	0·5	2·5	2·5
21b	1070	—	>60	>60	>60	>60	>60
21c	2078	389	2·5	0·5	0·5	2·5	2·5
21d	979	304	2·5	0·5	0·5	2·5	0·5
21e	1886	323	5	0·5	0·5	2·5	2·5
21f	409	120	5	2·5	2·5	5	2·5
21g	1037	—	>60	>60	>60	>60	>60
21h	1319	211	2·5	0·5	2·5	5	2·5
21i	95	26	10	2·5	10	10	5
21j	1040	—	>60	30	15	30	5
21k	300	43	10	2·5	5	10	0·5
21l	85	21	15	5	10	10	2·5

[a]Solubility in 30% methanol − 0.1 M sodium dihydrogen phosphate, pH 7.0.
[b]Time intervals screened were 0.5, 2.5, 5, 10, 15, 30, 45 and 60 min.

For example, the contact germicidal efficiency (CGE) of a number of esters of the chlorinated 2-amino-2-methyl-1-propranol (structures **21a-l**) are listed in Table 11. It is evident that the unchlorinated amino alcohol esters such as **21b** or **g** are inactive while the chlorinated derivatives at the relatively low concentration of 1-400 parts per million are very effective against a variety of bacteria.

It was found that the mechanism of action of these compounds involves inhibition of bacterial growth by inhibiting DNA, RNA and protein synthesis (Kohl *et al.*, 1980). It was established that the initial precursor was regenerated while the positive chlorine did interact primarily with SH containing enzymes as shown in Table 12. Thus, the predictable and controllable metabolism of the soft chloramines implies a definite advantage of these compounds over the hard lipophilic, aromatic C–Cl bond containing antimicrobials.

TABLE 12

Inhibition of enzyme activity by 3-chloro-4,4-dimethyl-2-oxazolidinone (**19**)

Concentration (M)	Inhibition[a] (%)				
	Malic dehydro-genase	Lactic dehydro-genase	Creatine phospho-genase	Fumarase	Ribo-nuclease
5.34×10^{-5}	16	10	0		0
1.07×10^{-4}	20	15	5	100	0
4.28×10^{-4}	54	40	30	100	0
8.56×10^{-4}	62	50	53	100	0
1.28×10^{-2}	100	100	85	100	0
1.72×10^{-2}	100	100	100	100	0

[a]No inhibition was found if the enzymes were pretreated with dithiothreitol at the concentration of **19**.

Another example for the activated soft compounds is the "soft alkylating agents". These compounds can formally be derived from simple alkanol esters of aliphatic or aromatic acids which then are activated by introducing a halogen atom to the α-carbon of the alcohol portion as shown by **22**.

These α-halo esters are relatively weak alkylating agents. Thus, it was assumed that many of them could have antitumor activity as their lower alkylating potency would allow their transport to tumor cells without indiscriminate alkylation. On the other hand, as activated esters, all these compounds are subject to hydrolytic cleavage and deactivation, hence their overall toxicity should be lower than that of conventional alkylating agents, which can only be deactivated by an alkylating process. A variety of α-halo esters were synthesized (Bodor and Kaminski, 1980), and their relative alkylating potency was determined by a competitive alkylation method, using

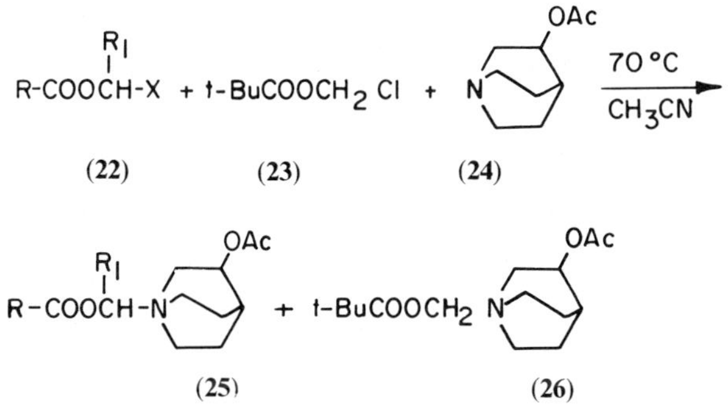

$$R\text{-}COOCH\text{-}X \ + \ t\text{-}BuCOOCH_2Cl \ + \ N\langle\text{OAc}\rangle \xrightarrow[CH_3CN]{70\,^\circ C}$$

$$\underset{R_1}{\ }$$

$$(22) \qquad\qquad (23) \qquad\qquad (24)$$

$$\underset{R_1}{R\text{-}COOCH\text{-}N}\langle\text{OAc}\rangle \ + \ t\text{-}BuCOOCH_2\ N\langle\text{OAc}\rangle$$

$$(25) \qquad\qquad\qquad (26)$$

SCHEME 8

as an arbitrary standard, chloromethyl pivalate (23), which is competing for the alkylation of a tertiary amine of low steric hindrance, 3-acetoxy quinuclidine (24) (Scheme 8). The analysis of the production composition allowed expressing the relative alkylating reactivity (RAR) as shown in Table 13.

TABLE 13

Relative alkylating reactivity (RAR) of selected soft alkylating agents

Compound	R	R_1	X	Product composition (%)		RAR(25/26)
				25	**26**	
22a	$CH_3(CH_2)_4$	H	Cl	35	65	0·54
22b	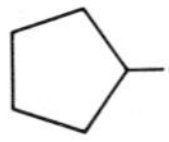 $\langle\rangle\text{-}CH_2$	H	Cl	40	60	0·67
22c	$C_6H_5CH_2$	H	Cl	73	27	2·70
22d	C_6H_5	H	Cl	40	60	0·67
22e	C_6H_5	H	Br	93	7	13·29
22f	$CH_3(CH_2)_4$	CH_3	Cl	—	>99	0

Evidently, the hindered **22f** is much less reactive than its lower homolog chloromethyl hexanoate **22a**. Biological studies revealed no activity of **22f**, while **22a** was active in the P388 leukemia test as shown in Table 14.

There is no reason to believe that chloromethyl hexanoate is the optimum structure in this large class of compounds. The activity is clearly due to the chloromethyl ester which is a small group, and thus its incorporation into transport molecules will not significantly alter the binding and transport properties of the carrier molecule, while the circulating free fraction can be deactivated by esterases, resulting in a more favorable separation of the desired activity from toxicity.

TABLE 14

Activity of the soft alkylating agent **22a** in P388 lymphocytic leukemia[a]

Dose (mg kg⁻¹)	Number of animals	% ILS[b]
400	5	109
200	6	127[c]
100	6	120
50	6	107

[a]One daily dose; total number of doses = 9.
[b]Percentage increase in median survival time as compared to the control group.
[c]Activity confirmed by second test.

2.3 THE ACTIVE METABOLITE PRINCIPLE

As it was shown in Scheme 1, most drugs undergo stepwise metabolic degradation yielding intermediates and structural analogs which have similar activity as the original drug molecule. For example, oxphenbutazone, a metabolite of phenylbutazone, 4-hydroxypropranolol (27), an active metabolite of propranolol and many other active drug metabolites belong to

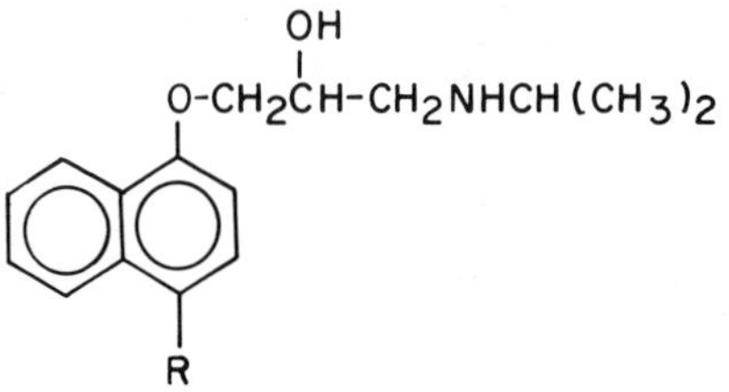

R = H   propranolol
  = OH   4-hydroxy-
            propranolol

(27)

this class. The main point is that these generally *oxidative metabolic trans-formations will put*, on the one hand, a *burden on the saturable and slow oxidative enzyme system*, but, even more importantly, will result in a *mixture of active compounds* which have different selectivity, pharmacokinetic, binding, distribution and elimination properties. The overall result is that depending on the presence of other compounds competing for the same enzyme system as well as on the activity and regulation of specific enzymes, a variety of *unpredictable* combinations of the active species will be present in different individuals at different times, rendering practically impossible the safe and effective dosing of these compounds. The pharmacokinetic and pharmacodynamic evaluation of these cases becomes impossible. A good illustration of such a situation is provided by bufuralol (28) which has three active metabolites (**29-31**) displaying different selectivities, and rather different pharmacokinetic properties (Francis *et al.*, 1976) as shown in Table 15.

TABLE 15

Metabolism and pharmacokinetic properties of bufuralol (**28**) and its metabolites (**29–31**)

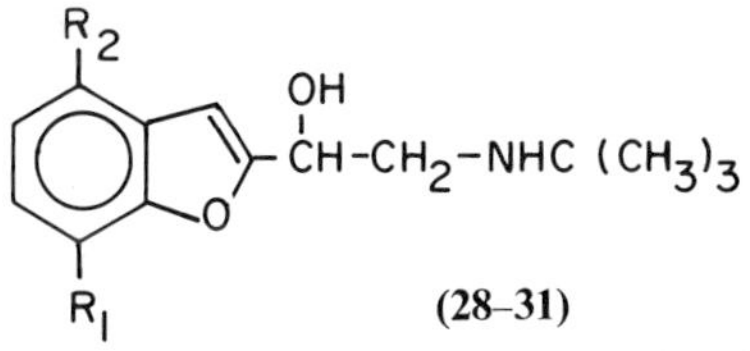

(28–31)

Compound	R_1	R_2	Concentration[a] (μg/ml)	$t_{\frac{1}{2}}$[b] (h)
28	$-CH_2CH_3$	H	22	4
29	$-CH(OH)CH_3$	H	19	7
30	$-COCH_3$	H	8	12
31	$-CH_2CH_3$	OH	>2	4

[a]Blood concentration at 9.5 h after administration to humans (20 mg oral dose).
[b]Biological half-life.

Evidently the relative *in vivo* concentrations of compounds **28–31** will vary with time, individual enzyme levels, indirect drug interactions, etc. Such situations are too complex for a correlation between blood levels and pharmacological activity to be found.

It is evident that this is a general problem. In most cases, it is not even clear which is the main active compound, the drug or its metabolite(s). In the latter case, the drug is only a prodrug provided it does not have substantial intrinsic activity. One additional major complication is that certain disease states involving renal insufficiency, edema or significant alterations in protein binding will substantially alter the elimination profile of the various metabolites. It is very important to realize, however, that in a large number of cases, based on our present knowledge, many metabolites can be predicted, and one does not have to wait for the classical metabolism studies to synthesize, identify and test these candidates.

According to the *basic soft drug design principles*, it *is preferable to use as the drug of choice an active species which undergoes a one-step, singular, predictable metabolic deactivation. Thus, the active metabolite theorem of the soft drug design states that whenever oxidative metabolic transformations of a drug take place, going through possibly toxic, highly reactive intermediates or through pharmacologically active species, if activity and pharmacokinetic considerations permit it, the drug of choice should be the active metabolite which is in the highest oxidized state.* This theorem can and certainly should be expanded to other metabolic transformations besides the oxidative ones.

Since it is now a generally accepted and even required step in drug development research to isolate and test at least the major metabolites, one should look for those active metabolites which appear to have significantly different pharmacokinetic properties particularly longer half-lives, and follow up on these leads to possibly replace the initial drug.

2.4 ENDOGENOUS SUBSTANCES AS NATURAL SOFT DRUGS

Endogenous substances such as steroid hormones (hydrocortisone, progesterone, testosterone, estradiol, etc.) or neurotransmitters (dopamine, GABA and others) can be considered *natural soft drugs*, since the body has developed efficient, fast metabolic ways for their disposition without going through highly reactive intermediates. Thus, their *metabolism is predictable* and it is certain that if used at concentrations close to their normal levels, they *will not cause unexpected toxicity.* Their use, rather than that of synthetic analogs, is highly desirable and would in fact be possible if their metabolism were not so fast and efficient and their transport so specific that they cannot efficiently be used as drugs. This situation can be possibly controlled by using *chemical delivery systems* (CDS) (Bodor and Farag, 1983a, 1983b) for these natural soft drugs. If one can achieve sustained, *local or site-specific delivery* of a *natural soft drug*, the overall gain in therapeutic index can be very substantial. Eventually, even a prodrug of a natural soft drug could be advantageous if it would control the delivery of the active species.

One example for this combined natural soft drug–chemical delivery system approach is given by the local (*topical*) *delivery of hydrocortisone*. Although hydrocortisone is an endogenous glucocorticoid, its topical applications that result in higher than normal *in vivo* levels can cause side effects such as dermal atrophy, thymus involution, and separation of adrenal, hypothalamus and pituitary functions (Kligman and Kaidbey, 1978). Formulations of hydrocortisone or derivatives of hydrocortisone that merely increase the efficiency of the delivery of this steroid cannot realistically be expected to alleviate these side effects. Improved separation of activity from toxicity (improved selectivity) should result from a derivative of hydrocortisone that is (1) inactive itself, i.e. a prodrug, but (2) accumulates in the skin and (3) hydrolyzes slowly to liberate the hormone with such a kinetics that its rate of systemic metabolism to inactive, easily excreted substances more closely matches its endogenous rate of release from the skin. These objectives were achieved using 3-spirothiazolidine derivatives such as the compounds described by

TABLE 16

Synthesized hydrocortisone 3-spirothiazolidines

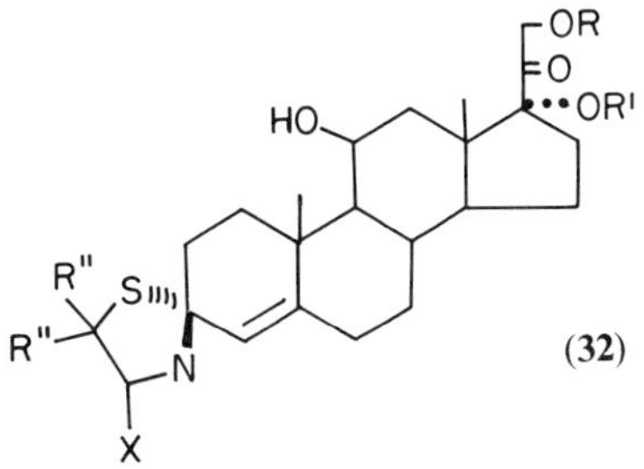

(32)

Compound	X	R	R′	R″
32a	$CO_2C_2H_5$	$COCH_3$	H	H
32b	H	$COCH_3$	H	H
32c	H	H	H	H
32d	$CO_2C_2H_5$	H	H	H
32e	$CO_2C_2H_5$	H	COC_4H_9	H
32f	$CO_2C_2H_5$	H	COC_2H_5	H
32g	H	H	COC_3H_7	H
32h	H	H	COC_2H_5	H
32i	H	H	$COCH_3$	H
32j	$CO_2C_2H_5$	H	$COCH_3$	H
32k	$CO_2CH_2CH_2OH$	$COCH_3$	H	H
32l	$CO_2C_2H_5$	$COCH_3$	H	CH_3
32m	$CO_2CO_{10}H_{21}$	$COCH_3$	H	H
32n	$CO_2C_6H_{13}$	$COCH_3$	H	H
32o	$CO_2C_4H_9$	$COCH_3$	H	H
32p	CO_2CH_3	$COCH_3$	H	H

formula **32** in Table 16 (Bodor *et al.*, 1982). These types of compounds, by eliminating the 4,5-unsaturated 3-ketone group, lack specific hydrocortisone binding and affinity properties. Some of the simple derivatives, namely, the ones derived from hydrocortisone 21-acetate (**34**) were also tested for their topical anti-inflammatory activity, and the results of their potency relative to hydrocortisone are given in Table 17. Hydrocortisone 17-butyrate (**35**) was included to confirm the obtained relative potencies. It is evident that the spirothiazolidines of hydrocortisone acetate are about 3–4 and 6–8 times more potent than hydrocortisone and hydrocortisone acetate, respectively. This implies that the active species, that is, hydrocortisone itself is released locally at the site of action in a somewhat better or more sustained way. The thymus involution studies on selected compounds such as the simple **32a** indicate that the spirothiazolidine derivative has less systemic side effects than hydrocortisone or hydrocortisone acetate, as shown in Table 18.

TABLE 17

Relative antiinflammatory activity[a] of selected cysteine based 3-spirothiazolidine derivatives of hydrocortisone

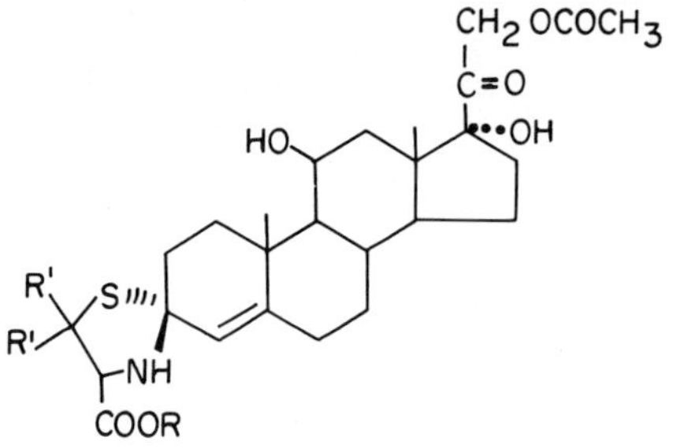

Compound	R	R'	ED_{50} (M)[b]	Potency relative to hydrocortisone
32p	CH_3	H	0·0035	3·1
32a	C_2H_5	H	0·0033	3·2
32o	C_4H_9	H	0·0027	4·0
32n	C_6H_{13}	H	0·0039	2·7
32m	$C_{10}H_{21}$	H	0·0036	3·0
32h	C_2H_5	CH_3	0·0055	1·9
33	Hydrocortisone		0·0107	1·0
34	Hydrocortisone 21-acetate		0·0203	0·5
35	Hydrocortisone 17α-butyrate		0·0011	10·0

[a]The test compounds were applied in acetone solution containing 2% croton oil on the anterior and posterior surface of the right ear. Three hours later, the mice (male DDY) were sacrificed and both ears were removed. Circular sections were punched out and drug effect expressed as percentage inhibition of inflammation compared to the control.

[b]Linear regression analysis of data obtained at 3×10^{-5}, 3×10^{-4}, 3×10^{-3} and 3×10^{-2} M.

TABLE 18

Thymus involution[a] in rats after topical application of steroids

Compound	mg of thymus 100 g of rat ± S.D.	% reduction in thymus[b]
Blank[c]	268 ± 25	
Vehicle	257 ± 59	
Hydrocortisone	168 ± 30	35
Hydrocortisone 21-acetate	167 ± 18	35
32a	204 ± 20	21
Hydrocortisone 17α-butyrate	206 ± 20	20

[a]All compounds were administered in a total of 50 µl as a 0.03 M acetone/IPM (90:10) solution to 10 rats, each.

[b]Compared to vehicle.

[c]Untreated rats.

TABLE 19

Steroid diffusion through fresh hairless mouse skin

Compound[a]	Mole % hydrocortisone[b] diffused $\pm$ S.D.[c] (hours after application)				
Hydrocortisone		$2\cdot1 \pm 0\cdot8$ (4)	$4\cdot1 \pm 1\cdot3$ (9)	$7\cdot5 \pm 1\cdot8$ (18)	$8\cdot4 \pm 3\cdot0$ (24)
Hydrocortisone 21-acetate		$1\cdot7 \pm 0\cdot6$ (4)	$3\cdot5 \pm 1\cdot3$ (9)	$6\cdot2 \pm 1\cdot3$ (18)	$14\cdot1 \pm 5\cdot9$ (24)
Thiazolidine (32a)	$0\cdot1 \pm 0\cdot05$ (2)	$0\cdot6 \pm 0\cdot1$ (4)	$1\cdot2 \pm 0\cdot2$ (7.5)	$1\cdot8 \pm 0\cdot3$ (12)	$3\cdot2 \pm 0\cdot7$ (24)

[a] 50 μl of 0.03 M acetone-IPM 90:10 was applied to the membranes.
[b] Only hydrocortisone was found on the receptor side of the membrane under HPLC conditions where hydrocortisone 21-acetate could have been detected. Samples for thiazolidine 32a were split and one-half was analyzed directly while the other half was treated with acid to hydrolyze any intact thiazolidine; there was no observable difference in the two results.
[c] $n = 3$.

TABLE 20

Ear[a] thinning in mice after topical application of steroids

Compound	Concentration (M)	First day Left	First day Right	Third day Left	Third day Right	Fifth day Left	Fifth day Right	% reduction in ear thickness
Hydrocortisone	3×10^{-3}	86 ± 5	86 ± 5	72 ± 4	88 ± 9	70 ± 4	89 ± 4	18·6
	1×10^{-3}	86 ± 5	86 ± 5	78 ± 4	85 ± 4	76 ± 4	88 ± 3	11·6
	3×10^{-4}	88 ± 6	88 ± 7	82 ± 5	89 ± 7	83 ± 6	91 ± 3	5·7
Hydrocortisone 21-acetate	3×10^{-3}	90 ± 7	87 ± 5			81 ± 6	86 ± 5	10·0
	1×10^{-3}	87 ± 4	84 ± 3			79 ± 5	83 ± 3	9·2
	3×10^{-4}	88 ± 3	87 ± 4			80 ± 5	83 ± 6	9·1
Thiazolidine (32a)	3×10^{-3}	88 ± 6	90 ± 6			82 ± 4	87 ± 6	6·8
	1×10^{-3}	87 ± 4	86 ± 5			78 ± 3	88 ± 7	10·3
	3×10^{-4}	89 ± 7	90 ± 7	74 ± 4	87 ± 5	84 ± 5	88 ± 6	5·6
Hydrocortisone 17-butyrate	1×10^{-3}	90 ± 4	92 ± 5			69 ± 4	86 ± 4	23·3
	3×10^{-4}	91 ± 5	90 ± 7			75 ± 4	87 ± 5	17·6
	1×10^{-4}	90 ± 5	89 ± 6			78 ± 5	90 ± 3	13·3
	3×10^{-5}	89 ± 6	89 ± 7			83 ± 7	89 ± 4	6·7
Hydrocortisone 17-valerate	3×10^{-3}	89 ± 5	88 ± 6			68 ± 3	82 ± 4	23·6
	1×10^{-3}	87 ± 5	89 ± 5			72 ± 4	88 ± 6	17·2
	3×10^{-4}	88 ± 5	88 ± 8			75 ± 7	89 ± 7	14·8
Triamcinolone acetonide	3×10^{-4}	87 ± 4	89 ± 6	70 ± 4	82 ± 2	66 ± 3	86 ± 5	24·1
	1×10^{-4}	84 ± 4	88 ± 6	73 ± 5	85 ± 6	70 ± 5	85 ± 5	16·7
Vehicle		90 ± 7	92 ± 5	89 ± 6	89 ± 3	91 ± 4	88 ± 4	

Ear thickness $\pm$ S.D.

[a]Left ears treated for 4 days with 10 μl of the steroid solution.

Percentage reduction in thickness $= 100 \times \dfrac{[\text{thickness of left ear (day 1)} - \text{thickness of left ear (day 5)}]}{[\text{thickness of left ear (day 1)}]}$

This decreased side effect implies a lower systemic delivery of the active species. In other words, the chemical delivery system discussed here somehow *enhances local but reduces systemic delivery* of the active species. Indeed, as shown in Table 19, significantly less hydrocortisone is delivered transdermally when using the spirothiazolidine **32a** than with either hydrocortisone or hydrocortisone 21-acetate. Based on these results as well as on the mechanism of stepwise hydrolysis of the thiazolidine ring to deliver the active 3-keto derivative (Sloan *et al.*, 1981a, 1981b), the enhanced local activity and reduced systemic toxicity can be explained by a binding through a disulfide bond of the intermediate **36** as shown in Scheme 9, and the bound **37** which now serves as the final form of the delivery system will hydrolyze releasing the active hydrocortisone. This local binding in the skin was confirmed by a similar type of behavior of the thiazolidine of progesterone as it will be discussed later. Thus, the overall result using this chemical delivery system

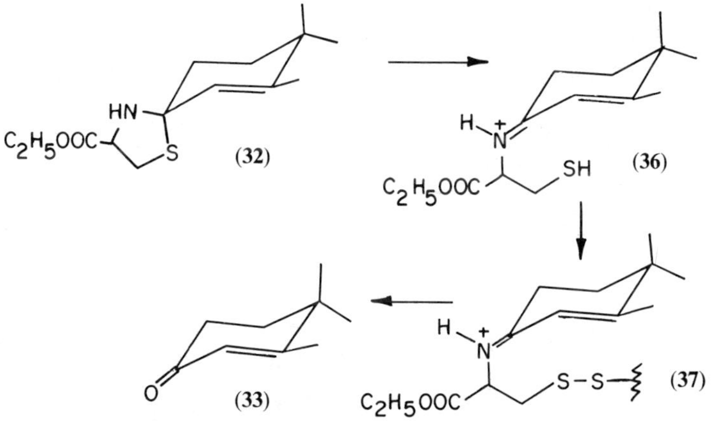

SCHEME 9

for hydrocortisone was a 3–4-fold increase in the antinflammatory ED_{50} and about a two-fold reduction in the toxicity–selectivity (thymus involution). Even the local toxicity, as reflected by the skin atrophy, was reduced, as shown in Table 20.

The improvement in the therapeutic index can thus be considered to be an average of eight-fold. The activity enhancement observed in the animal studies was also confirmed in the blanching studies using human volunteers (Bodor *et al.*, 1982). Similar types of derivatives for testosterone and progesterone were also synthesized (Bodor and Sloan, 1982).

In both cases, the double bond initially situated between carbons 4 and 5 could migrate during the preparation, and thus some of the 5,6 double bond analogs were also synthesized. It was found that the rate of hydrolysis and the regeneration of the active species are significantly slower from the 5,6 than from the 4,5 analogs. Also, in the case of progesterone, bis-thiazolidines as represented by **39** were also obtained besides the 3-spirothiazolidines **40** (Table 21A-C).

TABLE 21A

Thiazolidines of testosterone

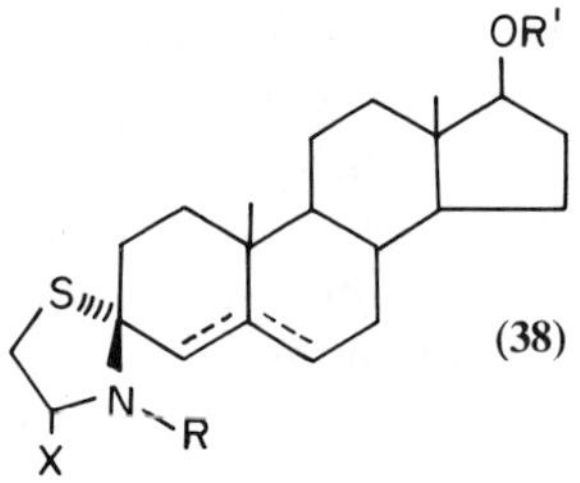

(38)

Compound	X	R	Δ	R′
38a	$CO_2C_2H_5$	H	5,6	COC_2H_5
38b	$CO_4C_2H_5$	H	4,5	COC_2H_5
38c	$C_2C_2H_5$	H	5,6	H
38d	$CO_2C_2H_5$	H	4,5	H
38e	$CO_2CH_2CH_2OH$	H	5,6	COC_2H_5
38f	$CO_2CH_2CH_2OH$	H	5,6	H
38g	H	H	5,6	COC_2H_5
38h	H	H	5,6	H
38i	H	CH_3	5,6	H

TABLE 21B

bis-Thiazolidines of progesterone

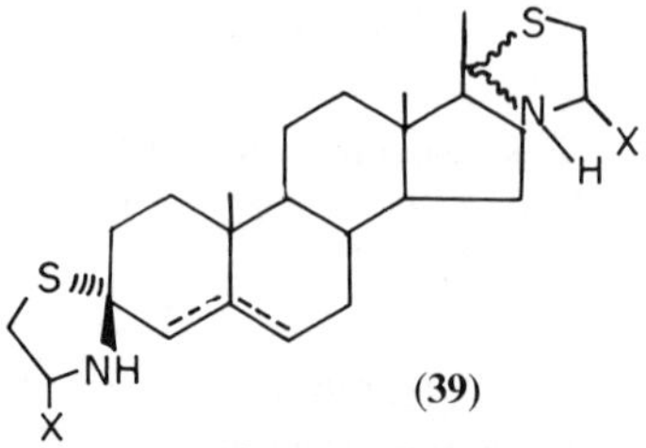

(39)

Compound	X	Δ
39a	$CO_2C_2H_5$	5,6
39b	$CO_2C_2H_5$	4,5
39c	$CO_2C_4H_9$	4,5
39d	$CO_2C_6H_{13}$	4,5 : 5,6(1 : 1)
39e	$CO_2C_{10}H_{21}$	4,5

TABLE 21C

Thiazolidines of progesterone

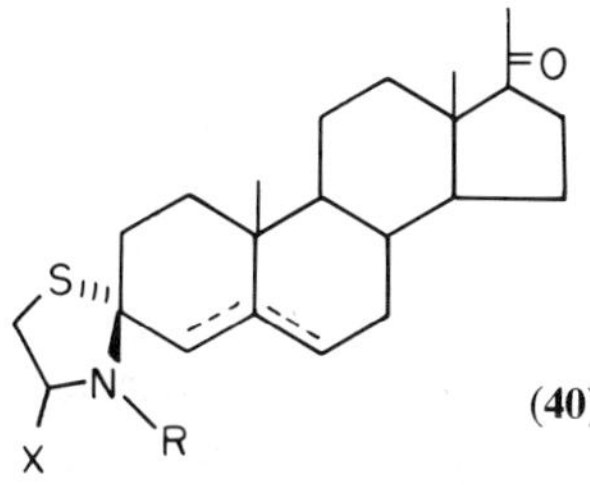

(40)

Compound	X	R	Δ
40a	$CO_2C_2H_5$	H	5,6
40b	$CO_2C_2H_5$	H	4,5
40c	H	H	5,6
40d	H	COH	5,6
40e	H	$COCH_3$	5,6
40f	H	$COCH_2NHCO_2CH_2C_6H_5$	5,6
40g	H	CH_3	5,6

Pharmacological studies indicate that none of the progesterone derivatives when given orally or subcutaneously had more than one-tenth the activity of a subcutaneous dose of progesterone in the Clauberg test. One derivative of testosterone, **38i**, was found to be more active than the parent steroid as shown in Table 22. The lack of activity of these derivatives can be attributed

TABLE 22

Androgenic test[a]

Compound	Total dose (mg)	Seminal vesicle weight (mg)	Ventral prostate weight (mg)
Testosterone	16·0	14·0 ± 2·0	38·5 ± 2·5
	32·0	13·4 ± 1·2[b]	45·7 ± 2·0
	64·0	28·9 ± 3·2	67·1 ± 2·5
38i	4·0	8·2 ± 0·4	39·9 ± 1·9
	8·0	9·9 ± 0·6	45·7 ± 2·5
	16·0	15·8 ± 0·8	50·9 ± 3·4
Vehicle		6·4 ± 0·3	8·3 ± 0·5

[a]The compounds were given orally as a suspension in sesame oil daily for 10 days starting on day of castration using 10 rats per dose.

[b]Unusually low value compared to data at same concentration in all other control experiments (17.0 ± 1.7 mg).

to their relatively slow plasma hydrolysis which was found to have $t_{\frac{1}{2}}$ values ranging from 15 hours for the mono and up to 160 hours for the bis-thiazolidines. The progesterone derivatives have, however, another potential use, that is, as a possible antiacne preparation (Bodor and Sloan, 1978, 1980). For this reason, **39a** was applied topically to hairless mice, and the residence time of the steroid in the skin was studied as compared to progesterone which was found to show activity in controlling acne (Girard *et al.*, 1980). The *in vivo* results show the remarkable ability of the thiazolidine **39a** to increase the relative amount of labelled steroid in the skin. It was again assumed that disulfide bond formation from the intermediate iminium salt enhances residence time and concentration of the progesterone derivative in the skin and at the same time will significantly reduce the transdermal delivery process.

TABLE 23

Dermal delivery of progesterone and **39a**

	Progesterone[a] (% dose) Mean ± SE[c]	**39a**[b] (% dose) Mean ± SE
Feces	16·65 ± 1·75	0·95 ± 0·13
Urine	7·00 ± 1·14	0·40 ± 0·09
Skin circle[d]	1·98 ± 0·10	4·52 ± 1·18
Intestine/fat	2·28 ± 0·47	0·09 ± 0·00
Liver	0·75 ± 0·06	0·08 ± 0·01
Blood	0·08 ± 0·02	0·28 ± 0·04
Kidney/spleen	0·06 ± 0·01	0·03 ± 0·01
Lung	0·04 ± 0·02	0·01 ± 0·00
Subtotal	28·74	6·36
Patch[e]	54·06 ± 1·6	83·46 ± 1·4
Total	82·80	89·82

[a]75 µl of a solution of 0.9 mg in 675 µl in ethanol-isopropyl myristate (90:10).
[b]75 µl of a solution of 1.85 mg in 675 µl ethanol-isopropyl myristate (90:10).
[c]$n = 6$.
[d]2-cm diameter plug of epidermis taken directly under the bandage patch (3 cm²).
[e]Includes the contents of an ethanolic wash of the skin circle after the bandage patch was removed.

The results are shown in Table 23. Very interesting results for the distribution of the thiazolidine derivatives were obtained when two of the progesterone derivatives were injected intravenously into the tail of rats. As shown in Table 24, a very significant portion of the dose was concentrated in the lung as compared to progesterone. These results did not seem to be artefactual and might have specific importance in site-specific delivery to the lungs. The reason for the high concentration can be related to the fact that in a number of

TABLE 24

Distribution of [4-^{14}C]progesterone, **39a** and **39d** in rats[a] 1 h after intravenous tail administration[b]

Compound	Dose (mg kg^{-1})	Dosage equivalents of progesterone (mg kg^{-1})	Organ	% dose/organ Mean ± SE
Progesterone	0·98	0·98[c]	Liver	16·25 ± 1·33
			Lungs	0·50 ± 0·07
			Blood	2·91 ± 0·39
			Feces	35·15 ± 2·97
39d	2·21	1·01[c]	Liver	14·22 ± 1·13
			Lungs	79·22 ± 4·14
			Blood	3·55 ± 0·51
			Feces	0·24 ± 0·06
39a	1·96	1·07[c]	Liver	14·39 ± 1.38
			Lungs	60·73 ± 1.12
			Blood	2·07 ± 0·49
			Feces	2·39 ± 0·27
39a	0·135	0·074[c]	Liver	40·57 ± 1·56
			Lungs	22·15 ± 1·62
			Blood	18·56 ± 2.68
			Feces	16·18 ± 4·5
39a	0·143	0·078[d]	Liver	34·41 ± 2.14
			Lungs	20·20 ± 1.76
			Blood	5·49 ± 0·56
			Feces	5·69 ± 0·94

[a] $n = 6$.
[b] 5 μl benzyl alcohol vehicle.
[c] Activity of progesterone 1 μCi mg^{-1}.
[d] Activity of progesterone 9.47 μCi mg^{-1}, $n = 4$.

species (rabbit, rat, hamster) some oxygenase activities are higher in the lung than in the liver. The proposed disulfide bond-type binding of these compounds involves oxidation.

2.5 SITE-SPECIFIC CHEMICAL DELIVERY SYSTEMS

The last example given in the previous section relates to an interesting finding of increased progesterone concentrations in the lungs when a bioreversible spirothiazolidine derivative was used. Based on the assumed oxidative binding mechanism of the intermediate iminium salt in the lung, this can be considered as a *site-specific delivery to the lungs*.

A more clear-cut example for site-specific delivery of a natural endogenous compound, adrenalin, is provided by using esters of adrenalone to deliver adrenalin. It was found some years ago (Bodor et al., 1978) that diester derivatives of adrenalone (41) have a high level of ocular sympathomimetic activity. Both mydriatic response and reduction in the intraocular pressure were observed using these compounds. This finding was most surprising, particularly because adrenalone itself (43, Scheme 8) has very low intrinsic sympathomimetic activity as even a 2% aqueous solution when instilled in the eye will not have any observable mydriatic activity (Weekers et al., 1955). The extent of the activity of the esters 41 was also surprising. Some of these compounds on a molar basis were more potent than the highly active prodrug form of adrenalin, dipivalyl adrenalin (Hussain and Truelove, 1976). The pharmacological basis for the observed activity was unclear in view of the low level of intrinsic activity of both adrenalone and the diester itself. The basic hypothesis for the activity was that 41 is transformed to adrenalin (46, Scheme 8) in the eye via a combined reduction-hydrolysis process (see Scheme 8).

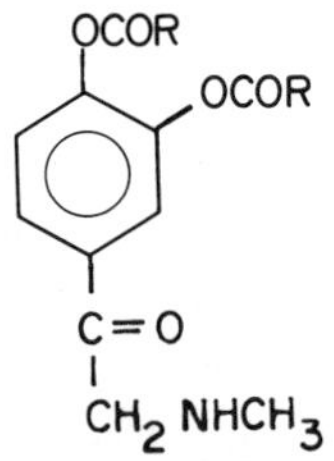

$$
\begin{array}{ll}
R = -CH_3 & 41a \\
\quad\ -C_2H_5 & b \\
\quad\ -C_3H_7 & c \\
\quad\ -i-C_3H_7 & d \\
\quad\ -(CH)_4CH_3 & e \\
\quad\ -CH_2CH(CH_3)_2 & f \\
\quad\ -CH_2C_6H_5 & g
\end{array}
$$

(41)

In most of the studies dealing with the transport and the disposition of topically applied ophthalmic agents, the anterior segment has been considered to be the target area (Patton, 1980). Few of these studies, however, consider the quantitative distribution and metabolism of the drug in ocular tissues and structures. In many instances only drug levels in aqueous humor are determined, and from these data conclusions are often made concerning transport efficiency and bioavailability. In the case of the delivery system of the type 41, the analysis of tissue concentrations within the eye and the determination of the major site of biotransformation of these compounds are critical to the evaluation of the drug of action. Analysis of the aqueous humor alone would not accurately reflect the various processes that determine adrenalone activity. A highly sensitive analytical procedure was developed to ascertain the concentration and disposition of adrenalone derivatives (41)

TABLE 25

Tissue concentration of adrenalone (**43**) and adrenalin (**46**) following topical administration of diisovaleryl adrenalone (**41f**)[a]

	Concentration of adrenalone			Concentration of adrenalin		
	15 min (μg g^{-1})	30 min (μg g^{-1})	60 min (μg g^{-1})	15 min (μg g^{-1})	30 min (μg g^{-1})	60 min (μg g^{-1})
Cornea	4·47 ± 1·14	7·75 ± 1·92	2·27 ± 0·84	ND[b]	ND	ND
Aqueous humor	0·33 ± 0·09	0·87 ± 0·27	0·52 ± 0·12	ND	ND	ND
Iris/ciliary body	0·42 ± 0·14	2·61 ± 0·72	1·11 ± 0·86	0·09 ± 0·05	0·58 ± 0·35	0·04 ± 0·01

[a]Dose of **41f** equivalent to 0.05% of **46**, to the volume instilled: 50 μl.
[b]ND—no detection of adrenalin at limit of quantitation 0.035 μg g^{-1} tissue.

and their possible metabolites in the various ocular tissues and fluids (Bodor and Visor, 1984). The method combining HPLC with electrochemical detection has allowed determination of the concentrations of various compounds in the compartments of the eye as achieved following *in vivo* administration of the delivery system **41**. One of the more potent diesters, diisovaleryl adrenalone (**41f**), was selected for these studies. The results are presented in Table 25. Tissue concentrations of adrenalone can be seen to increase and decrease quite rapidly. The highest levels were found in the cornea, and this is characteristic of its role as both the major barrier to penetration and its capacity to act as a drug reservoir. The concentration of adrenalone in the aqueous humor follows the same time course as that determined in other tissues, but the levels are significantly lower. The iris–ciliary body tissues were found to have a fairly large concentration of adrenalone, with peak levels coinciding with those of the aqueous humor and cornea. The most interesting and significant finding of these experiments was the detection and quantitation of the potent adrenergic agonist, adrenalin, in the uveal tissues. The presence of a significant quantity of adrenalin exclusively in the iris–ciliary body tissue in the same time frame as the peak levels of adrenalone is indicative of drug biotransformation. The bioactivation of adrenalone esters, either the diester or the monoester forms, by a reduction process appears to account for the detection of adrenalin as a metabolite of adrenalone. Control animals did not have any detectable quantities of endogenous adrenalin present (detection limit = 200 pg). Based on evidence reported in the literature (Shichi and Nebert, 1980; Das and Shichi, 1981) and on our own experiments, the iris–ciliary body tissue appears to be one of the major sites of drug metabolism in the eye. It is not surprising, therefore, that adrenalin is found there and only there. On the other hand, the rapid disappearance of the adrenalin produced is probably related to significant levels of monoamine oxidase (MAO) and catechol *O*-methyltransferase (COMT) activity in these tissues. The role of COMT and MAO in the inactivation of catecholamines is well known, and the presence of these enzyme systems may limit the amount of detectable adrenalin due to rapid metabolism before the tissue can be extracted. The question of stereospecificity of the adrenalone reductase and its specificity for the diester form or the catecholamine itself is unclear. However, the low intrinsic activity of the D-enantiomer implies that a considerable proportion (and maybe all) of the adrenalin was produced in the L-form. In an important supportive experiment, a 2% concentration of adrenalone was studied; this is 40 times higher than the dose equivalent used when testing the diester. Tissue concentrations were determined as in the case of **41**, indicating high levels in the cornea and significant concentrations in the iris–ciliary body (Table 26). However, no activity was observed, supporting again the assumption that adrenalone is not a good substrate

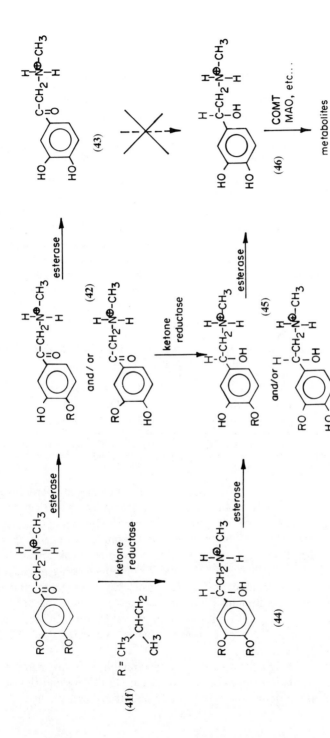

SCHEME 10. Proposed mechanism of bioactivation of diacyl adrenalone derivatives in the uveal tract.

TABLE 26

Tissue concentration of adrenalone following its topical administration (30 min)[a]

Cornea	0.52 ± 0.13 μg g^{-1}
Aqueous humor	0.04 ± 0.03 μg g^{-1}
Iris/ciliary body	0.13 ± 0.09 μg g^{-1}

[a]Determined at 30 min after administration by HPLC with electrochemical detection (potential 0.7 V).
A solution of 2% adrenalone-HCl was used. *No* adrenalin could be detected.

for the reductive enzyme. In addition, when a 0.05% solution of the diisovaleryl adrenalin (44) was administered, adrenalin (46) concentrations were comparable in the iris–ciliary body, but much higher in the cornea and the aqueous humor (compare Tables 27 and 25). Thus, it appears that the diester and the monoesters (42) of adrenalone may be the preferred substrates for the reductase as shown in Scheme 10, summarizing the bioactivation of 41.

TABLE 27

Tissue concentrations of adrenalin (46) following topical administration
of diisovaleryl adrenalin (44)[a]

Cornea	5.72 ± 0.50 μg g^{-1}
Aqueous humor	0.14 ± 0.04 μg g^{-1}
Iris/ciliary body	0.29 ± 0.09 μg g^{-1}

[a]Determined at 30 min after administration by HPLC with electrochemical detection (potential 0.7 V). Dose equivalent to 0.05% of parent compound (adrenalin).

These investigations clearly indicate that the diester derivatives of adrenalone are not simply prodrugs, but rather comprise an *efficient chemical delivery system that is site-specifically activated*. This type of system is superior to other chemical approaches, for example, adrenalin prodrugs (Hussain and Truelove, 1976), because of fast and predictable metabolism of the transport form, formation of the active component only at the site of action and, thus, avoidance of toxic effects resulting from non-target tissue exposure. An adrenalin prodrug such as 44 delivers the drug to all compartments of the eye. In addition, due to substantial drainage, it will deliver it systemically while the *chemical delivery system* 41 will deliver it *only to the site of action*.

The detection of significant quantities of adrenalin as a major metabolite implies that enzymatic carbonyl reduction occurs in the eye and this activity can be useful in the design of other bioreversible transport systems.

It is evident that the concept of developing methods for site-specific delivery of biologically active agents is highly desirable to improve efficacy and decrease toxicity. The *site-specific and sustained release of drugs to the brain* is even more difficult. The delivery of drugs to the brain is often seriously limited by transport and metabolism factors and, more specifically, by the functional barrier of the endothelial brain capillary wall called the blood–brain barrier (BBB) (Rapaport, 1976). It is generally accepted that the ability of the molecule to cross the blood–brain barrier is a function of its partition coefficient between lipid and water. Lipid-insoluble or highly ionized compounds fail to achieve a cerebrospinal fluid (CSF) over plasma distribution ratio of 1, unless they are actively transported (Fishman, 1964). This is due to the fact that the rate of entry is much slower than the rate of exit from the CSF. The approach of derivatizing the compound and forming a prodrug that exhibits improved physicochemical properties for the transport through the blood–brain barrier should be treated with caution. Indeed, while one can improve delivery of the drug to the brain, the prodrug may simultaneously exhibit improved transport to other tissues and depots, thus increasing the incidence of systemic side effects. In addition, one has to keep in mind that these prodrugs, in analogy with lipidic compounds which do pass the blood–brain barrier, can be kept at *therapeutically useful levels in the brain only if there is a constant circulating concentration*. In other words, one has to keep the whole body loaded with the compound, and generally at relatively high concentrations. This is a serious limitation in many cases due to peripheral toxicity. Delivering drugs exclusively or preferentially to the brain is very difficult, and, until recently, no simple and general method to achieve this goal had been known. A general method based on a dihydro-pyridine-pyridinium-type redox delivery system for brain-specific sustained release of the drugs was recently developed (Bodor *et al.*, 1981) which can be summarized as shown in Scheme 11.

According to this Scheme, a drug [D] is either coupled to a tertiary carrier [C] and then quaternized, or coupled to a quaternary carrier [QC]$^+$ directly, and the obtained [D–QC]$^+$ is reduced chemically to the lipophilic dihydro form [D-DHC]. Alternatively, the drug [D] can directly be coupled with the dihydro carrier [DHC]. After *in vivo* administration of this [D-DHC] compound, it is quickly distributed (k_0) throughout the body, including the brain. The dihydro form [D-DHC] is then oxidized in the brain ($k_1{}^1$) and in the body ($k_1{}^2$) (e.g. by NAD/NADH systems) to the original [D-QC]$^+$ (ideally inactive) quaternary salt. (Superscript 1 refers to processes in the brain, while superscript 2 indicates similar processes in the body. These latter processes are assigned an overall rate (e.g. $k_1{}^2$ for oxidation), although the actual process takes place with different rates in the various organs.) Due to its ionic hydrophilic character, [D-QC]$^+$ should be eliminated rapidly

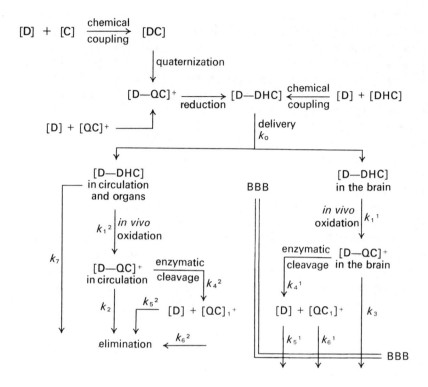

SCHEME 11

from the brain ($k_2 \gg k_3$; $k_2 \gg k_7$). Enzymatic cleavage of the [D-QC]$^+$ that is *trapped in the brain* will result in a sustained delivery of the drug species [D], followed by its normal elimination (k_5^1) and metabolism. A properly selected carrier, [QC]$^+$, will also be eliminated rapidly from the brain ($k_6^1 \gg k_3$). Due to the facile elimination of [D-QC]$^+$ from the general circulation, only small amounts of the drug are released in the body ($k_2 \gg k_4^2$), hence [D] will be released primarily in the brain ($k_4^1 > k_3$). The overall result, ideally, will be a *brain-specific sustained release of the target drug.*

A quick analysis of the concept indicates that this is not a simple prodrug type design, but rather a "chemical delivery system" (CDS). That is, the [D-QC]$^+$ species can be considered a prodrug of [D], but the reduced [D-DHC] form, which is actually delivered, is not a prodrug; rather, it is a special pro-prodrug with additional properties resulting in a site-specific and sustained release.

One additional, very significant aspect of the present redox delivery system relates to toxicity: it is expected to significantly reduce systemic toxicity by accelerating the elimination of the drug-quaternary carrier system from the general circulation. On the other hand, even the central toxicity should be reduced by providing a low-level sustained release of the active species in the brain. One main factor in this whole picture is the choice of the quaternary carrier, which must be of low toxicity alone and in combination with the drug.

It is important to note that this method will provide the desired level of a drug in the CNS without requiring high circulatory concentrations. The drug blood level has virtually no effect on the brain levels, once the last oxidation step and the "lock-in" process have taken place.

This general approach was first applied for phenylethylamine (**47**) which was transformed into the chemical delivery system **48** where the redox carrier is the dihydrotrigonelline ⇄ trigonelline redox system.

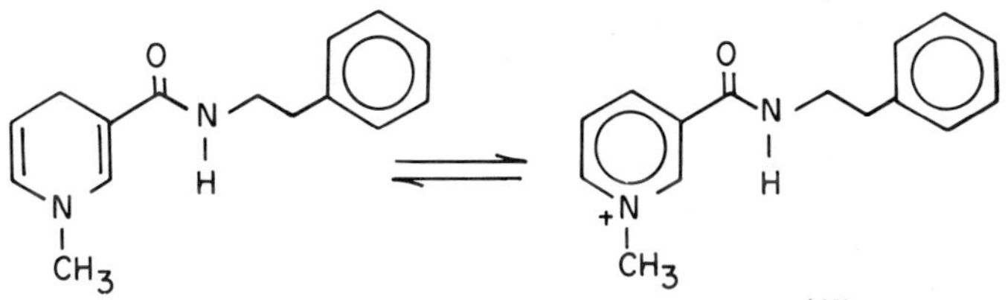

(**48**)   (**49**)

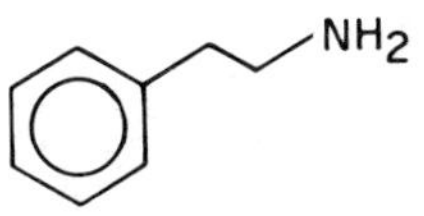

(**47**) 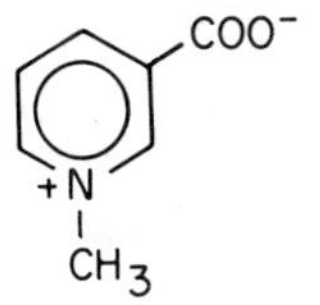   (**50**)

The lipidic form **48** is oxidized to the quaternary from **49** with relative ease in various biological fluids as shown in Table 28. The corresponding *in situ* oxidation secures not only trapping in brain of this oxidized form but a continuous buildup of its cerebral concentration with simultaneous decline in blood concentration.

At about 1 hour following administration, the *in vivo* results indicate a very high brain concentration of the precursor **49** locked in the brain and almost completely eliminated from the blood. These features are illustrated in Fig. 1. The descending portion of the brain concentrations in Fig. 1 corresponds to a half-life of 2.35 hours. The rate of conversion of **49** to phenylethylamine and trigonelline was found to have a half-life of 3 hours

TABLE 28

Rates of oxidative conversion in biological fluids[a] of 1-methyl-3-(N-phenethyl-carbamoyl)-1,4-dihydropyridine **48** to the corresponding quaternary pyridinium salt **49**.

		48 → 49		
Medium	n	$k \times 10^{-4}$ (s⁻¹)	r	$t_{\frac{1}{2}}$ (min)
Human plasma	13	1.80 ± 0.34	0.998	64.2 ± 12.1
Whole blood	5	8.40 ± 0.94	0.952	13.7 ± 1.9
Brain homogenate	8	4.12 ± 0.28	0.996	28.2 ± 2.0
Liver homogenate	7	8.13 ± 0.96	0.999	14.4 ± 2.1

[a] At 37°C, undiluted heparinized human whole blood, 20% fresh human plasma, and 2% rat brain and liver homogenates were used. The conversion of **48** to **49** was followed by the changes in their characteristic UV spectra ($\lambda_{max} \simeq 350$ nm for **48**; 262 nm for **49**), against appropriate reference samples.

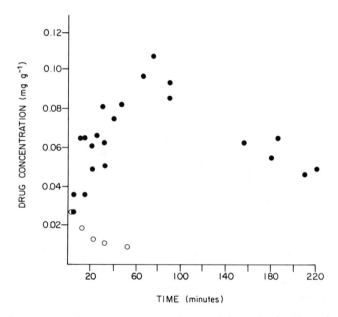

FIG. 1. The concentration of 1-methyl-3-(N-phenethylcarbamoyl) pyridinium (ion) (**49**) in the brain (●) and the blood (○) of rats following administration of 1-methyl-3-phenethylcarbamoyl-1,4-dihydropyridine (**48**). Protocol: A group of 22 male Sprague–Dawley rats of average weight of 300 ± 50 g were anesthetized with Inovar, and the freshly prepared dihydro compound (**48**) was injected through the external jugular as a solution in Me_2SO (0.5 g ml⁻¹) at a dose of 125 mg kg⁻¹ animal body weight. After appropriate time periods, the blood and brain were analyzed for **49** by HPLC.

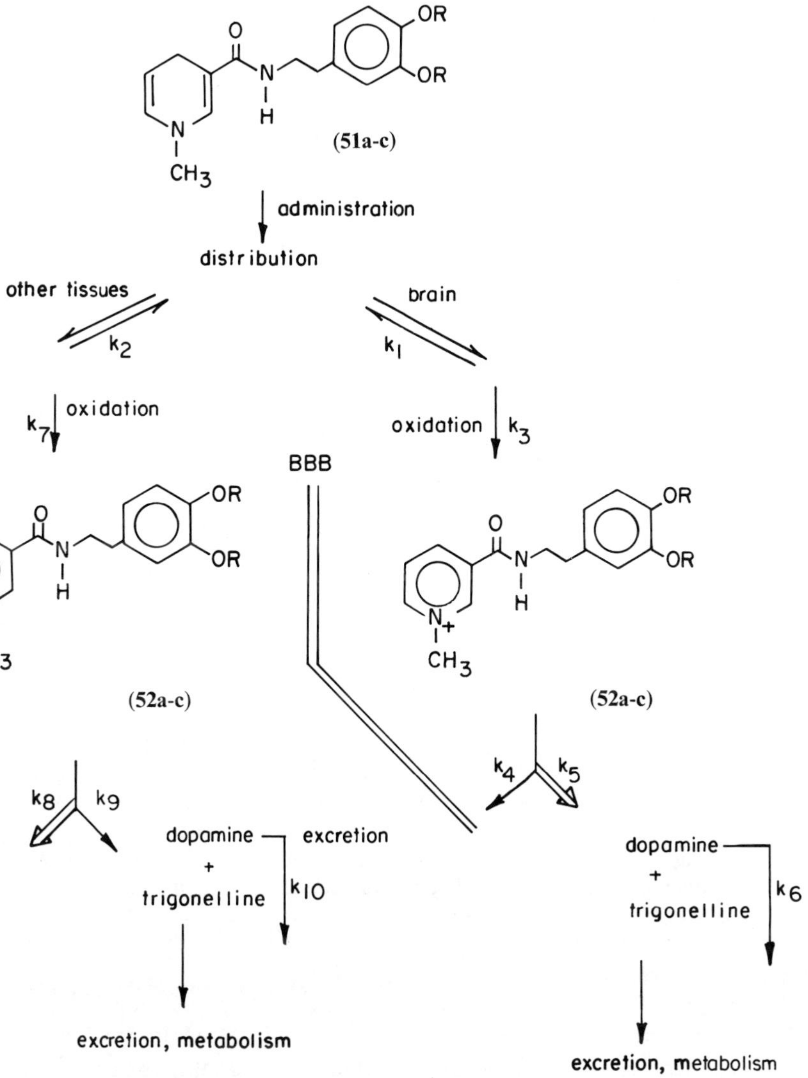

^{a} a, R = H; b, R = COCH$_3$; R = CO(CH$_3$)$_5$.

SCHEME 12

using fresh rat brain homogenate. Thus, the descending portion in Fig. 1 corresponds mainly to the sustained delivery of phenylethylamine in the brain. All criteria set forth in the previous scheme were met, since one i.v. injection of a drug coupled to a dihydropyridine carrier system resulted in an accumulation of the corresponding drug quaternary carrier in the brain followed by a sustained release of the drug in the brain, while the drug quaternary carrier was rapidly eliminated from the blood. When the quaternary derivative **49** was administered at equivalent dose levels, no amount could be detected in the brain of rats.

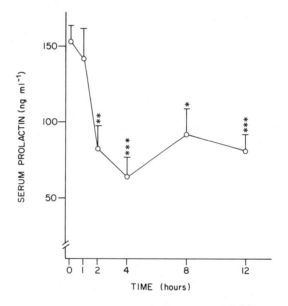

FIG. 2. Effect of compound **51** administered i.v. at a 1 mg kg^{-1} dose level on the serum prolactin levels in rats. Error bars represent S.E. of mean, $*p < 0.025$; $**p < 0.01$; $***p < 0.005$ versus control. Each print represents the average of six animals. For details see Bodor and Farag (1983a).

A similar type of delivery system was used for the sustained delivery of dopamine to the brain and/or the anterior pituitary while providing much lower concentrations in the peripheral circulation and other tissues. According to the following scheme, the designed delivery system for dopamine, compound **50**, would result in high and sustained concentrations of the precursor **51a** in the brain while this quaternary form was very quickly eliminated from the rest of the body (Scheme 12). The locked-in form **52a** resulted then in a sustained slow release of dopamine to the anterior pituitary which resulted in a very substantial and prolonged inhibition of prolactin release as shown in Fig. 2. It is important to note that the carrier precursor form **51a** does not have intrinsic dopaminergic activity. On the other hand, when injected as such it will cause only very brief reduction in the prolactin release which will return to the normal value within 1 hour.

The redox-type chemical delivery system to the brain was also applied to a very important class of compounds, namely that of steroids. This application is important for several reasons. There are a number of clinical situations in which the delivery of sex hormones to the brain is desirable. These include sexual dysfunctions like impotency as well as in contraception. In addition, steroids are relatively large molecules, and this application does extend the CDS to larger substrates. The first compound to be used was testosterone. In developing a CDS for this hormone, the blood–testes barrier (BTB) (Kormano, 1967a, 1967b; Fawcett et al., 1970; Dym and Fawcett, 1970) was also taken into consideration. Like the BBB, this barrier acts to exclude compounds from the semeniferous tubules but, unlike the BBB, it is not the result of a vascular component. Most recent theories indicate that this impermeable barrier is due to tight adjunctions in the sertoli cells which surround the spermatogenic apparatus. In any case, the BTB and the BBB are very similar in their gross effects. The dihydropyridine-pyridinium salt redox system should be effective in concentrating testosterone in the testes as well as in the brain. The testosterone-CDS **54** was obtained (Scheme 13) (Bodor and Farag, 1984) and administered systemically to female rats.

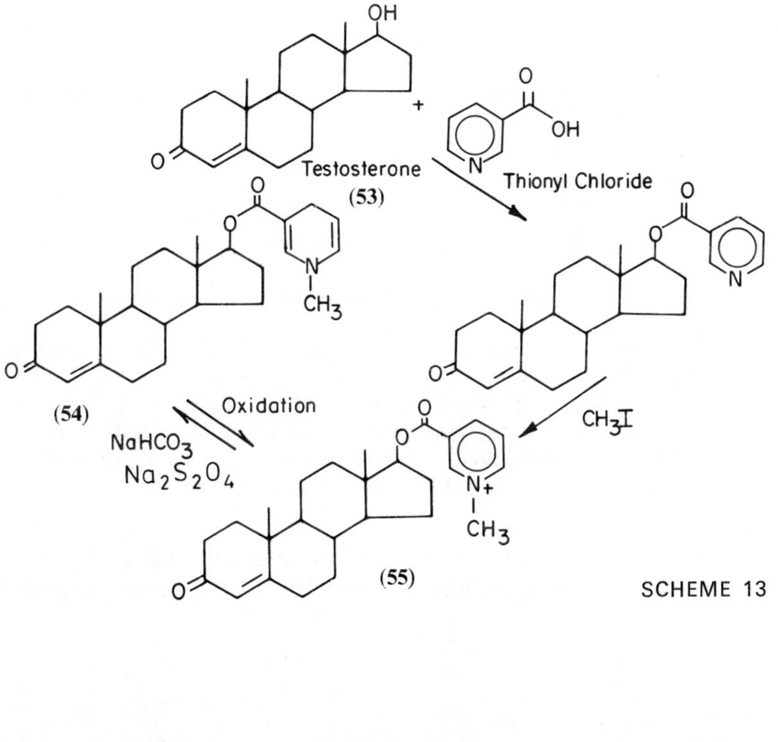

SCHEME 13

The quaternary compound **(55)** was found in high concentrations in the brain where it is retained with an efflux $t_{\frac{1}{2}}$ of 5·7 hours. Conversely, the quaternary salt after systemic injection was rapidly lost from the peripheral circulation, in the same way as it was lost when formed peripherally (half-life of efflux in the order of 50 minutes). Furthermore, it was possible in this case to show delivery of testosterone itself to the brain; when liberated *in situ*, the hormone shows a very slow efflux with a half-life of about 20 hours. This may be due, firstly, to its sustained formation from the precursor, and secondly to high-affinity binding to globulins. If testosterone itself is given in equimolar amounts, it is rapidly lost from both the brain and the blood. These data are summarized in Fig. 3, indicating that the method allows a constant low level delivery of testosterone to the brain.

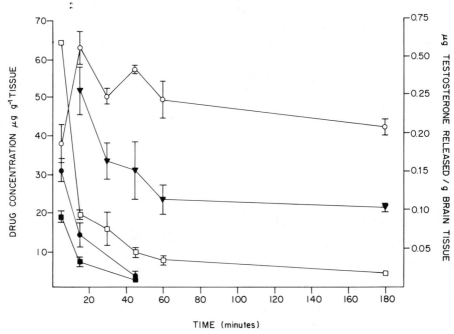

FIG. 3. Concentrations versus time of testosterone 17-nicotinate-*N*-methyl cation, calculated as iodide, in brain (○) and in blood (□), and concentration of released testosterone (ng g⁻¹) in brain (▼), all following administration of the corresponding dihydropyridine derivative **(54)**. Also, concentrations of testosterone in brain (●) and blood (■) following administration of testosterone. Female Sprague–Dawley rats were used.

The above redox delivery system has great potential for a variety of drugs to be delivered in a sustained manner to the brain. Its potential is quite high for the treatment of various diseases caused by neurotransmitter disorders or brain tumors.

Again, it has to be emphasized that the main objective of all these site- and organ-specific delivery systems is to separate activity and toxicity and, thus, to improve the therapeutic index of the drugs.

2.6 THE INACTIVE METABOLITE APPROACH

The inactive metabolite approach is one of the most promising and most versatile methods for developing safe soft drugs. The main objective of this type of design is again to include the *design of the metabolism of the active species*. However, there is a basic variation in that the actual activity and toxicity of the metabolite is known, and the design process also allows for the metabolic pathway to be operative once the drug has performed its role. Accordingly, the *principles of the inactive metabolite approach are*:

1. *Start* the design process with a known *inactive metabolite* of a drug which is used as the lead compound.
2. Design the structures and then perform chemical modifications on this metabolite to obtain *structures which resemble* (isosteric and/or isoelectronic) *the drug from which the lead inactive metabolite* was derived. This is the activation stage.
3. Design the structure of the new soft analog in such a way that its *metabolism will yield the starting inactive metabolite* in one step and without going through toxic intermediates (predictable metabolism).
4. *Control the transport and binding properties* as well as the rate of metabolism and pharmacokinetics by molecular manipulations in the first, activation stage (controllable metabolism).

The easiest way to understand this approach is by analyzing the toxicity of DDT (**56**) and its analogs and metabolites (Scheme 14) (Abou-Donia and Menzel, 1968). DDT undergoes stepwise dehalogenation forming among others the acidic metabolite **60**. This metabolite is inactive and it is of relatively low toxicity. This is the form which can be excreted as a water-soluble species. Thus, **60** should be an ideal lead compound for the inactive metabolite approach. Indeed, its ethyl ester (**61**) was found to have good activity, but significantly lower toxicity and very much lower carcinogenicity than either DDT or Kelthane (**57**), as indicated in Table 29. The reason for this much reduced toxicity of **61** is clearly its ability to be deactivated to an excretable metabolite (**60**) in one hydrolytic step. The active soft pesticide **61** is formally derived from the inactive metabolite **60** and the metabolism of compounds of type **61** is predictable and controllable.

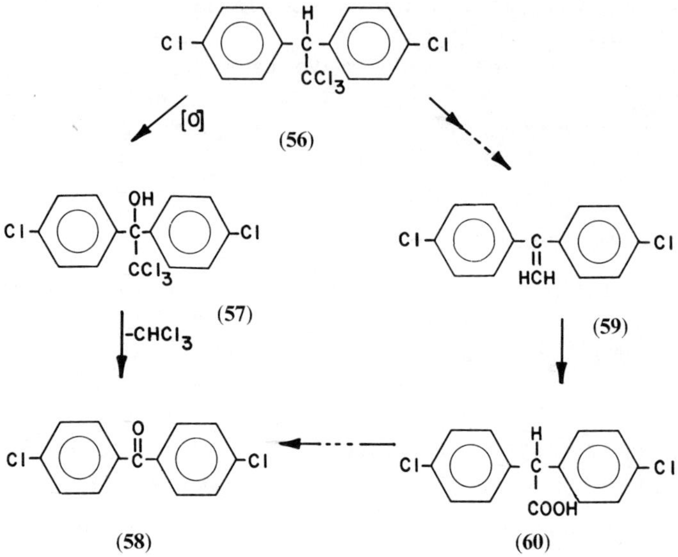

SCHEME 14

TABLE 29

Toxicity of some pesticides

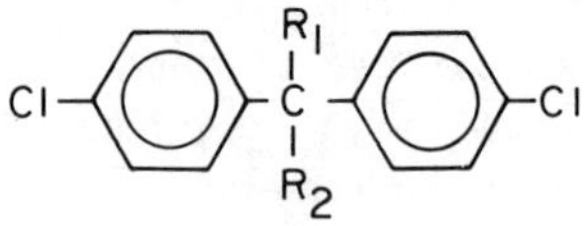

Compound	R_1	R_2	Name	LD_{50} (mg kg^{-1}) oral	Carcinogenic concentration (ppm)
56	–H	–CCl$_3$	DDT	120–200	300
57	–OH	–CCl$_3$	Kelthane	800–1400	300
61	–OH	–COOC$_2$H$_5$	Chlorobenzylate	1500–3200	6000

On a more general basis, the metabolism of a large number of drugs was analyzed by us and many useful inactive metablites were found. For example, major antiinflammatory steroidal agents undergo, among others, oxidative metabolic degradation of the dihydroxyacetone side chain. Thus, the proto-type hydrocortisone (33) will be oxidized stepwise to the ketoaldehyde

(62a), the 20-oxo-21-oic acid (62b) and the cortienic acid (62c), in addition to a variety of A-ring reduced products.

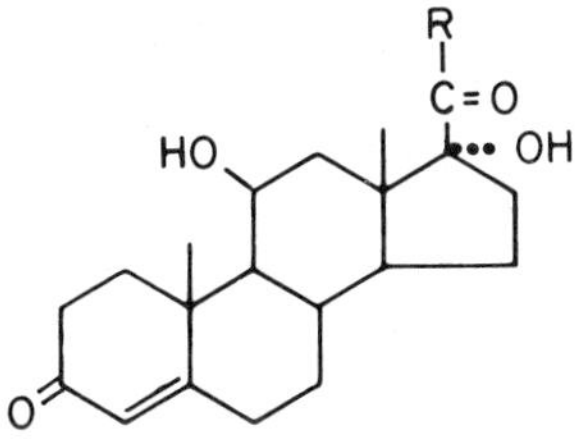

Nr.	R
33	CH_2OH
62a	CHO
62b	COOH
62c	OH

The acidic metabolites 62b and 62c are inactive and can be used as lead compounds to design isosteric and/or isoelectronic analogs of 17α- and 21-substituted hydrocortisone and its various more potent analogs, for example, fluorinated derivatives. Thus, in the general design of structures 63 and 64, the objective was to have the 17α- and 21-groups contribute to affinity and binding as they do in 65, or to have the whole side chain (including the 17α- + 17β-substituent combinations) isosteric-isoelectronic with that in 65.

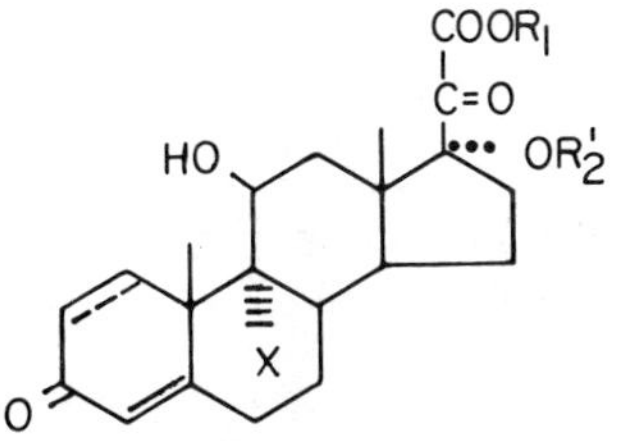

(63)

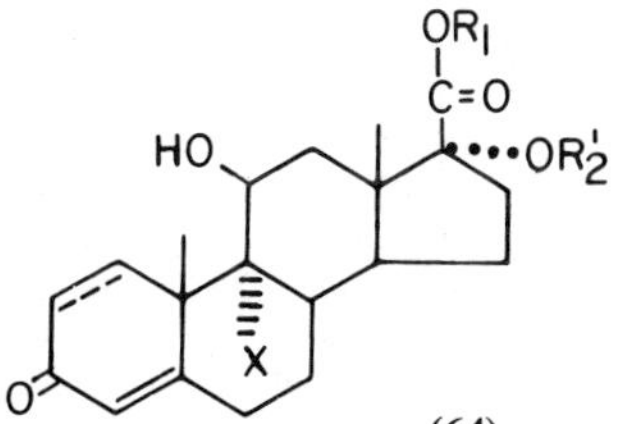

(64)

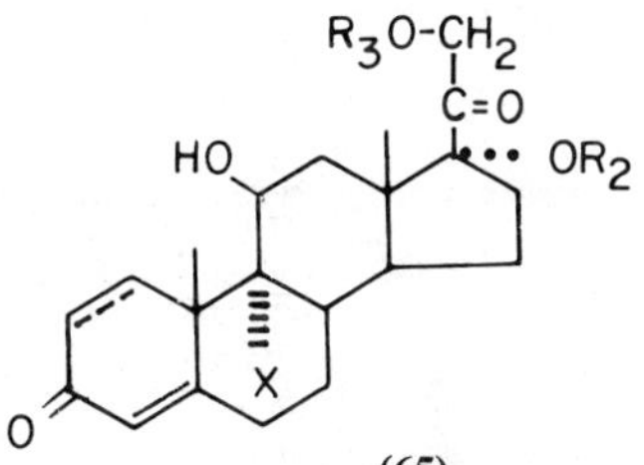

(65)

Examples of active topical antiinflammatory steroids which fall into this class are fluocortin butyl (66) (Mützel, 1977) and $17\alpha,17\beta$-diesters of cortienic acid (67) (Laurent et al., 1975).

TABLE 30

Effect of locally administered selected "soft steroids" and reference steroids on granulation tissue formation caused by implantation of cotton pellets in rats[a]

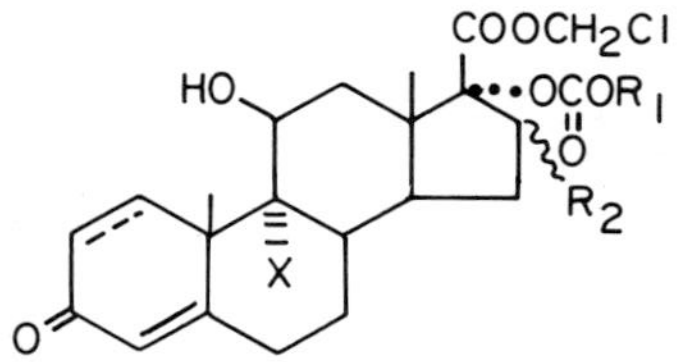

Test compound	Dose (μg per pellet)	Number of test animals	Body weight gain (g)	Granulation inhibition (%)	Thymus weight[b] mg	Decrease (%)
None (control)		10	32·4 ± 1·4		445 ± 20	
69 $R_1 = -CH$ $\overset{CH_3}{\underset{CH_3}{\big|}}$; $R_2 = H$; $X = H$	100	8	34·9 ± 2·7	13·8	452 ± 29	
	300	8	33·9 ± 1·6	37·3	469 ± 25	
	1000	8	34·0 ± 2·6	70·3	464 ± 30	
	3000	8	32·4 ± 2·3	75·0	459 ± 24	
70 $R_1 = -CH$ $\overset{CH_3}{\underset{CH_3}{\big|}}$; $R_2 = H$; $X = H$; Δ^1	30	8	32·4 ± 1·2	37·2	523 ± 26*	
	100	7	35·0 ± 1·5	49·4	537 ± 31*	
	300	8	34·4 ± 1·1	53·1	525 ± 28*	
	1000	8	29·4 ± 1·5	77·2	423 ± 26	

No.	R groups / Name	Dose	n				
71	$R_1 = -C_2H_5$; $R_2 = \alpha\text{-}CH_3$; $X = F$; Δ^1	0.3	8	32.4 ± 1.1	29.4	492 ± 26	
		1	8	$37.3 \pm 1.5^*$	55.2	$519 \pm 22^*$	
		3	8	34.3 ± 1.1	66.3	472 ± 16	
		10	8	36.1 ± 1.1	72.8	521 ± 35	
		30	8	31.3 ± 1.4	74.9	505 ± 26	
72	$R_1 = -CH\begin{smallmatrix}CH_3\\ \\CH_3\end{smallmatrix}$; $R_2 = \beta\text{-}CH_3$; $X = H$; Δ^1	1	7	33.0 ± 1.7	45.3	$526 \pm 30^*$	
		3	8	30.4 ± 1.1	66.9	471 ± 20	
		10	8	33.0 ± 1.5	63.2	474 ± 25	
		30	8	31.8 ± 1.7	75.5	489 ± 26	
35	Hydrocortisone 17-butyrate	300	6	$26.2 \pm 1.7^*$	58.1	$353 \pm 37^*$	(20.7)
		1000	6	$26.2 \pm 1.2^{**}$	56.5	$99 \pm 7^{***}$	(77.8)
		3000	6	$6.7 \pm 2.2^{***}$	65.5	$58 \pm 5^{***}$	(87.0)
		10000	6	$-2.0 \pm 2.4^{****}$	66.5	$46 \pm 7^{***}$	(89.7)
73	Betamethasone valerate	100	7	$24.9 \pm 1.9^{***}$	49.4	$364 \pm 24^*$	(18.2)
		300	8	$22.3 \pm 1.2^{***}$	59.0	$264 \pm 29^{***}$	(40.7)
		1000	7	$5.3 \pm 1.0^{***}$	53.1	$77 \pm 5^{***}$	(82.7)
		3000	8	$6.6 \pm 1.4^{***}$	47.0	$63 \pm 3^{***}$	(85.8)

[a]The steroid was dissolved in acetone and injected into cotton pellets. The pellets were dried and implanted beneath the skin of each rat. Six days later, the weight of dried pellets was determined.
[b]Changes in body weight and thymus weight are indicative of systemic effects.
*$p < 0.05$.
**$p < 0.01$.
***$p < 0.001$.

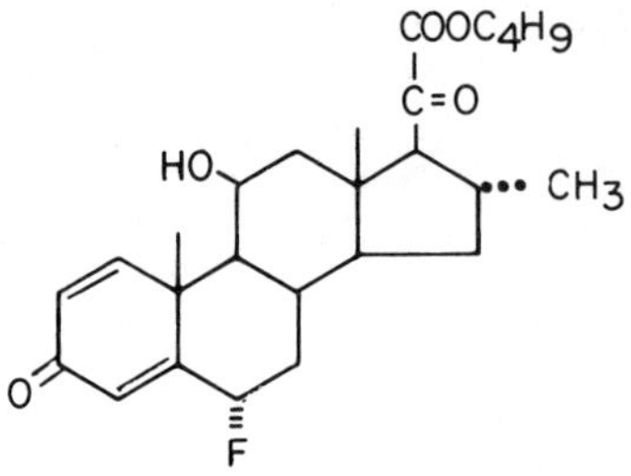

(66) 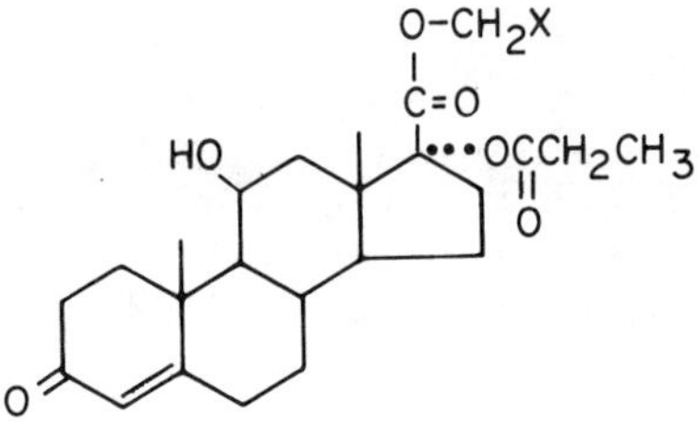   (67)

Special attention is given to the most recent 17α-carbonates (Bodor, 1981a, 1981b; Bodor et al., to be published), as represented by the general formula **68**. A large number of analogs belonging to this new class of steroids were designed according to isosteric/isoelectronic principles based on molecular modeling and molecular orbital calculations (Bodor and Phillips, to be published), as well as metabolism and binding considerations.

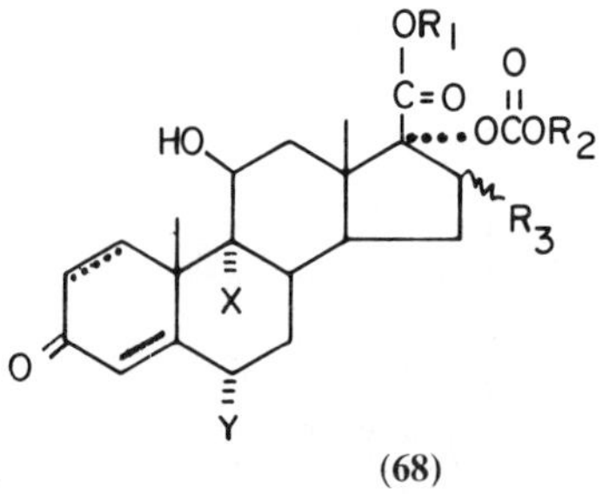

R_1, R_2 = alkyl, haloalkyl, alkoxyalkyl aryloxyalkyl, etc.

R_3 = H, OH, CH_3

X and Y = H or halogen

(68)

When tested for their activity and toxicity characteristics some of the new soft steroids showed truly dramatic improvement in the therapeutic index. Of more than 120 analogs synthesized and tested in this class, four were selected; they are compared in Table 30 with two highly used topical cortical steroids, hydrocortisone 17-butyrate (35) and betamethazone valerate (73).

It can be seen that the soft steroids are very potent and that the 9α-fluoro,16α-methyl derivative **71** shows good activity at a much lower dose than reference steroids while having no systemic effect (no change in body weights or in the very sensitive thymus weight test). The reference steroids show a very high systemic activity, up to 90% reduction in thymus weight after 6 days. Relative potencies of a few selected soft steroids in the cotton pellet granuloma assay are compared to that of hydrocortisone 17-butyrate

TABLE 31

Relative potencies[a] of selected soft steroids in the local cotton pellet granuloma assay

Compound (see Table 30)	ED_{40} (µg per pellet)	Relative potency	ED_{50} (µg per pellet)	Relative potency	ED_{60} (µg per pellet)	Relative potency
73	307 (238–394)	1	460 (360–623)	1	690 (523–1023)	1
70	47 (15–85)	6·5	119 (60–202)	3·9	301 (178–627)	2·3
71	0·47 (0·23–0·75)	653	1·07 (0·66–1·59)	430	2·44 (1·65–3·86)	283
72	0·25 (0·004–0·886)	1228	0·97 (0·08–2·31)	474	3·75 (1·25–7·68)	184
74 $R_1 = C_2H_5$; $R_2 = \beta\text{-}CH_3$; $X = F$; Δ^1	2·31 (1·07–6·38)	133	6·45 (2·96–44·58)	71	18·01 (6·47–393·8)	38
75 $R_1 = n\text{-}C_3H_7$; $R_2 = \alpha\text{-}CH_3$; $X = F$; Δ^1	0·58 (0·20–1·01)	529	1·20 (0·67–2·88)	383	2·49 (1·37–13·32)	277
35 Hydrocortisone 17-butyrate	—	—	—	—	1015 (724–26866)	0·7

[a] ED_{40}, ED_{50}, ED_{60} indicate inhibition of 40, 50 and 60%, respectively, of the granulation tissue.

TABLE 32

Effects of systemically administered[a] (s.c.) soft steroids and reference steroids on body weight and thymus weight in rats

Compound (see Table 30)	Dose (mg kg⁻¹ day⁻¹)	Number of test animals	Body weight gain (g)	Thymus weight (mg)	Inhibition (%)
None (control)		10	18.9 ± 0.6	550 ± 24	
71 $R_1 = C_2H_5$; $R_2 = \alpha\text{-}CH_3$; $X = F$; Δ^1	10	7	14.2 ± 1.9	533 ± 31	3.1
76 $R_1 = CH{<}^{CH_3}_{CH_3}$; $R_2 = \alpha\text{-}CH_3$; $X = F$; Δ^1	10	7	$2.7 \pm 1.9^{***}$	$234 \pm 31^{***}$	57.5
77 $R_1 = CH{<}^{CH_3}_{CH_3}$; $R_2 = \beta\text{-}CH_3$; $X = F$; Δ^1	10	7	$5.3 \pm 1.4^{***}$	$260 \pm 26^{***}$	52.7

318

78 $R_1 = C_2H_5$; $R_2 = \beta$-CH_3; $X = F$; Δ^1	10	7	2.4 ± 1.8***	266 ± 20***	51.6
75 $R_1 = n$-C_3H_7; $R_2 = \alpha$-CH_3; $X = F$; Δ^1	10	7	2.7 ± 1.7***	277 ± 25***	49.6
79 Clobetasol 17-propionate	0.003	8	18.2 ± 0.6	537 ± 28	2.4
	0.01	8	15.5 ± 1.1*	498 ± 15	9.5
	0.03	8	12.3 ± 1.3**	363 ± 22***	34.0
	0.1	8	-0.4 ± 1.3***	149 ± 9***	72.9
	0.3	8	-14.3 ± 1.3***	63 ± 3***	88.5

aDaily s.c. injections for three days; 48 h after last injection, the animals were sacrificed and the thymi weighed. Male Sprague—Dawley rats, weighing 185 g (162–209 g), were used.

*$p < 0.05$.
**$p < 0.01$.
***$p < 0.001$.

319

TABLE 33

Therapeutic indices of representative "soft steroids" as compared to reference steroids

Compound (see Table 30)	$ED_{50}{}^a$	Relative potency	$TED_{40}{}^b$	Relative potency	Therapeutic index^c
69	460 (360–623)	1	31·0 (23·9–41·9)	1/24	24
70	119 (60–202)	4	16·2 (11·2–23·2)	1/12	48
80 $R_1 = CH_3$; $R_2 = \alpha\text{-}CH_3$; $X = F$; Δ^1	2·38 (1·60–3·78)	202	46·0 (36·0–62·1)	1/36	7270
35 Hydrocortisone 17-butyrate	480 (313–892)	1	1·3 (1·1–1·5)	1	1
73 Betamethasone 17-valerate	100	5	0·3 (0·24–0·36)	4	1

^{a}Anti-inflammatory activity in the cotton pellet granuloma (μg per pellet).
^{b}Thymus inhibition effect subcutaneously (mg kg^{-1}).
^{c}The ratio of the relative potency for the ED_{50} to the relative potency for the TED_{40}; hydrocortisone 17-butyrate has been assigned arbitrarily a value of 1.

TABLE 34

Human vasoconstrictor activity[a] of selected "soft steroids" and reference compounds

| Compound | Compound structure | | | | | | Vasoconstrictor activity[b] | | | | | |
| | | | | | | | 2 h | | | 4 h | | |
	R_1	R_2	R_3	X	Y	Δ^1	0·0%	0·01%	0·001%	0·1%	0·01%	0·001%
81	CH_2Cl	C_2H_5	H	H	H	—	2·4	2·1	0·6	2·1	1·8	0·6
69	CH_2Cl	$CH(CH_3)_2$	H	H	H	—	1·8	1·3	0·1	1·7	1·1	0·3
82	CH_2Cl	CH_3	H	H	H	+	1·7	1·6	1·0	2·1	2·0	1·4
78	CH_2Cl	C_2H_5	β-CH_3	F	H	+	1·8	1·6	0·4	1·6	1·5	0·7
83	CH_2F	C_2H_5	α-CH_3	F	H	+	2·3	2·1	0·7	2·4	2·4	1·0
84	CH_2F	n-C_3H_7	α-CH_3	F	H	+	2·2	2·0	0·7	2·4	2·1	0·8
85	CH_2Cl	i-C_3H_7	α-CH_3	F	F	+	1·6	1·0	0·4	2·4	1·6	0·8
86	CH_2Cl	C_2H_5	α-CH_3	H	F	+	2·4	1·8	0·5	2·8	2·4	0·7
87	CH_2Cl	n-C_3H_7	α-CH_3	H	F	+	1·2	0·7	0·2	2·3	1·1	0·2
88	CH_2Cl	i-C_3H_7	α-C_3H_3	H	F	+	1·2	0·7	0·0	2·1	1·1	0·1
90	CH_2Cl	CH_3	α-CH_3	H	F	+	1·8	1·8	1·2	2·4	2·4	2·0
79	Clobetasol propionate						2·4			2·7		
73	Betamethasone valerate						2·3	1·9	0·8	2·6	2·4	1·1

[a] Occlusion time 4 h.
[b] Reading 2 and 4 h after removal of occlusion—scale: 0–3. Average of 6 volunteers.

321

in Table 31. The truly dramatic difference in the toxicity between these soft steroids and some reference steroids is also demonstrated following systemic, subcutaneous administration for 3 days, as indicated in Table 32. Significantly higher doses of the soft steroids cause much less toxic systemic effects than the reference clobetasol 17-propionate. Table 33 compares the therapeutic indices based on relative antiinflammatory versus thymus inhibition potency of representative soft steroids with reference steroids. The improvement is obviously very significant.

Human testing of a large number of these soft steroids confirmed their high local activity, as shown in Table 34.

Recently, the inactive metabolite approach was applied to some β-blockers. Metoprolol (91) is a selective β_1-adrenoreceptor antagonist. Its metabolism was extensively studied in man, dog and rat (Borg *et al.*, 1975; Ablad *et al.*, 1975), including patients with impaired renal function (Hoffmann *et al.*, 1980). As shown in Scheme 15 there are four oxidized metabolites among which the O-demethylmetoprolol (92) and α-hydroxymetoprolol (93) have a selective β-blocker activity, which is 5–10 times smaller than that of 91 (Borg *et al.*, 1975; Regardh and Hoffmann, 1979), while the acids 94 and 95

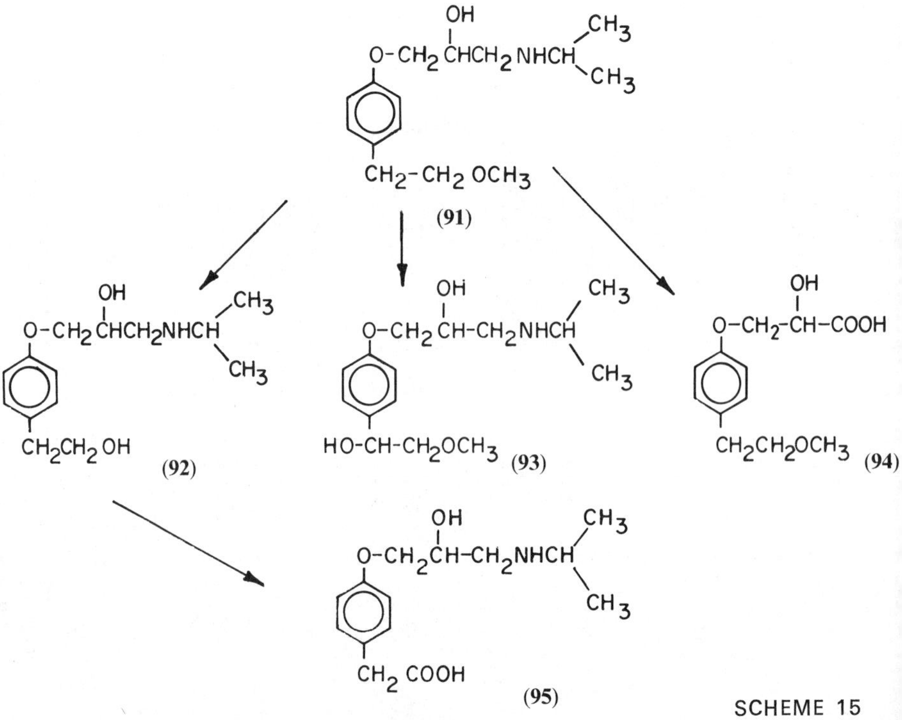

SCHEME 15

are inactive. The phenylacetic derivative **95**, a major urinary metabolite, is an ideal lead compound for our inactive metabolite approach since, according to a principle of the soft drug design, oxidative metabolism is to be avoided. Thus, a series of esters of **95** were prepared and expected to have β-blocking activity. A single hydrolytic process should deactivate the compounds yielding the starting inactive metabolite, and no oxidative activation or deactivation is expected to take place. The following compounds were synthesized and studied (**96–103**).

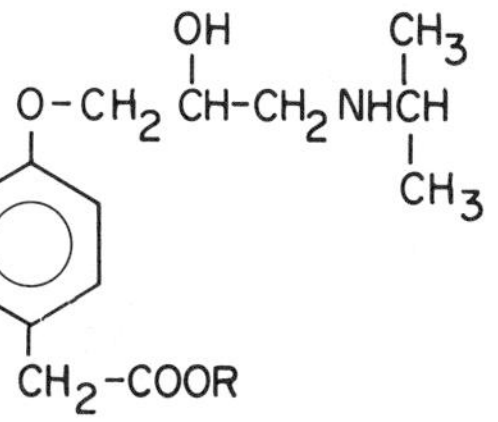

	R
95	H
96	ethyl
97	n-propyl
98	i-propyl
99	n-butyl
100	benzyl
101	cyclohexyl
102	2,6-dimethylcyclohexyl
103	3,3,5,5-tetramethylcyclohexyl
104	N-t-butyl analog of **99**

The hydrolytic stabilities of these esters were determined at pH 12, and the results are listed in Table 35. The hydroxyl ion-catalyzed hydrolysis of these various esters does not show any unexpected results, the rates being generally controlled by the relative steric hindrance at the ester portion. Compound **102** was obtained as a 1:2 mixture of two isomers separable by HPLC and thus showed biphasic kinetics. In contrast, the relative hydrolysis rates in human plasma are quite unexpected (Table 36). The isopropyl ester (**98**) is hydrolyzed up to 100 times more slowly than most of the other esters. Surprisingly, the isomer of **102**, more stable in basic conditions, did not hydrolyze detectably in plasma. As expected, the presence of the *t*-butyl group on the amine did not affect the hydrolysis rates (compare **99** with **104**). It is evident, however, that except for **98**, all esters hydrolyze rapidly in the plasma. The rate of hydrolytic deactivation is probably faster in the whole

TABLE 35

Chemical hydrolysis of β-blocker esters: observed pseudo first-order hydrolytic rate constants (k), standard errors (S.E.), half-lives ($t_{\frac{1}{2}}$) and initial concentrations (C_0) in 0·01 N sodium hydroxide at pH 12·0, ionic strength 0·10 M (NaCl) and 27·3 ± 0·2°C.

Compound	$k \pm$ S.E. (min^{-1})[a]	$t_{\frac{1}{2}}$ (min)	C_0 (M)
96	0·117 ± 0·001	5·91	4·5 × 10^{-4}
97	0·103 ± 0·001	6·73	4·6 × 10^{-4}
98	2·07 ± 0·03 × 10^{-2}	33·5	9·8 × 10^{-4}
99	9·27 ± 0·07 × 10^{-2}	7·48	5·0 × 10^{-4}
100	0·208 ± 0·004[a]	3·33	2·2 × 10^{-4}
101	4·96 ± 0·03 × 10^{-2}	14·0	1·7 × 10^{-4}
102	$\begin{cases} 9·71 \pm 0·27 \times 10^{-4} \\ 1·09 \pm 0·06 \times 10^{-2} \end{cases}$	$\begin{matrix} 7·14 \\ 63·3 \end{matrix}$	$\begin{matrix} 8·3 \times 10^{-5} \\ 2·8 \times 10^{-5} \end{matrix}$
103	1·56 ± 0·04 × 10^{-2}	44·4	3·0 × 10^{-5}
104	7·19 ± 0·04 × 10^{-2}	9·64	8·1 × 10^{-4}

[a]Average of three runs ± SEM.

TABLE 36

Enzymatic hydrolysis of β-blocker esters: observed first order hydrolytic rate constants (k), standard errors (S.E.), half-lives ($t_{\frac{1}{2}}$) and initial concentrations (C_0) in human plasma at 37·0 ± 0·1°C. The hydrolytic rate constants were obtained by following the disappearance of the compounds by HPLC.

Compound	$k \pm$ S.E. (min^{-1})	$t_{\frac{1}{2}}$ (min)	C_0 (M)
96	0·238 ± 0·010[a]	2·91	1·6 × 10^{-3}
97	0·143 ± 0·005	4·86	2·5 × 10^{-3}
98	0·414 ± 0·001 × 10^{-2}	1·67 × 10^2	1·1 × 10^{-3}
99	0·612 ± 0·016	1·13	1·4 × 10^{-3}
100	0·236 ± 0·007[a]	2·93	1·4 × 10^{-3}
101	1·46 ± 0·15[b]	0·47	5·8 × 10^{-4}
102	$\begin{cases} -^{c} \\ 1·64 \pm 0·14 \times 10^{-2} \end{cases}$	$\begin{matrix} - \\ 42·2 \end{matrix}$	$\begin{matrix} 5·9 \times 10^{-4} \\ 2·0 \times 10^{-4} \end{matrix}$
103	0·566 ± 0·027	1·22	9·3 × 10^{-4}
104	0·351 ± 0·019	1·98	1·5 × 10^{-3}

[a]Average of three runs ± SEM.
[b]Average of four runs ± SEM.
[c]Essentially no change in the peak height over a period of 3 hours.

body, as is often the case due to the high esterase activity of the liver. Since the acid **95** is inactive and is the only product forming from these compounds, the only way that significant β-antagonist activity can be observed is if the plasma concentration of the active species and *in vivo* activity are not directly related. This is quite possible as the pharmacological activity triggered by receptor binding can last much longer than the presence of the active species in plasma. Five compounds, **98, 99, 100, 103** and **104**, were selected for *in vivo* studies in rats and compared to propranolol. In the first study, an agonist, isoproterenol, was given 1 hour after administration of the potential blocker and the changes in the heart rate and blood pressure were recorded continuously. As shown in Fig. 4, the esters **103** and **99** effectively controlled the heart rate although their *in vitro* plasma half-life was of the order of 1 minute.

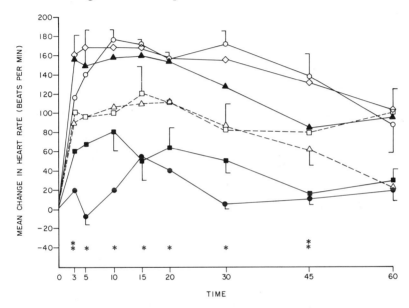

FIG. 4. Mean change in heart rate following administration of isoproterenol (25 μg kg^{-1} s.c.). Each group was pretreated with either compound **98** (○); **100** (△); **103** (■); **99** (□); **104** (◇); (±) propranolol (●) or the control vehicle (▲). Each agent was administered 60 minutes prior to isoproterenol. A one-way analysis of variance (f29, 6) revealed no significant differences in resting heart rates prior to administration of isoproterenol: 345 ± 19; 405 ± 22; 372 ± 19; 340 ± 14; 307 ± 7; 320 ± 23 and 333 ± 17 beats per minute, respectively. However, significant differences in the mean heart rate response among the 7 groups were observed: *$p < 0.005$; **$p < 0.025$. Comparisons between groups were made by the Newman–Keuls procedure with significance set at the 95% confidence interval. During the first 20 minutes, the group administered compound **103** was significantly different from both control- and compound **104**-treated groups. The propranolol-treated group was significantly different for the first 30 minutes. Additionally, the group administered compound **103** and the propranolol-treated group were significantly different from the groups treated with compound **99** and **104** at 10 through 45 minutes following administration of isoproterenol. All data shown as mean ± standard error of the mean.

(*In vivo* hydrolysis rates cannot be measured accurately since the drugs were administered i.p., and the *in vitro* half-life is already very short.) The selected compound **103** was studied for the extent of its activity. The results obtained for challenges 15, 60 and 90 minutes after administration of isoproterenol are shown in Fig. 5. It appears that at 15 and 60 minutes there is significant activity on heart rate which, however, disappears at 90 minutes. Similar studies of the compounds indicate that all these compounds have minimal effect on the blood pressure.

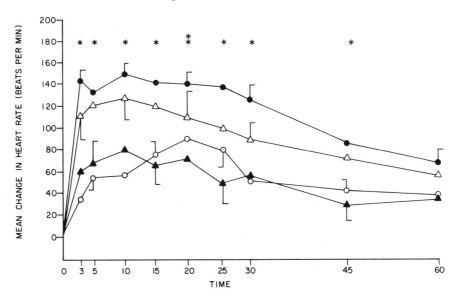

FIG. 5. Mean change in heart rate response in groups pretreated with control vehicle (●); or compound **103**, at 15 (○), 60 (▲) or 90 (△) minutes prior to administration of isoproterenol (25 μg kg⁻¹ s.i.) at time zero. Resting heart rates were similar in all 4 groups prior to administration of isoproterenol; 342 ± 12; 375 ± 14; 372 ± 19 and 385 ± 17 beats per minute, respectively. One-way analysis of variance (f40, 3) revealed a significant difference in response between the 4 groups during the 45 minutes following administration of isoproterenol: $^*p < 0.005$; $^{**}p < 0.025$. Comparison between groups demonstrated an attenuated heart rate response when compound **103** was administered either 15 or 60 minutes prior to the administration of isoproterenol. Data shown as mean ± standard error of the mean.

Additional *in vivo* cardiovascular experiments were performed in the dog, a good model for experiments of this type. Based on the results obtained on rats on the tetramethyl cyclohexyl ester **103**, the simpler homologs **101** and **102** were also tested and compared to the simple ethyl ester **96**. All four compounds showed β₁-antagonist activity, the cyclohexyl ester **101** being the most potent in blocking the cardiac effects of isoproterenol. The other three agents had a comparable ability to block isoproterenol induced tachycardia (Fig. 6).

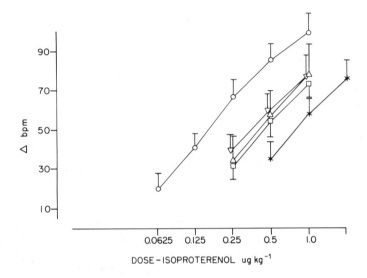

FIG. 6. The β-adrenergic blocking activities of selected "soft" compounds (O——O control; ▽——▽ **103**; △——△ **96**; □——□ **102** and ★——★ **101**) on the heart rate of dogs. Each compound was given i.v. at 1 mg kg^{-1} dose and increase in heart rate (△ bpm) was recorded. Baseline values were all around 117 ± 6 bpm. Error bars represents S.E. of mean.

The time course of the β-adrenergic blockade on heart rate was different for the four compounds. While **96** produced an antagonism which dissipated fairly reproducibly between 45 and 60 minutes after administration, the duration of action of **102** and **103** was much more variable and generally longer. It is interesting to note that, like in rats (Fig. 5, compound **103**), the maximum blockade in dogs was not seen at the earliest time following administration but after 45 or 60 minutes (see Table 37). Compound **101** had the longest duration of action as approximately 90 minutes were required for return to control values of heart rate responsiveness to isoproterenol (Table 37). None of the agents had any significant effect upon the diastolic depressor response to isoproterenol.

In conclusion, ester-type soft β-adrenergic blocking agents designed and synthesized based on an acidic inactive metabolite of metoprolol have been shown to possess significant β-blocking activity. The time of the peak β-blocking activity and the duration of action do not show any correlation

TABLE 37

Peak antagonist activity[a] and duration of action[b] of selected "soft" β-adrenergic blocking agents

Compound	Maximal blockade[a]		Duration[b]	
	Range (min)	Mean (min)	Range (min)	Mean (min)
96	(15–15)	15	45–60	~50
101	(15–30)	20	75–90	~85
102	(15–60)	38	45–90	~65
103	(30–60)	40	45–90	~70

[a]Time necessary to reach maximal blockade (15 min measurements). Data were obtained from dose—response curves before and after 1 mg kg^{-1} of each agent.
[b]Time after each β-adrenergic blocking agent (1 mg kg^{-1}) at which response to isoproterenol had returned to control levels.

with the *in vitro* plasma hydrolysis rates. Actually, the longest acting compound (101) has the shortest plasma hydrolytic half-life (less than 1 minute). The fast, predictable hydrolytic deactivation of the circulating active species must result in reduced overall toxicity and less probable drug interactions.

Based on these results as well as on theoretical considerations, we have to emphasize one very important concept in separating activity and toxicity and providing easier, controllable medication. And this is that despite all the attempts to develop a variety of long-acting drugs, actually the best direction to develop long-acting and safe drugs is the use of *short-acting compounds which are then delivered in a sustained, controllable manner*. This is particularly true for compounds like 102, which have a peak activity at about 45–60 minutes and then rapidly disappear. In addition, the short blood half-life would assure that instead of high circulating concentrations of relatively stable compounds one would have practically no amount of the active species circulating besides what is necessary to produce the desired activity. By adjusting the input rates to the metabolism kinetics and peak activity time, ideal controlled medication would result.

3 Conclusion

Designing drugs of low toxicity or having the *highest therapeutic index* must be the primordial objective of drug designers. Two major directions were summarized previously, *the soft drug design* and the *site-specific chemical drug delivery systems*. The field of design of safer drugs based on the soft drug approach has opened a number of general ways leading to very successful separation of the drug activity and toxicity. This highly logical approach has just started to gain recognition as one of the most important and integral parts of the drug design process. The methods of applying the basic concept can differ and can involve the usual basic structure–activity relationships or using computer optimized structures, etc. The main point is that in order to avoid many toxic effects of drugs, the design of drug metabolism should be involved at a very early stage of the drug design process.

The other basic approach, site-specific chemical delivery systems, is also based on enzymatic reactions. Successive enzymatic reactions can specifically optimize the presence and activity of the active species at or around the site of action. Rather than looking for organ- and site-specific enzyme systems which will possibly activate certain precursors only at the site of action, the examples strongly suggest combination of basic principles of physico-chemistry, enzyme activity and kinetics, and receptor based pharmacological studies as well as drug metabolism in order to achieve successful site-specific drug delivery.

Acknowledgements

I would like to express true gratitude to my very able former and present co-workers who helped me to develop many of the ideas in the soft drug design and site-specific drug delivery. These include, among others, Drs J. Kaminski, R. Woods, K. Sloan, Y. Oshiro, H. Farag, T. Loftsson, G. Visor, W. Caldwell, M. Brewster, T. Sato, as well as R. Little, N. Gildersleeve, S. Selk, M. Matsuo, and T. Nakamura. Financial support by the National Institutes of Health, Otsuka Pharmaceutical Company, Key Pharmaceutical Company and Pharmatec, Inc. is gratefully acknowledged. Special thanks are extended to Laurie Johnston and Joan Martignago for their help in the preparation of the manuscript.

References

Ablad, B., Borg, K. O., Johansson, G., Regardh, C. G. and Solvell, L. (1975). *Life Sci.* **16**, 693–704.
Abou-Donia, M. B. and Menzel, D. B. (1968). *Biochem. Pharmacol.* **17**, 2143–2161.
Albert, A. (1982). *Chem. Austral.* **49**, 412.
Ariëns, E. J. (1977). *In* "Biological Activity and Chemical Structure" (J. A. Kerverling Buisman, ed.), pp. 1–35. Elsevier, Amsterdam.
Ariëns, E. J. (1981). Presentation at the Second IUPAC-IUPHAR Symposium, "Strategy in Drug Research". Noordwijkerhout, The Netherlands, August 25–28.

Ariëns, E. J. and Simonis, A. M. (1977). *In* "Drug Design and Adverse Reactions" (H. Bundgaard, P. Juul and H. Koford, eds), pp. 317–330. Munksgaard, Copenhagen.

Ariëns, E. J. and Simonis, A. M. (1982). *In* "Strategy in Drug Research" (J. A. Keverling Buisman, ed.), pp. 165–178. Elsevier, Amsterdam.

Bartsch, H., Margison, G. P., Malaveille, C., Camus, A. M., Brun, G., Margison, J. M., Kolar, G. F. and Wiessler, M. (1977). *Arch. Toxicol.* **39**, 51–63.

Bodor, N. (1977a). *In* "Design of Biopharmaceutical Properties through Prodrugs and Analogs" (E. B. Roche, ed.), pp. 98–135. Academy of Pharmaceutical Sciences, Washington, D.C.

Bodor, N. (1977b). U.S. Patent 4,061,722, December 6.

Bodor, N. (1981a). *In* "Drug Metabolism and Drug Design: Quo Vadis?" (M. Briot, W. Cautreels and R. Roncucci, eds), pp. 217–251. Centre de Recherches Clin-Midy, Montpellier, France.

Bodor, N. (1981b). *Drugs of the Future* **6**, 165–182.

Bodor, N. (1982a). *In* "Strategy in Drug Research" (J. A. Keverling Buisman, ed.), pp. 137–164. Elsevier, Amsterdam.

Bodor, N. (1982b). *Trends Pharmacol. Sci.* **3**, 53–56.

Bodor, N. (1982c). *In* "Optimization of Drug Delivery" (H. Bundgaard, A. B. Hansen and H. Kofod, eds), pp. 156–174. Munksgaard, Copenhagen.

Bodor, N. and Farag, H. H. (1983a). *J. Med. Chem.* **26**, 528–534.

Bodor, N. and Farag, H. H. (1983b). *J. Med. Chem.* **26**, 313–318.

Bodor, N. and Farag, H. H. (1984). *J. Pharm. Sci.* **73**, 385–389.

Bodor, N. and Freiberg, L. (1981). U.S. Patent 4,262,765, April 28.

Bodor, N. and Kaminski, J. J. (1980). *J. Med. Chem.* **23**, 566–569.

Bodor, N. and Oshiro, Y. (1983). Jap. Patent 21201, February 10.

Bodor, N. and Simpkins, J. W. (1983). *Science* **221**, 65–67.

Bodor, N. and Sloan, K. B. (1978). U.S. Patent 4,069,322, January 17.

Bodor, N. and Sloan, K. B. (1980). U.S. Patent 4,239,757, December 16.

Bodor, N. and Sloan, K. B. (1982). *J. Pharm. Sci.* **71**, 514–520.

Bodor, N. and Visor, G. (1984). *Pharm. Res.*, **4**.

Bodor, N., Kaminski, J. J. and Roller, R. G. (1978). *Int. J. Pharmaceut.* **1**, 189–196.

Bodor, N., Kaminski, J. J. and Selk, S. H. (1980a). *J. Med. Chem.* **23**, 469–474.

Bodor, N., Woods, R., Raper, C., Kearney, P. and Kaminski, J. J. (1980b). *J. Med. Chem.* **23**, 474–480.

Bodor, N. Farag, H. H. and Brewster, M. E. (1981). *Science* **214**, 1370–1372.

Bodor, N., Sloan, K. B., Little, R. J., Selk, S. H. and Caldwell, L. (1982). *Int. J. Pharmaceut.* **10**, 307–321.

Borg, K. O., Carlsson, E., Hoffmann, K. J., Jonsson, T. E., Thorin, H. and Wallin, B. (1975). *Acta Pharmacol. Toxicol.* **36** (Suppl. V), 125–135.

Das, N. D. and Shichi, H. (1981). *Exp. Eye Res.* **33**, 525–533.

Dym, N. and Fawcett, D. W. (1970). *Biol. Reproduct.* **3**, 308–326.

Fawcett, D. W., Leav, L. V. and Heidger, P. M. (1970). *J. Reproduct. Fertil.* (Suppl.) **10**, 105–122.

Fishman, R. A. (1964). *Am. J. Physiol.* **206**, 836–844.

Francis, R. J., East, P. B., McLaren, S. J. and Larman, J. (1976). *Biomed. Mass Spectrom.* **3**, 281–285.

Geiger, W. B. and Alpers, H. (1964). *Arch. Int. Pharmacodyn. Ther.* **148**, 352–358.

Gillette, J. R. (1963). *In* "Progress in Drug Research" (E. Jucker, ed.), Vol. 6, pp. 11–73. Birkhauser Verlag, Basel.

Gillette, J. R., Mitchell, J. R. and Brodie, B. B. (1974). *Ann. Rev. Pharmacol.* **14**, 271–288.

Girard, J., Barbier, A. and Lafille, C. (1980). *Arch. Dermatol. Res.* **269**, 281–290.

Hoffmann, K. J., Regardh, C. G., Aurell, M., Evrik, M. and Jordo, L. (1980). *Clin. Pharmacokin.* **5**, 181–191.

Hussain, A. and Truelove, J. E. (1976). *J. Pharm. Sci.* **65**, 1510–1512.

Kaminski, J. J., Bodor, N. and Higuchi, T. (1976a). *J. Pharm. Sci.* **65**, 553–557.

Kaminski, J. J., Bodor, N. and Higuchi, T. (1976b). *J. Pharm. Sci.* **65**, 1733–1737.

Kaminski, J. J., Huycke, M. M., Selk, S. H., Bodor, N. and Higuchi, T. (1976c). *J. Pharm. Sci.* **65**, 1737–1742.

Klingman, A. M. and Kaidbey, K. H. (1978). *Cutis* **22**, 232–244.

Kilmer-McMillan, F. S., Reller, H. M. and Snyder, R. H. (1964). *J. Invest. Dermatol.* **43**, 363–377.

Kohl, H. H., Wheatley, W. B., Worley, S. D. and Bodor, N. (1980). *J. Pharm. Sci.* **69**, 1292–1295.

Kormano, M. (1967a). *Acta Physiol. Scand.* **71**, 125–126.

Kormano, M. (1967b). *Histochemistry* **9**, 327–338.

Kosugi, M., Kaminski, J. J., Selk, S. H., Pitman, I. H., Bodor, N. and Higuchi, T. (1976). *J. Pharm. Sci.* **65**, 1743–1746.

Kutty, K. M., Jacob, J. C., Hutton, C. J., Davis, P. J. and Peterson, S. C. (1975). *Clin. Biochem.* **8**, 379–383.

Kutty, K. M., Redheendran, R. and Murphy, D. (1977). *Experientia* **33**, 420–422.

Laurent, H., Gerhards, E. and Weichert, R. (1975). *Angew. Chem., Int. Ed.* **14**, 65–69.

Mannering, G. J. (1981). *In* "Concepts in Drug Metabolism" (P. Jenner and B. Testa, eds), Part B, pp. 53–166. Dekker, New York.

Mützel, W. (1977). *Arzneim.-Forsch.* **27**, 2230–2233.

Nelson, S. D., Mitchell, J. R., Dybing, E. and Sasame, H. A. (1976). *Biochem. Biophys. Res. Commun.* **70**, 1157–1165.

Orton, T. C. and Lowery, C. (1977). *Br. J. Pharmacol.* **60**, 319P.

Patton, T. F. (1980). *In* "Ophthalmic Drug Delivery Systems" (J. R. Robinson, ed.), pp. 28–54. American Pharmaceutical Association, Washington, D.C.

Rapoport, S. E. (1976). "Blood Brain Barrier in Physiology and Medicine". Raven Press, New York.

Regardh, C. G., Ek, L. and Hoffmann, K. J. (1979). *J. Pharmacokin. Biopharm.* **7**, 471–479.

Sinkula, A. A. and Yalkowsky, S. H. (1975). *J. Pharm. Sci.* **64**, 181–210.

Shichi, H. and Nebert, D. (1980). *In* "Extrahepatic Metabolism of Drugs and Other Foreign Compounds" (T. E. Gram, ed.), pp. 333–363. Spectrum Publications, Jamaica, New York.

Sloan, K. B., Bodor, N. and Zupan, J. (1981a). *Tetrahedron* **37**, 3463–3466.

Sloan, K. B., Bodor, N. and Little, R. J. (1981b). *Tetrahedron* **37**, 3467–3471.

Weekers, R., Delmarcell, Y. and Gastin, J. (1955). *Am. J. Ophthalmol.* **40**, 666–672.

SUBJECT INDEX

A

Acenocoumarol, 65, 83
Acetaldehyde, 118, 119, 144, 187
Acetylcholine, 272, 276, 277
Acetylcholinesterase, 126
Acetyl-coenzyme A, 137
β-N-Acetyl-D-hexosaminidase, 127
Acetylnorcholine, 276
N-Acetyltransferase, 35, 137–139
α_1-Acid glycoprotein, 61–64, 68–69, 71–73, 77, 78, 81–83, 86–89
Acrylamide, 142
Activated soft compounds, 281–286
Active metabolite principle, 286–288
Acylamide hydrolases, 129
Acylases, 139–141
Acyl-CoA synthetases, 139
Adenosine, 186
S-Adenosylmethionine, 131
Adenylate cyclase, 27, 186, 235
Adipocytes, 222
Adrenalin, 132, 145, 212–214, 216, 217, 221, 222, 241–243, 298–300, 302
Adrenal medulla, 100
Adrenalone, 298–300
Adrenalone esters, 301, 302
Adrenals, 103
Adrenergic synapse, 212
α-Adrenoceptors, 71, 210–213, 219, 221–234, 236, 239, 244, 247, 248
α_1-Adrenoceptors, 210–222, 226, 228, 229, 232, 233, 235–244, 247, 248
α_2-Adrenoceptors, 210–226, 228–230, 231–243, 245, 247, 248
β-Adrenoceptors, 27, 71, 210, 229, 232, 248
β_1-Adrenoceptors, 211, 217, 248, 322
β_2-Adrenoceptors, 211, 217, 248
Adrenochrome, 112
Agonism, concept of, 24
Ah locus, 34
Alcoholics, 36
Alcoholism, 187
Alcohol dehydrogenase, 35, 117
Alcohols, 117, 135, 146, 187

Aldehyde dehydrogenase, 119
Aldehyde oxidase, 109, 121
Aldehyde reductases, 118
Aldehydes, 109, 145
Aldose reductase, 118
Alprenolol, 70
Amidases, 126, 128–130
Amidephrine, 214
Amikacin, 61
α-Aminoacylpeptide hydrolases, 129
para-Aminobenzoic acid, 138
γ-Aminobutyric acid (GABA), 128, 185, 288
Aminochromes, 122
2-Amino-6,7-dihydroxytetrahydronaphthalene (6,7-ADTN), 96, 127, 191
5-Aminolaevulinate dehydratase (ALA-dehydratase), 154
5-Aminolaevulinate synthetase (ALA-synthetase), 153
2-Amino-2-methyl-1-propyl carboxylates, 283
Aminopyrine, 112, 138, 176, 178
Amitriptyline, 88
Amphetamine, 101, 165, 190
Amygdala, 121
Anaesthetics, 180
Androgens, 72, 171
Androsta-1,4,6-triene-3,17-dione, 172
Androstenedione, 171, 172, 173
Angiotensin II, 243
Antagonism, concept of, 24
Antibiotics, 89
Anticholinergic agents, 271–278
Anticoagulants, 89
Antiinflammatory drugs, 89
Antimicrobial agents, 281
Antiperspirants, 270
Apomorphine, 191
Arachidonic acid, 111
AR-C 239, 215
Arene oxides, 120, 124
Aroclor 1254, 161, 163
Aromatase, 171–173
Aromatic amines, 112, 137
Aromatic L-amino acid decarboxylase, 123
Artificial intelligence, 15, 40, 44

CUMULATIVE INDEX OF AUTHORS

CUMULATIVE INDEX OF TITLES